QUICK
REFERENCE *to*
CRITICAL
CARE

FOURTH EDITION

Nancy H. Diepenbrock, RN, CCRN
MedEvac Critical Care Transport Nurse
Aspirus Wausau Hospital
Wausau, Wisconsin

Wolters Kluwer | Lippincott Williams & Wilkins
Health

Philadelphia • Baltimore • New York • London
Buenos Aires • Hong Kong • Sydney • Tokyo

Acquisitions Editor: *Elizabeth Nieginski/Bill Lamsback*
Product Manager: *Laura Scott/Annette Ferran*
Design Coordinator: *Joan Wendt*
Illustration Coordinator: *Brett MacNaughton*
Manufacturing Coordinator: *Beth Welsh*
Prepress Vendor: *Aptara, Inc.*

4th edition

9 8 7 6 5 4 3 2 1

Printed in China

Library of Congress Cataloging-in-Publication Data
Diepenbrock, Nancy H.
  Quick reference to critical care / Nancy H. Diepenbrock. — 4th ed.
  p. ; cm.
Includes bibliographical references and index.
ISBN 978-1-60831-464-5 (alk. paper)
  1. Critical care medicine—Handbooks, manuals, etc. I. Title.
[DNLM: 1. Critical Care—Handbooks. WX 39]
RC86.8.D54 2012
616′.028—dc22

                                            2010042486

Speak tenderly to them.
Let there be kindness in your face,
In your eyes, in your smile,
In the warmth of your greeting.
Always have a cheerful smile.
Don't only give your care,
But give your heart as well.
Mother Teresa

This book is dedicated to those loving individuals
who not only give tender care
but give their hearts
every day.

CONTRIBUTING AUTHOR

Tracy McGaw, RN, CCRN, CNRN
Clinical Educator
University of Texas Southwestern Medical Center at Dallas
Dallas, Texas

Critical Care Staff Nurse
Baylor Regional Medical Center at Grapevine
Grapevine, Texas

Kristena Calderhead, RN, CCRN, MSNEd, APN
Instructor
Chamberlain College of Nursing
Columbus, Ohio

Theresa Cartier, RN, MSN, CCRN
Nursing Instructor
University of Pittsburgh Medical Center (UPMC)
Shadyside School of Nursing
Pittsburgh, Pennsylvania

Jack E. Dean, MSN, RN
Advanced Practice Nurse
University of Pittsburgh Medical Center (UPMC)
Pittsburgh, Pennsylvania

Carol Lynn
Assistant Professor
Ivy Tech Community College
Madison, Indiana

Karen S. March, PhD, RN, CCRN, ACNS-BC
Professor, Department of Nursing
York College of Pennsylvania
York, Pennsylvania

Heidi McCoy, RN, MSN
Instructor
University of Nebraska Medical Center
Lincoln, Nebraska

PREFACE

This is the fourth edition of *Quick Reference to Critical Care,* and during the 10 years since its original publication, the text has been expanded, modified, revised, and revamped. Yet in all that time, the original goal has remained unchanged: to provide quick, easy-to-find answers for the frequent "lapse-of-memory" questions that arise daily at the bedside. No healthcare worker can "remember it all" and the aim of this backpack-sized book is to provide a "memory jogger" to answer the question at hand *now.* It does *not* provide in-depth information (the reader is encouraged to research the topic at a later time in a more detailed text), but rather gives short, to-the-point explanations that facilitate *immediate* problem solving. Alphabetical arrangement of topics (within each body system) allows the reader to locate subjects easily and quickly, and meticulous cross-referencing prevents answers from getting lost because of a discrepancy in terms. Indexing is extensive and thorough, providing yet another way for the user to rapidly access a specific subject. The book contains a host of abbreviations (list provided following index) as well as numerous "remember" points, diagrams, figures, and illustrations. Visit *http://thePoint.lww.com/ Diepenbrock4e* for Internet resources.

This edition in particular has undergone some exciting renovations. Color has been added, making headings easier to locate and figures and tables easier to read. New up-to-date information has been included in every section. Of particular note, Part 9 (Labs) has been totally revised to make it more user-friendly, and Part 10 (Imaging) has been expanded to reflect the increased use of these procedures in daily practice. The book continues to arrange subjects first by body system, then alphabetically within the system:

Part 1: Neurologic
Part 2: Cardiovascular
Part 3: Pulmonary
Part 4: Gastrointestinal and Urinary
Part 5: Renal
Part 6: Endocrine
Part 7: Hematologic and Immune
Part 8: Drugs, Doses, Tables
Part 9: Labs
Part 10: Imaging
Part 11: Miscellaneous

ACKNOWLEDGMENTS

The effort put into the fourth edition of *Quick Reference to Critical Care* has been astronomical and most definitely not accomplished on my own. There are many people to thank, first and foremost being my contributing author, Tracy McGaw (and her husband, mentor, and friend, Steven). Without Tracy's help, this edition would have been close to impossible.

Likewise, there are many to thank for their guidance, opinions, and expertise in their areas of practice: Deb Karow, Marilyn Byrne, Camille Sheldon, Allison O'Donnell, Marcia Castella, Dr. Gary Jones, Claudia Quittner, Damon Watkins, and William Tharpe.

Lastly, I thank my editors: Elizabeth Nieginski, Executive Acquisitions Editor; Annette Ferran, Senior Product Manager; and Laura Scott, Associate Product Manager, for their over-the-top efforts in assisting me in this endeavor. They were continually supportive and enthusiastic, and somehow managed to make a very complicated and difficult task go smoothly.

CONTENTS

PART 1

Neurologic System

ACCOMMODATION

Accommodation is the adaptation of eyes for near vision. It is demonstrated by having patient focus on object at arm's length. When object is brought toward patient, the pupils should converge and constrict. This cannot be done on a comatose patient.

ACOUSTIC NEUROMA *(see Tumors, Neurogenic, p. 61)*

ADENOMA *(see Tumors, Neurogenic, p. 63)*

AMYOTROPHIC LATERAL SCLEROSIS *(see also Spinal Cord, p. 53)*

ALS, commonly known as Lou Gehrig's disease, is a chronic progressive neurodegenerative disease of unknown cause that adversely affects the upper and lower motor neurons (wasting and weakness of muscles is related to lower motor damage, whereas spasticity and exaggerated weakness is related to upper motor neuron damage). Over time, motor neuron destruction leads to the inability to innervate and control voluntary muscle fibers. The result is muscle weakness and atrophy with eventual total loss of muscle function leading to respiratory failure and death. The disease does not affect the individual's sensory or cognitive abilities.

ANATOMY: ARTERIAL BLOOD SUPPLY TO BRAIN

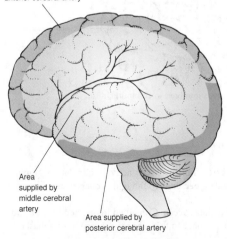

Area supplied by anterior cerebral artery

■ Arterial blood supply to the brain.

Area supplied by middle cerebral artery

Area supplied by posterior cerebral artery

1

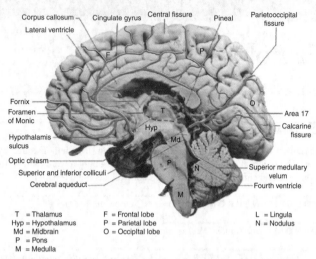

T   = Thalamus   F = Frontal lobe   L = Lingula
Hyp = Hypothalamus   P = Parietal lobe   N = Nodulus
Md = Midbrain   O = Occipital lobe
P   = Pons
M   = Medulla

■ Major blood vessels to brain. (Used with permission from Hendelman, W. J. [2000]. *Atlas of functional neuroanatomy.* Boca Raton, FL: CRC Press.)

ANATOMY: BRAIN STRUCTURES AND FUNCTION
(see also Tumors, Neurogenic, p. 61)

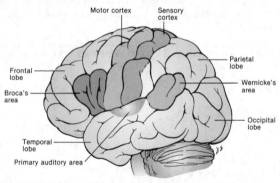

■ Cerebrocortical areas involved in communication.

FRONTAL
- Located in front of skull
- Plan for future
- Speech
- Prefrontal: Controls respiration, gastrointestinal (GI) activity, circulation, pupillary reactions, and emotions; helps regulate personality, thought processes, intellect, math ability, and concentration
- Broca's area: Controls ability to articulate speech. Contained in one hemisphere and is almost always dominant in the left. Damage to this area may cause motor aphasia.

(continued)

- Written speech area: Controls ability to write words. Regardless of whether patient is right or left handed, this area is usually situated in the left cerebral hemisphere.

PARIETAL
- Located up near crown of head
- A primary sensory area; receives sensory stimuli from other parts of the body and defines them according to size, shape, weight, texture, consistency, position sense, touch, and pressure.
- Processes visual-spatial information in nondominant lobe

TEMPORAL
- Located around temples
- Second weakest bone in skull
- Deals with sound
- Wernicke's area: Works to understand spoken word and written language
- Auditory speech: Integrates sound into pitch, quality, and loudness
- Postcranial area: Controls body's sensory areas

OCCIPITAL
- Located at bottom and back of head
- Visual: Integrates visual stimulation for size, form, motion, and color

CORPUS CALLOSUM
- Located in center of brain
- A thick area of nerve fibers connecting one hemisphere to the other
- Prevents chaos between hemispheres

CEREBELLUM
- Located at base of cerebrum
- Divided into two hemispheres, each composed of gray and white matter; governs walking, balance, coordination, and muscular memory

REMEMBER:

A lesion in the cerebellum presents signs and symptoms (e.g., ataxia) on the same side of the body (the ipsilateral side).

MIDBRAIN
- The top part of the brain stem
- CN III and CN IV exit here; the pathway for cerebral hemispheres and the center for auditory and visual reflexes

PONS
- The middle part of the brain stem
- CN V through CN VIII exit here; maintains a bridge between midbrain and medulla
- Controls respiratory function

MEDULLA
- The bottom part of the brain stem; attaches to spinal cord
- CN IX through CN XII exit here; transmits information for coordination of head and eye movements, and contains cardiac, vasomotor, and respiratory centers

(continued)

THALAMUS
- White matter located deep in the center of the brain near the brain stem
- Responsible for the sense of movement and position, and the ability to recognize size, shape, and quality of objects
- Also responsible for the routing of all sensory stimuli to their destinations, including the cerebral cortex, which receives them and translates them into appropriate responses

HYPOTHALAMUS
- Located between the pituitary gland and the brain stem
- Regulates appetite, sexual arousal, thirst, temperature, hormonal secretions, water metabolism, and visible physical expressions in response to emotions (blushing, clammy hands, dryness of mouth)
- Also the center for the autonomic nervous system

PITUITARY GLAND
- Located "front and center" of brain
- Considered the "master gland" because of the number of hormones and functions it controls. The pituitary receives the "OK" from the hypothalamus to secrete hormones via the pituitary stalk (infundibulum).
- Anterior lobe secretes growth stimulating hormone (GSH), adrenocorticotropin hormone (ACTH), thyroid stimulating hormone (TSH), follicle stimulating hormone (FSH), and luteinizing hormone (LH).
- Posterior lobe secretes antidiuretic hormone (ADH) and oxytocin.

NOTES

ANATOMY: CRANIAL LAYERS

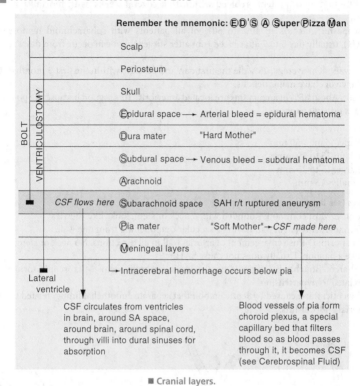

Remember the mnemonic: **E** **D**'S **A** **S**uper **P**izza **M**an

	Scalp	
	Periosteum	
	Skull	
Epidural space	→ Arterial bleed = epidural hematoma	
Dura mater	"Hard Mother"	
Subdural space	→ Venous bleed = subdural hematoma	
Arachnoid		
CSF flows here **S**ubarachnoid space	SAH r/t ruptured aneurysm	
Pia mater	"Soft Mother" → *CSF made here*	
Meningeal layers		
→ Intracerebral hemorrhage occurs below pia		

BOLT / VENTRICULOSTOMY

Lateral ventricle

CSF circulates from ventricles in brain, around SA space, around brain, around spinal cord, through villi into dural sinuses for absorption

Blood vessels of pia form choroid plexus, a special capillary bed that filters blood so as blood passes through it, it becomes CSF (see Cerebrospinal Fluid)

■ Cranial layers.

ANEURYSMS: CEREBRAL *(see also Embolization, p. 26; Subarachnoid Hemorrhage, p. 60; Vasospasm, p. 64)*

SUBARACHNOID GRADING SCALE

Numerous subarachnoid grading scales have been proposed; however, the Hunt and Hess scale is the most widely used (see figure).

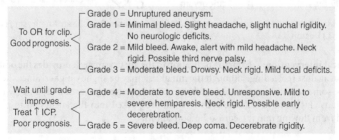

To OR for clip. Good prognosis.
- Grade 0 = Unruptured aneurysm.
- Grade 1 = Minimal bleed. Slight headache, slight nuchal rigidity. No neurologic deficits.
- Grade 2 = Mild bleed. Awake, alert with mild headache. Neck rigid. Possible third nerve palsy.
- Grade 3 = Moderate bleed. Drowsy. Neck rigid. Mild focal deficits.

Wait until grade improves. Treat ↑ ICP. Poor prognosis.
- Grade 4 = Moderate to severe bleed. Unresponsive. Mild to severe hemiparesis. Neck rigid. Possible early decerebration.
- Grade 5 = Severe bleed. Deep coma. Decerebrate rigidity.

■ Hunt and Hess scale.

(continued)

Rebleed risk: Peak incidence occurs 24 to 48 hours after initial bleed. Approximately 30% to 40% of patients rebleed within first several weeks, with mortality rate of 42%.

Vasospasm: Occurs in 40% to 60% of all patients with subarachnoid hemorrhage (SAH), usually day 5 to 7 after bleed (not after surgery) but can occur from day 1 to day 21.

Survival: On average, 25% die the first day, and 50% die within the first 3 months; 50% of survivors have major deficits.

Sites: About 85% of aneurysms are located anteriorly. This is good because the posterior area is difficult to access.

Size:
- Super giant: >50 mm
- Giant: 25 to 50 mm
- Large: 15 to 25 mm
- Small: <15 mm

Types (see figures):
- Berry: Most common. Rounded with a neck or stem, looks like "berries."
- Saccular: Any aneurysm having a saccular outpouching from one wall.
- Fusiform: Diffuse enlargement of arterial wall in all directions. No neck or stem; looks like a balloon. Usually does not cause SAH.
- Charcot-Bouchard: Origin is basal ganglia or brain stem. Microscopic formations related to hypertension.
- Mycotic: Rare; caused by septic emboli that separate endothelial lining; related to bacterial endocarditis.

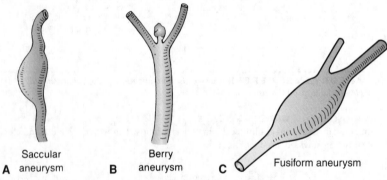

Saccular
A aneurysm

Berry
B aneurysm

C Fusiform aneurysm

■ Saccular, berry, and fusiform aneurysms. (Part C: Adapted from Brain Aneurysm Foundation, Inc., Boston, MA.)

Surgical intervention: Clipping or ligation of the aneurysm neck provides the best protection against rebleeding, although the initial risk may be slightly higher. Since the early 1990s, some cerebral aneurysms have been treated using embolization (coiling), wherein platinum Guglielmi detachable coils (GDCs) are packed into the aneurysm to prevent blood from flowing into it (see also Embolization).

(continued)

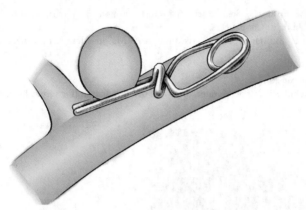

■ Clipping a cerebral aneurysm. (From Springhouse. [2008]. *Visual nursing*. Philadelphia: Lippincott Williams & Wilkins.)

Embolization: Since the early 1990s, an endovascular technique called "coiling" has also been used. It involves the interventional radiologist guiding a catheter from the femoral artery, up through the aorta, and into the cerebral vasculature, via either the carotid or the vertebral artery, until it reaches the cerebral aneurysm. Tiny platinum coils are then threaded through the catheter into the aneurysm to pack it tightly and close off blood flow into it, thereby preventing rupture. This process is called embolization. The coil itself has a memory effect (similar to a slinky toy) that allows it to form a coil of a given radius, thickness, and softness. Coils are manufactured in a variety of sizes from 2 mm in diameter or more, and in different lengths. They also come in two thicknesses, 10/1000 and 18/1000, and two stiffnesses, soft and regular. Occasionally, it is necessary to put more coils in later to complete treatment.

ANGIOGRAPHY, CEREBRAL

Cerebral angiography is a diagnostic tool that produces images of the blood vessels of the brain with the added benefit of interventional capabilities during the procedure, if required. As with any angiogram, access is gained via the femoral or brachial arteries. A catheter is then threaded through this access to the carotid arteries, where contrast medium is injected directly into the arterial vasculature of the brain (known as "shooting the carotids"). Digital subtraction angiography (DSI) removes bone and tissue from the image, leaving only the dye-filled blood vessels for optimal visualization and interpretation. Postprocedure care includes observance of routine angiogram complications, as well as an added neurological assessment. Complications of this procedure include artery/arterial wall damage or dislodgement of debris such as plaque or a clot, which may result in a stroke.

APNEUSTIC BREATHING *(see Respiratory Patterns in Part 3, p. 203)*

ARTERIOVENOUS MALFORMATION

Arteriovenous malformations (AVMs) are congenital brain lesions composed of tangled, dilated vessels that form an abnormal communication between arterial and venous systems. Intracranial "steal" occurs when the AVM is large, related to blood being diverted from one area of brain tissue because of lower vascularization in another area.

(*continued*)

Signs and symptoms: Seizure activity is most common. Hemorrhage and/or headache occurs in about 50% of patients.

Treatment: Similar to aneurysms, though AVMs pose less risk of bleed with intervention.

- Embolization
- Surgical excision
- Gamma knife, linear accelerator, or proton beam radiation (for surgically inaccessible AVMs)

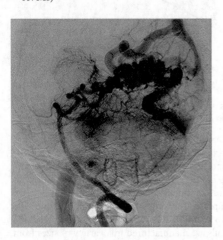

■ Arteriovenous malformation. (Courtesy of UT Southwestern University Hospital—Zale Lipshy, Dallas, Texas.)

ASTROCYTOMA *(see Tumors, Neurogenic, p. 62)*

AUTONOMIC DYSREFLEXIA *(see Dysreflexia, p. 24)*

BABINSKI'S REFLEX

Positive response for Babinski's reflex is fanning of toes and extension of great toe with stimulation of plantar surface of foot. It is normal in babies but abnormal in adults. Response is related to upper motor neuron lesion and is seen on opposite side of cerebral damage.

Negative response is flexion of foot and is normal in adults.

BASILAR SKULL FRACTURE

Injury to the olfactory (first cranial) nerve is common with fracture, along with otorrhea or rhinorrhea. Drainage sample may be positive for glucose, though this is not always a reliable sign. Allow cerebrospinal fluid (CSF) to drain freely, keeping in mind that draining CSF due to a torn dura puts the patient at high risk for meningitis. Avoid NG, nasal suction, Valsalva's maneuver, and cough. Raccoon eyes (ecchymotic areas around the eye orbits), epistaxis, visual defects, and anosmia are indicative of anterior fossa fracture, whereas Battle's sign (ecchymosis over the mastoid bone 24 to 48 hours after injury), conductive hearing loss, and facial nerve palsy are indicative of posterior fossa fracture.

BATTLE'S SIGN *(see Basilar Skull Fracture, p. 8)*

BIOT'S RESPIRATIONS *(see Respiratory Patterns in Part 3, p. 203)*

BISPECTRAL INDEX MONITORING
(see also Ramsey Scale, p. 49; Riker Sedation-Agitation Scale, p. 50)

A processed EEG parameter used to measure the hypnotic effects of anesthetic and sedative agents on the brain. A sensor is placed on the patient's forehead, and the BIS monitor translates information from the EEG into a single number (i.e., 100 = wide awake;
0 = absence of brain activity). Use of the BIS monitor does not replace the use of the
peripheral nerve stimulator. Riker's sedation-agitation scale is frequently used in conjunction with BIS monitoring to document the patient's level of sedation.

ELECTRODE PLACEMENT
After wiping the forehead with alcohol and drying with gauze, position the electrodes.
In most cases, either side can be used, but if the patient has had a stroke, place it on the
unaffected side.
- Place electrode #1 at the center of forehead, about 1½ inches above the bridge of nose.
- Place electrode #4 directly above and adjacent to the eyebrow.
- Place electrode #3 on the temple, between the outer canthus of the eye and hairline.
- Electrode #2 will then be in proper position to be secured.

MONITORING
After connecting cable, each electrode needs to self-test and "pass" before monitoring can
begin. Watch the signal quality index (SQI) bar for EEG activity.

ASSESSMENT

BIS Reading	Clinical State	EEG
0	**Unresponsive**	Flat
1–40	**Deep hypnotic state** <20, only possibility of intact protective reflexes and limited respiratory drive <40, protective reflexes possibly intact, may respond to deep stimulation	<20, approaching burst suppression <40, increased proportion of suppressed EEG
41–60	**Moderate hypnotic state** Deep sedation; low probability of consciousness; unresponsive to verbal stimuli, low risk of recall	Normalized low-frequency activity (determined by proprietary method)
61–90	**Light hypnotic state** Responds to loud verbal and deep tactile stimuli (< responsiveness with index near 60)	60–70, beta augmentation 70–80, synchronized high-frequency activity (beta augmentation)
91–100	**Awake**	Normal EEG

TROUBLESHOOTING
- Replace sensors every 24 hours.
- When disconnecting sensor, press release button on interference cable.
- Increased EEG activity may artificially increase BIS score; be sure to check SQI.

(continued)

- False BIS highs may also be due to:
  1. High-frequency power contained in pacemakers, ECG signals, warming blankets, or oscillating ventilators;
  2. Muscle shivering, tightening, or patient motion;
  3. Neuromuscular blocking agents that may be wearing off;
  4. REM sleep;
  5. Pain.
- BIS lows may be due to:
  1. Neuromuscular blockade

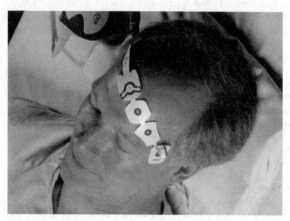

■ Bispectral index monitoring electrode placement. (Courtesy of Aspect Medical Systems, Inc., Newton, MA.)

BLOOD-BRAIN BARRIER
(see also Anatomy: Cranial Layers, p. 5; Choroid Plexus, p. 16)

Blood-brain barrier refers to the special permeability of brain capillaries and choroid plexus that limits transfer of certain substances into extracellular fluid of CSF of brain. H_2O, CO_2, O_2, and glucose cross easily. It is important because the blood-brain barrier is often damaged or infected when tissue is injured; damage leads to increased permeability.

BRAIN ATTACK *(see Stroke, p. 57)*

BRAIN DEATH CRITERIA* *(see also Organ Donation in Part 11, p. 387)*

Brain death diagnosis is made in the absence of hypothermia (temperature <32.2°C) and central nervous system depressants. Patient must be:

1. **Areflexic** except for simple spinal cord reflexes; pupillary, extraocular, corneal, gag, and cough reflexes are absent.
2. **Without spontaneous respiration as determined by apnea test.** To do an apnea test: Preoxygenate patient. Disconnect ventilator, and give O_2 at 8 to 12 L/min by tracheal

Criteria are from the President's Commission for the Study of Ethical Problems in Medicine and Biomedical Research.

(continued)

cannula. Observe patient for spontaneous respirations. After 10 minutes, draw blood for arterial blood gases (ABGs). PCO_2 must be >60 mm Hg for an accurate test. Reconnect the ventilator. Patient is considered apneic if PCO_2 is >60 mm Hg and there is no respiratory movement. If hypotension and/or arrhythmia develops, reconnect ventilator. Consider other confirmatory tests.

3. **Considered to have an irreversible condition.** Duration of observation depends on clinical judgment: 12 hours is recommended when an irreversible condition is well established and no test is confirmatory; 24 hours is recommended for anoxic brain damage and no test is confirmatory.
4. **Positive for flat electroencephalogram (EEG) (if performed).**
5. **Positive for absence of blood flow by cerebral radionuclide scan or arteriogram (if performed).**

BRAIN STEM *(see also Cranial Nerve Exam, p. 80)*

Brain stem collectively includes midbrain, pons, and medulla. It is an area that controls basic functions dealing largely with involuntary activities: blood pressure, heart rate, and respiration. Brain stem is "bottommost" in skull. Brain stem "trouble" can be identified by means of cranial nerve tests (see Cranial Nerve Exam).

BRAIN STRUCTURES AND FUNCTION
(see Anatomy: Brain Structures and Function, p. 2)

BRAIN TUMORS *(see Tumors, Neurogenic, p. 61)*

BREATHING PATTERNS *(see Respiratory Patterns in Part 3, p. 203)*

BROWN-SÉQUARD SYNDROME

Syndrome is due to incomplete lesion to one side of spinal cord, related to penetrating trauma. Assess for vibration sense, proprioception, and light touch.

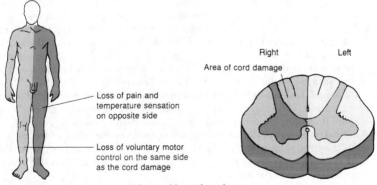

Right   Left
Area of cord damage

Loss of pain and temperature sensation on opposite side

Loss of voluntary motor control on the same side as the cord damage

■ Brown-Séquard syndrome.

REMEMBER:

Whichever side the lesion is on (right or left), the lesion causes that side to lose motor function. The opposite side loses pain and temperature sensation.

BRUDZINSKI'S SIGN *(see also Kernig's Sign, p. 42)*

In response to passive flexion of neck, hip and knees will flex. This is due to irritating exudate around roots in lumbar region. It is a sign indicative of meningitis or for bleeding into the subarachnoid space.

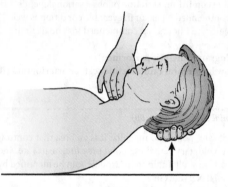

■ Brudzinski's sign. (From Hickey, J. V. [2009]. *Neurological and neurosurgical nursing* [6th ed.]. Philadelphia: Lippincott Williams & Wilkins.)

CALORIC TEST *(see also Doll's Eyes, p. 23)*

Designed to evaluate the eighth cranial nerve and the oculovestibular reflex in an awake patient, and the integrity of the brain stem on a comatose patient. It is considered to be one component in the evaluation of brain death, but is contraindicated in patients with cervical injury or a ruptured tympanic membrane. The patient is supine with the head of the bed up 30°. Instill 5 to 10 mL of water tympanically. Normal response depends on whether iced water or warm water is used, and whether patient is awake or unconscious.

- **A normal iced caloric test result on an awake patient** (indicating eighth cranial nerve and oculovestibular reflex intact) is an initial conjugate movement of the eyes toward the side being irrigated. After about 30 seconds, the lateral gaze changes to a rapid nystagmus, pulling the eyes back to midline.
- **A normal iced caloric test result on an unconscious patient** is conjugate, tonic eye movement toward the irrigated ear (indicating brain stem is intact). In effect, the brain has the capacity to say, "Hey, what's that?" and tells the eyes to check it out. This is considered a good sign. It is normal in a lethargic or unconscious patient for the response to the nystagmic component (that follows the lateral movement) to be diminished or absent, since this portion is controlled by the cerebral cortex.
- **An abnormal iced caloric test result in an unconscious patient** is associated with a poor prognosis. There may be absent or dysconjugate eye movement to the side being irrigated (indicating loss of brain stem control), and absent nystagmus.
- **A normal warm water caloric test result on an awake patient,** while seldom used in the ICU setting, is opposite that of cold calorics. The instillation of warm water will result in conjugate eye deviation away from the side being irrigated, followed by a rapid nystagmus toward the irrigated ear.

REMEMBER:

The mnemonic COWS (cold opposite, warm same). It refers to the water temperature used and the nystagmic portion of the reflex.

(continued)

It is also possible to irrigate both ears at once. Cold irrigation will produce a slow downward deviation of the eyes, whereas warm irrigation will result in a slow upward deviation.

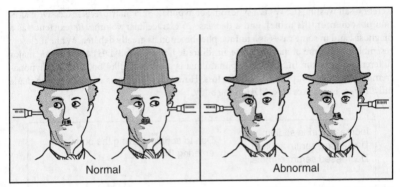

Normal   Abnormal

■ Cold caloric test on unconscious patient. (From Marino, P. L. [2007]. *The ICU book [3rd ed.]*. Philadelphia: Lippincott Williams & Wilkins.)

CENTRAL HERNIATION *(see Herniation, p. 32)*

CENTRAL NEUROGENIC HYPERVENTILATION
(see Respiratory Patterns in Part 3, p. 203)

CEREBRAL PALSY

Cerebral palsy is a disease resulting from brain damage in a newborn, and the exact cause is difficult to determine. At highest risk are the premature or babies who have a congenital malformation. Diagnosis usually involves a period of waiting (frequently up to 18 months) for the definite and permanent appearance of specific motor problems, that is, spasticity (inability of a muscle to relax) or athetosis (inability to control the movement of a muscle). Damage is fixed and rarely shows progression or regression. While there is no specific cure or standard therapy, drugs are often used for seizure and spasm control, and braces are used for muscle imbalance. Life expectancy varies with the severity of the disease.

CEREBRAL PERFUSION PRESSURE *(see also Increased Intracranial Pressure p. 35; Intracranial Pressure Monitoring, p. 37)*

Cerebral perfusion pressure (CPP) refers to the pressure difference across the brain between incoming mean arterial pressure (MAP) and the opposing intracranial pressure (ICP) (see table).

Cerebral Perfusion Pressure		
CPP	**=**	**MAP Minus ICP***
Average		80–100 mm Hg
Minimum for perfusion		50 mm Hg
Brain death		<30 mm Hg

*If ICP is negative, consider it zero when calculating CPP.

CEREBRAL SALT WASTING *(see also Syndrome of Inappropriate Antidiuretic Hormone in Part 6, p. 273)*

Cerebral salt wasting (CSW) is a syndrome of hyponatremia, natriuresis (excessive excretion of sodium in the urine), and a decrease in extracellular volume. Its existence as a diagnosis, and in some cases as a unique phenomenon, is greatly debated. While it closely resembles syndrome of inappropriate antidiuretic hormone (SIADH), there is one major differentiating factor. In SIADH, hyponatremia is a result of dilution. In CSW, hyponatremia is the result of primary sodium loss. However, a diagnosis of CSW can be made only if there is not excessive ADH in the body.

Increased urine sodium Decreased serum sodium Decreased serum osmolality	Due to sodium leaving the body and entering the urine
Decreased plasma volume Decreased body weight	Water will follow sodium out of the body
Increased BUN	Body is becoming dehydrated

■ CSW findings.

How exactly a neurologic insult leads to CSW is not yet clearly understood. It is thought that atrial natriuretic factors (ANF), substances released from the atria, play a part. ANF is also thought to cause diuresis, vasodilation, and suppression of the renin-aldosterone system.

CSW needs to be differentiated from SIADH because the treatments are the exact opposite of one another. In SIADH, the low sodium is treated with fluid restriction (to alleviate the dilutional state). In CSW, the treatment is to administer fluids (oral and hypertonic [3%] or isotonic IVs). This will replace the sodium that has already been excreted. The repletion should not be done faster than 0.7 mEq/L/hr for a maximum total daily change not to exceed 20 mEq/L. Fludrocortisone, a mineralocorticoid drug, is an adjunct to sodium and fluid replacement for CSW. It enhances sodium reabsorption in the renal tubules, allowing the body to retain more sodium.

CEREBROSPINAL FLUID *(see also Anatomy: Cranial Layers, p. 5; Halo Sign, p. 31; Lumbar Puncture, p. 42; Spinal Cord, p. 53)*

CSF is made in lateral ventricles by choroid plexus. It is constantly produced and constantly absorbed. It circulates from ventricles in brain, around subarachnoid space and spinal cord. It is absorbed through villi into dura mater. Approximately 400 to 500 mL of CSF is made daily, or about 20 mL/hr. About 15 to 25 mL is located in each ventricle. It is characteristically clear and colorless (xanthochromic CSF is a sign of bleeding in area), with pressure of 80 to 180 mm H_2O while patient is side lying.

Abnormal lab values for CSF (the following are "rules of thumb" only):

- Red blood cells (RBCs). Finding RBCs in the CSF indicates hemorrhage somewhere in the central nervous system, e.g., from torn or ruptured blood vessels from injury or ruptured aneurysm. This can also be due to a bloody spinal tap.

(continued)

- Increased cells. Increased cells may indicate infection somewhere in the central nervous system. For example, polymorphonuclear leukocytes and increased lymphocytes may occur with viral infections and tuberculosis. If extremely large numbers of cells are present, the CSF may appear cloudy.
- Lowered blood sugar. This often results from bacterial infections of the central nervous system or from SAH. A normal glucose value for CSF is 60% of serum glucose.
- Lowered chloride level. Drop in chloride often results from bacterial infections of the central nervous system.
- Increased protein level. Rise in protein usually occurs in the presence of a brain tumor or degenerative disease.

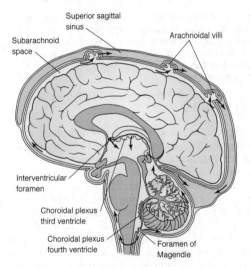

Superior sagittal sinus

Arachnoidal villi

Subarachnoid space

Interventricular foramen

Choroidal plexus third ventricle

Choroidal plexus fourth ventricle

Foramen of Magendie

■ Flow of cerebrospinal fluid from the time of its formation from blood in the choroid plexuses, until its return to the blood in the superior sagittal sinus.

CHEYNE-STOKES RESPIRATION
(see Respiratory Patterns in Part 3, p. 203)

CHIARI MALFORMATIONS

These are a group of abnormalities of the craniocervical junction characterized by the hindbrain descending down through the foramen magnum. The malformation is divided into three types (see figure on the next page).

(continued)

NOTES

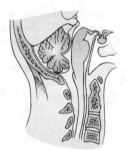 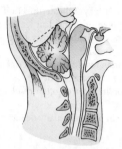 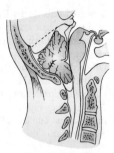

Type I. Descent of cerebellar tonsils through foramen magnum.

Type II. Marked descent of hindbrain structures (pons, medulla, and fourth ventricle) through foramen magnum. Often associated with myelomeningocoele.

Type III. Hindbrain herniation into a high cervical meningocoele.

■ Chiari malformation. (Reprinted with permission from Palmer, J. [1996]. *Manual of neurosurgery*. New York: Churchill Livingstone.)

The abnormality is rare, affecting only 1 in 10,000 to 15,000, with males more commonly affected than females. Average age for diagnosis is estimated at 30 to 40 years for adults and 11 years for children. There is a wide variance in how these patients present clinically, probably accounting for frequent delays in diagnosis. Treatment generally requires surgical intervention consisting of either (1) local decompression or (2) diversion. Local decompression consists of removing the base of the back of the skull and the posterior portions of the uppermost vertebrae. This will widen the opening of the foramen magnum. Once the bone has been removed, the membrane (dura) overlying the cerebellum and spinal cord is opened. A tissue graft is then "spliced" into the dura to provide even more room for the easy passage of CSF. Less often, diversion is used, by draining the cavity within the spinal cord with a diverting shunt tube. This can be directed from the spinal cord cavity to either the chest or the abdominal wall.

CHORDOMA *(see Tumors, Neurogenic, p. 61)*

CHOROID PLEXUS

The choroid plexus is a special capillary bed located in the brain that filters blood and is responsible for the production of cerebral spinal fluid.

CHVOSTEK'S SIGN *(see also Trousseau's Sign, p. 61)*

Chvostek's sign is a twitch of facial muscles, upper lip, and eye following a sharp tap to facial nerve (seventh cranial nerve) anterior to the ear, just below the temple. It is related to a decreased serum calcium level.

CIRCLE OF WILLIS

The circle of Willis is an anatomic juncture representing an anastomosis of four major vessels: posterior cerebral, anterior cerebral, internal carotid, and posterior/

(continued)

anterior communicating. The "circle" is the most common site for an intracranial aneurysm.

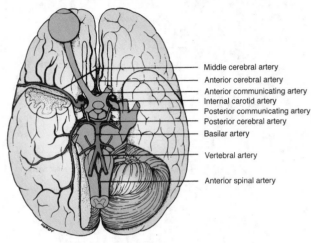

- The circle of Willis seen from below the brain.

Anterior circulation includes:
- 2 internal carotids (ICA)
- 1 anterior communicating (Acomm, AcoA)
- 2 anterior cerebrals (ACA)
- 2 posterior communicating (Pcomm, PcoA)
- 2 middle cerebrals (MCA)
- 2 ophthalmics (OA)
- 2 anterior choroidals

Posterior circulation includes:
- 2 vertebrals (verts)
- 2 posterior cerebrals (PCA)
- 1 basilar (BA)
- 2 superior cerebellars (SCA)
- 2 posterior inferior cerebellars (PICA)
- 2 anterior inferior cerebellars (AICA)
- Many pontines

(*continued*)

NOTES

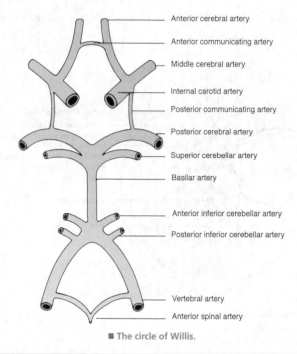

Anterior cerebral artery

Anterior communicating artery

Middle cerebral artery

Internal carotid artery

Posterior communicating artery

Posterior cerebral artery

Superior cerebellar artery

Basilar artery

Anterior inferior cerebellar artery

Posterior inferior cerebellar artery

Vertebral artery

Anterior spinal artery

■ The circle of Willis.

CLUSTER BREATHING (*see Respiratory Patterns in Part 3, p. 203*)

COILING (*see Embolization, p. 26*)

COMA (*see also Caloric Test, p. 12*)

Coma is a state defined as being unconscious, unarousable, and unresponsive to touch or sound. Coma is caused by one of two things:

1. Damage to both cerebral hemispheres
2. Damage to ascending reticular activating system in brain stem

The caloric test differentiates between the two (see Caloric Test).

CONSENSUAL REFLEX

A normal reflex, the consensual reflex is demonstrated by constriction of opposite pupil when light stimulates one eye.

REMEMBER:

Consensus = both agree.

CORNEAL REFLEX

The corneal reflex tests the fifth cranial nerve, the trigeminal. Touch cornea with wisp of cotton or place a drop of artificial tears in eyes and observe for blink reflex, or apply pressure

(*continued*)

to supraorbital ridge and observe for facial grimacing (reflex is decreased or absent on same side as hemiplegia).

CRANIAL NERVES

The 12 pairs of symmetrically arranged cranial nerves are attached to the brain and exit through a foramen at its base. The site where the fibers composing the nerve enter or leave the brain surface is usually termed the superficial origin of the nerve; the more deeply placed group of cells from which the fibers arise or around which they terminate is called the nucleus of origin.

To remember the names of the 12 nerves, remember the mnemonic "On old Olympian towering tops, a Finn and German viewed some hops." But because the names of so many of the nerves begin with the same letter, also remember the mnemonic "Little people can only imitate big champions." This gives the second letter (or third, if both second letters are the same) of the nerve. To remember the type of nerve, remember the mnemonic "Some say marry money, but my brother says (it is) bad business marrying money" (s = sensory; m = motor; b = both sensory and motor).

Twelve Cranial Nerves

Mnemonic		Cranial Nerves and Function	Type (S = Sensory, M = Motor, B = Both)
First Letter	**Circled Letter**		
On	(little)	I **O(l)factory.** Smells.	S (some)
Old	(people)	II **O(p)tic.** Sees; Snellen Chart.	S (say)
Olympian	(can)	III **O(c)ulomotor.** Moves eyes, with 4 and 6. Constricts pupils, accommodates.	M (marry)
		REMEMBER: CN III = pilars. Open eyes.	
Towering	(only)	IV **Tr(o)chlear.** Moves eyes, with 3 and 6. Downward, inward.	M (money)
Tops	(imitate)	V **Tr(i)geminal.** Sensations from face, cornea, teeth, tongue, nasal, oral mucosa. Chews (see also Corneal Reflex).	B (but)
A	(big)	VI **A(b)ducens.** Moves eyes, with 3 and 4. Laterally.	M (my)
Finn		VII **Facial.** Moves eyes, salivation, taste (anterior 2/3 of tongue).	B (brother)
		REMEMBER: CN VII = hook. Closes eyes.	

(continued)

Twelve Cranial Nerves (Continued)

Mnemonic		Cranial Nerves and Function	Type (S = Sensory, M = Motor, B = Both)
And	(champions)	VIII **A©oustic.** Hears. Regulates balance (see also Caloric Test, Rinne Test, Weber's Test).	S (says) (it is)
German		IX **Glossopharyngeal.** Taste (posterior 1/3 of tongue), swallow, gag, pharyngeal sensation, salivation. Reflex control of BP, pulse, respirations.	B (bad)
Viewed		X **Vagus.** Sensation and movement of pharynx, larynx, thoracic and abdominal viscera.	B (business)
Some		XI **Spinal Accessory.** Turns head, lifts shoulders.	M (marrying)
Hops		XII **Hypoglossal.** Moves tongue.	M (money)

CRANIAL NERVE EXAM

Cranial Nerve Assessment

Cranial Nerve	Assessment	Comments
I Olfactory	**Sense of smell** Usually deferred	Deficits noted in only a few cases, usually with lesion in the parasellar area or a basilar skull fracture (anterior fossa)
II Optic	**Vision** Monitor while working with patient; observe for difficulty with ADLs Ask patient to identify how many fingers are being held up or to read menu or newspaper Use Rosenbaum Pocket Vision Screener to assess vision in each eye Monitor for visual field cuts by checking upper and lower quadrants while patient focuses on your nose	Common deficits, often related to a basilar skull fracture (anterior fossa), can cause blindness in one eye, bitemporal hemianopia, or homonymous hemianopia
III Oculomotor	**Pupil constriction; elevation of upper eyelid** Assess size, shape, and direct light reaction of pupils	Changes are common with a number of progressing neurologic problems
III Oculomotor IV Trochlear VI Abducent	**Extraocular movement** Tested together in conscious, cooperative patient; ask patient to follow a pencil tip through the six cardinal eye movements	Deficits are common; inability to move the eyes in one or more directions; or strabismus

(continued)

Cranial Nerve Assessment (Continued)

Cranial Nerve	Assessment	Comments
V Trigeminal	**Sensation to face; mastication muscles** Often deferred If assessed, patient must be cooperative and able to accurately report facial sensation to stimulation	Deficits found in trigeminal neuralgia and sometimes with acoustic neuroma Corneal reflex assessed in trigeminal neuralgia; can assess reflex in unconscious patient
VII Facial	**Muscles for facial expression; efferent limb of corneal reflex** In cooperative patient, ask him or her to smile, show teeth, puff cheeks, wrinkle brow; observe for symmetry of face In a comatose patient, tickle each nasal passage, one at a time, by inserting a cotton-tipped applicator; observe for facial movement	Total unilateral facial weakness, called Bell's palsy Unilateral from below the eye and down, seen in stroke Note the difference between central and peripheral facial involvement Deficits often seen in basilar skull fracture, posterior fossa
VIII Acoustic	**Hearing and balance** Usually deferred May note deficit while working with patient in the posterior fossa	Deficits with acoustic neuroma, cerebellopontine angle tumors, Meniere's disease, and skull fracture
IX Glossopharyngeal X Vagus	**Palate, pharynx, vocal cords, and gag reflex;** tested together because of overlap In conscious patient, have patient open mouth and say "ah," assess gag reflex In unconscious patient, assess gag reflex	Deficits common in posterior fossa lesions Gag reflex is a brain stem reflex and has prognostic value in unconscious patient
XI Spinal accessory	**Shrug shoulders and move head side to side** Usually deferred	Deficits common in posterior fossa lesions
XII Hypoglossal	**Movement of tongue** In conscious patient, ask him or her to stick out the tongue	Deficits common in posterior fossa lesions

CRANIOPHARYNGIOMA (see Tumors, Neurogenic, p. 62)

CREUTZFELDT-JAKOB DISEASE

Creutzfeldt-Jakob disease (CJD) is a degenerative neurologic disease that is rapid and fatal, similar to "mad cow" disease (bovine spongiform encephalopathy, or BSE). Though the two are similar, no correlation of a relationship between them is evident. The onset of CJD manifests itself as confusion and then it progresses rapidly to coma and death, usually within 2 years, often within 1 year. The disorder is seen in adults with an average age of 60 years. Because it is infectious, standard precautions should be taken with invasive procedures or contaminated body fluids, especially spinal fluid or brain tissue.

CSF (see Cerebrospinal Fluid, p. 14)

CUSHING'S REFLEX *(see also Cushing's Triad, p. 22)*

When CSF pressure and the pressure within the intracranial cerebral arteries start to equilibrate, the cerebral arteries become compressed and begin to collapse. This compromises cerebral blood flow. Cushing's reflex is activated, and the arterial pressure rises to a level higher than the CSF pressure, allowing cerebral blood flow to be reestablished and ischemia to be relieved. The blood pressure is maintained at a new, higher level, and the brain is protected from further loss of adequate blood flow. Cushing's reflex causes the symptoms of Cushing's triad.

CUSHING'S TRIAD *(see also Cushing's Reflex, p. 22)*

The triad refers to three signs caused by Cushing's reflex:

1. Bradycardia
2. Hypertension (with widened pulse pressure)
3. Bradypnea (often irregular)

It is indicative of an advanced increase in intracranial pressure, that is, the brain's "last gasp." The triad and the reflex are late findings, and irreversible neurologic damage may have already occurred by the time they are recognized.

CVA *(see Stroke, p. 57)*

DECEREBRATE

Decerebration is demonstrated by extension of involved extremities with outward pronation of the wrists and hands. Legs are stiffly extended at the knees with the feet plantar flexed. This indicates disruption of motor fibers in the midbrain and brain stem and is a more ominous sign than decortication.

REMEMBER:

"Without cerebrum" or "extension."

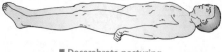

■ Decerebrate posturing.

DECORTICATE

Decortication is demonstrated by flexion of the upper extremities and extension and internal rotation of the lower extremities on the side of the lesion. It is seen in patients with interruption of cortical nerve fibers but intact pathways through the brain stem.

REMEMBER:

"To the core" or "without cortex."

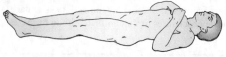

■ Decorticate posturing.

DELIRIUM TREMENS *(see CIWA Score in Part 11, p. 375)*

DERMATOMES *(see Epidural Analgesia, p. 28)*

DIABETES INSIPIDUS *(see Diabetes Insipidus in Part 6, p. 264)*

DOLL'S EYES *(see also Caloric Test, p. 12; Cranial Nerve Exam, p. 20)*

Also known as the oculocephalic reflex/response, Doll's eyes testing is used on a comatose patient to check for an intact brain stem. It should never be performed on a suspected neck injury.

With eyelids held open, briskly turn the head either horizontally side-to-side (cranial nerves III, VI) or vertically up and down (cranial nerve III only).

Reflex normal (positive doll's eyes, brain stem intact): Eyes move in the opposite direction of the head turn and then slowly drift back to the midline as if to fixate on a stationary object.

REMEMBER:

"It's good to be a doll!" (A positive thing!)

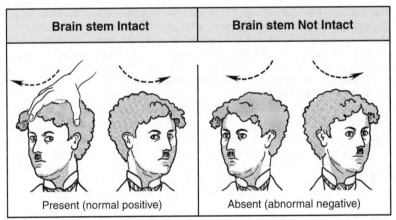

Brain stem Intact	Brain stem Not Intact
Present (normal positive)	Absent (abnormal negative)

■ Doll's eyes. (From Marino, P. L. [2007]. *The ICU book* [3rd ed.]. Philadelphia: Lippincott Williams & Wilkins.)

Reflex abnormal (negative doll's eyes, brain stem dysfunction from the pons to midbrain level): Eyes do not move in the sockets and instead follow the direction of head movement, remaining stationary with respect to the head.

REMEMBER:

"Barbie is brain dead!" (Painted eyes on Barbie doll remain fixed and stare in whatever direction head is turned.)

An abnormal finding is usually followed by a cold caloric test.

DOPPLER STUDIES *(see Transcranial Doppler Studies, p. 60)*

DRIFT

Ask the patient to close eyes and extend arms up with palms facing inward ("catch the rain" or "deliver a pizza"). Have patient count backward from 10 while maintaining elevated arms. Downward drift of one or both arms or pronation of palms indicates a positive drift and is indicative of mild hemiparesis.

DYSREFLEXIA

Dysreflexia is a state unique to spinal cord injured patients at T5 and above, sometimes seen in patients with injury at T6 to T10. The cascade of events is triggered when an irritating stimulus (such as an overfilled bladder) is introduced to the body below the level of the injury. Since the impulse cannot reach the brain due to the injury, the body responds by initiating a reflex to increase the sympathetic portion of the autonomic nervous system. This results in spasms, narrowing of the blood vessels, and a rise in blood pressure. Nerve receptors in the heart and blood vessels detect this rise, and in an effort to control it, the brain sends a message to the heart causing the heartbeat to slow down and the blood vessels above the level of the injury to dilate. However, since the brain cannot deliver the same message to the receptors below the level of the injury, the blood pressure is unable to be regulated, and life-threatening hypertension ensues. Other common symptoms include headache, flushing, red blotches on skin above the level of the injury, and sweating above the level of the injury, due to vasodilation. Cold, clammy skin and goose bumps below the level of the injury are due to vasoconstriction. Nausea, as well as a metallic taste in the mouth, are due to vagal parasympathetic stimulation. Treatment must be initiated promptly and is aimed primarily at alleviating the precipitating stimulus, though often antihypertensives must be prescribed.

ECIC BYPASS

Extracranial/Intracranial. Literally, it is a CABG to the head, usually reserved for patients with symptomatic large vessel occlusive disease not amendable to direct surgical repair (i.e., most vertebrobasilar lesions, intracranial ICA or MCA stenosis, and complete ICA occlusion). Saphenous vein grafts are sometimes used because of the high flow that can be provided, but superficial temporary artery, middle cerebral artery (STA-MCA) bypass is also used.

ELECTROENCEPHALOGRAM (EEG) MONITORING
(see also Seizures, p. 51)

An EEG is a noninvasive procedure used to evaluate electrical activity of the brain. Neurons produce predictable electrical energy patterns as a result of normal activity. The electrical pattern is detected via electrodes placed at designated locations on the cranium. The amplitude of the impulses is converted to a traceable waveform, much like chest electrodes produce an EKG tracing of the heart. A typical EEG recording has a duration of 20 to 40 minutes, plus prep time to apply the multiple electrodes. EEG may be used in the critical care setting to monitor for nonconvulsive seizures or to monitor the sedation level of chemically induced coma

(continued)

(i.e., increased ICP). EEG may also be useful as a diagnostic tool in suspected brain death.

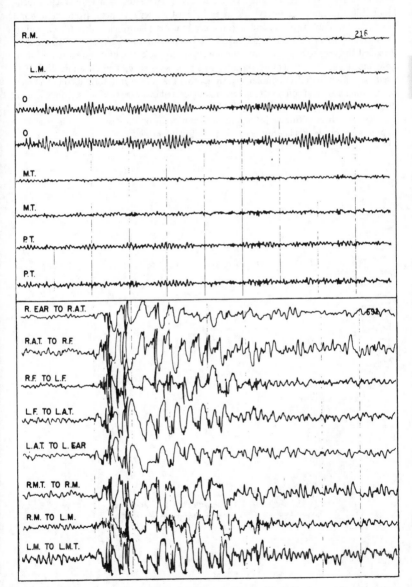

■ Comparison of a normal electroencephalogram (*top*) with that of an epileptic patient during a tonic-clonic seizure (*bottom*). Note the sharp, spiky waves recorded during the seizure. (From Hickey, J. V. [2009]. *Neurological and neurosurgical nursing* [6th ed., p. 107]. Philadelphia: Lippincott Williams & Wilkins.)

EMBOLIZATION *(see also Aneurysms, p. 5)*

Since the early 1990s, cerebral aneurysms have also been treated by an endovascular technique called coiling. The interventional radiologist guides a catheter from the femoral artery, up through the aorta, and into the cerebral vasculature via either the carotid or the vertebral artery until it reaches the cerebral aneurysm. Tiny platinum GDCs are then threaded through the catheter into the aneurysm to pack it tightly and close off blood flow into it, thereby preventing rupture. This process is called embolization. The GDC itself has a memory effect (similar to a slinky toy) that allows it to form a coil of a given radius, thickness, and softness. Coils are manufactured in a variety of sizes, from 2 mm in diameter or more, and different lengths. They also come in two thicknesses, 10/1000 and 18/1000, and three stiffnesses, standard, soft, and ultra soft. Occasionally, it is necessary to put more coils in at a later time to complete treatment.

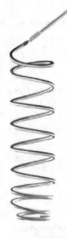

■ GDC 2-diameter coil. (Courtesy of Boston Scientific/Target, Fremont, CA.)

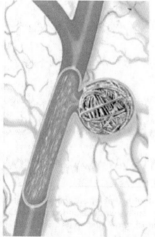

■ Coils deployed in aneurysm. (Courtesy of Boston Scientific/Target, Fremont, CA.)

EPENDYMOMA (see Tumors, Neurogenic, p. 62)

EPIDURAL ANALGESIA

Epidural catheter is placed in the "potential" space along the spinal column, located between the dura mater and the ligamentum flavum. The catheter may be placed in the lumbar or thoracic spine, but L1 to L5 is most common. It provides excellent pain relief without affecting motor function and without diminishing the sensations of touch, temperature, and proprioception.

Opiates are injected into the epidural space and bind to fat. Fat carries the opiates across the dura mater into the subarachnoid space and binds to opiate receptors in the spinal cord. Transmission of pain impulses is thus inhibited.

PRECAUTIONS

Patients who have an epidural catheter in place currently, or within the past 24 hours, and some patients who have received a spinal injection, **should not** receive any form of anticoagulation (heparin, enoxaparin, warfarin, fondaparinux, argatroban) without the approval of the provider who injected/placed the catheter. Anticoagulation in this patient population can lead to a spinal hematoma, which may cause permanent paralysis.

Common Epidural Medications			
	Fentanyl	**Hydromorphone (Dilaudid)**	**Morphine**
Dose:	50–100 μg	0.5–2 mg	5–10 mg
Onset:	4–10 min	13 min	23 min
Relief:	20 min	25 min	45 min
Duration:	4–5 hr	1–12 hr	12–18 hr
Soluble:	High lipid solubility = binds quickly to fat = rapid onset	Moderate	Low lipid solubility (water soluble) = less rapid binding, slower onset, and longer duration; also has greater potential for side effects

ADMINISTRATION OF ANALGESIA

Most frequently given as a continuous infusion (rather than an intermittent bolus) and frequently combined with a local anesthetic (bupivacaine or ropivacaine) to increase the analgesic effect of the drug and reduce the side effects. Note, however, that local anesthetics may cause hypotension and motor block. Reports of a tingling sensation around the mouth and/or tremors may indicate intravascular injection and local systemic anesthetic toxicity. The physician should be notified immediately, as seizures may occur.

Note: Many institutions require personnel to be certified before being allowed to administer drugs epidurally.

1. Draw up (filtered needle) the ordered amount of preservative-free opiate and preservative-free normal saline in 10-mL syringe.
2. Using empty 3-mL syringe, assess placement of catheter by slowly aspirating for 30 seconds. More than 1 mL of fluid indicates intrathecal placement. Presence of blood indicates vascular placement. Terminate procedure.

(continued)

3. If no aspirate, or aspirate is <1 mL, administer medication, maintaining sterility of cap.

Note: If injection is difficult, reposition the patient supine with spine flexed. This increases the intervertebral space and decreases compression on the catheter.

4. Monitor and record BP and pulse at least every 30 minutes for 2 hours. Patient should be monitored by continuous pulse oximetry.

REMEMBER:

The absolute DO NOT list for epidural catheters:

1. Do not use alcohol swabs. Alcohol (which acts as a preservative) is toxic to the spinal cord.
2. Do not flush an epidural catheter.
3. Do not use medication not specifically labeled for epidural use.
4. Do not use any tubing with injection ports.
5. Do not disconnect an epidural catheter.
6. Do not send a patient to MRI with an epidural catheter.
7. Do not cut the catheter.
8. Do not start other narcotics or sedatives while the epidural is infusing without first contacting the provider.

POTENTIAL ADVERSE EFFECTS

- Respiratory depression (<1%). An early sign is pupil constriction, followed by a decrease in the rate and depth of breathing. Naloxone (Narcan), an opiate antagonist, is usually given at 0.1 to 0.2 mg IVP, every 2 to 3 minutes. The half-life of Narcan, however, is only 30 minutes. Thus, redosing may be required should symptoms recur.
- Urinary retention (15% to 90%). This is related to the local anesthetic effect opioids produce on sympathetic and sensory pathways, which innervate the bladder. A urinary catheter should be placed and intake/output closely monitored.
- Pruritus (30% to 100%). Relief is not usually achieved with antihistamines. Low-dose naloxone (Narcan) infusion (0.25 to 1 mcg/kg/hr) can be given without the loss of the analgesic effect of the opioid.
- Nausea, vomiting (30% to 100%). Results from stimulation of the chemoreceptor trigger zone in the lower brain stem. Antiemetic agents will frequently provide relief.
- Cardiovascular effects. A result of sympathetic blockade and increased parasympathetic activity, hypotension, and decreased heart rate are generally mild and well tolerated. However, they can be pronounced in patients with hypovolemia or heart failure and may require IV fluid boluses as well as small doses of vasopressors.

DERMATOMES

Since drugs injected via an epidural catheter produce a band-like distribution of analgesia, this "level" of analgesia can be assessed through the use of dermatomes. This is accomplished by applying a cold alcohol pad or skin-refrigerant spray first to one side of the body and then to the other, for comparison. Start at the lower extremity, and touch random points on the limb, moving upward. When the patient states that the sensation changes from cool to cold, compare the findings to a dermatome chart. This will identify the anatomical level of analgesia.

(continued)

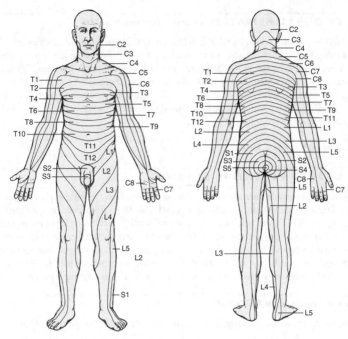

■ Dermatomes. (From Stedman's Medical Dictionary [27th ed.]. Baltimore: Lippincott Williams & Wilkins, 2000.)

Dermatomes	Spinal Nerve Roots
Back of head (occiput)	C2
Neck	C3
Neck and upper shoulder	C4
Lateral aspect of shoulder	C5
Thumb, radial aspect of arm, index finger	C6
Middle finger, middle palm, back of hand	C7
Ring and little finger, ulnar forearm	C8
Inner aspect of arm and across shoulder blade	T1 and T2
Nipple line	T4
Lower costal margin	T7
Umbilical region	T10
Inguinal (groin) region	T12 and L1
Anterior thigh and upper buttocks	L2
Anterior knee and lower leg	L3 and L4
Outer aspect of lower leg, dorsum of foot, great toe	L5
Sole of foot and small toes	S1
Posterior middle thigh and lower leg	S2
Medial thigh	S3
Genitals and saddle area	S4 and S5

EPIDURAL HEMATOMA *(see also Herniation, p. 32)*

Epidural hematoma is usually related to trauma, brain stem contusion, or basilar or temporal bone fracture. It is caused by a mass influx of blood into the epidural space. Signs are rapid onset of decreased LOC, ipsilateral (same-side) fixed pupil, increased intracranial pressure, and contralateral hemiparesis. Watch for uncal herniation (see Herniation). Epidural hematoma is treated by surgical evacuation. Lumbar puncture is contraindicated in an expanding lesion because it can cause herniation and is usually inaccurate (CSF needs to flow freely to be accurate).

EPILEPSY *(see Seizures, p. 51)*

EVOKED POTENTIAL STUDIES

Evoked potential studies are recordings of the central nervous system electrical output, measured after a specific sensory stimulus is delivered. This differs from spontaneous potentials as noted with an EEG. Three types of evoked potential studies are common for assessing response between sensory organs and the brain. Visual evoked potentials test the visual pathways, auditory evoked potentials test the auditory pathways, and somatosensory evoked potentials test peripheral nerve pathways, via the spinal cord. Evoked potentials are used to clinically diagnose a wide variety of central nervous system disorders, such as multiple sclerosis.

FORAMEN MAGNUM

Foramen magnum means "large hole" and is the point at which brain stem becomes spinal cord.

GAMMA KNIFE

Gamma knife is a type of stereotactic radiosurgery used most commonly for brain metastases or for benign tumors such as acoustic neuromas, meningiomas, or pituitary adenomas. Tumor control is achieved in >95% of the cases. Multiple doses of radiation, frequently delivered one after the other all in one treatment in one day, are given to the patient who has been fitted with a lightweight frame to hold the head still during the procedure. The term gamma "knife" is a misnomer, since no incision is made and the skull is never opened. Treatment generally takes less than 2 hours, and patients are discharged from the hospital the same day. Side effects are rare, other than a mild headache or nausea.

GLASGOW COMA SCALE

A "perfect" score = 15. Score <8 requires transport to a facility with a neurosurgery team. All patients (if alive) receive a minimum score of 3 "just for showing up."

Scoring of eye opening:
- 4 Opens eyes spontaneously when nurse approaches
- 3 Opens eyes in response to speech (normal or shout)
- 2 Opens eyes only to painful stimuli (e.g., squeezing of nail beds)
- 1 Does not open eyes to painful stimuli

(continued)

Scoring of best motor response:
- 6 Can obey a simple command, such as "Lift your left hand off the bed"
- 5 Localizes to painful stimuli and attempts to remove source
- 4 Purposeless movement in response to pain
- 3 Flexes elbows and wrists while extending lower legs to pain
- 2 Extends upper and lower extremities to pain
- 1 No motor response to pain on any limb

Scoring of best verbal response:
- 5 Oriented to time, place, and person
- 4 Converses, although confused
- 3 Speaks only in words or phrases that make little or no sense
- 2 Responds with incomprehensible sounds (e.g., groans)
- 1 No verbal response

From Hickey, J. V. (2009). *Clinical practice of neurological and neurosurgical nursing* (6th ed.). Philadelphia: Lippincott Williams & Wilkins.

GLIOBLASTOMA *(see Tumors, Neurogenic, p. 62)*

GLIOMA *(see Tumors, Neurogenic, p. 62)*

GLYCOLYSIS

Glycolysis provides energy in the form of adenosine triphosphate (ATP) by anaerobically metabolizing glucose. Glucose is a "cheap" source of ATP for the brain. Therefore, during hypoxia, the rate of glucose breakdown (glycolysis) is increased. Remember, the brain does not need insulin to use glucose; a constant supply of both O_2 and glucose is what it needs for metabolism. Because the brain has no glucose store, it therefore depends on a constant blood supply.

GUILLAIN-BARRE SYNDROME

Guillain-Barre syndrome, also known as infectious polyneuritis, is a demyelination of lower motor neurons affecting the spinal and cranial nerves (peripheral nervous system). It is an ascending paralysis and is usually symmetric, with no alteration of consciousness. It may occur after a viral infection, usually of the upper respiratory tract. The most serious complication is respiratory arrest (decreased work ability of diaphragm and breathing muscles). Signs are decreased vital capacity and increased protein in CSF. Urinary tract infection is a common complication.

HALO SIGN *(see also Cerebrospinal Fluid, p. 14)*

Leaking CSF can sometimes be identified by a characteristic "halo" sign, or a yellowish ring, surrounding the drainage on dressings or linens. The leak may arise from otorrhea (leakage of CSF from the ear), rhinorrhea (leakage of CSF from the nares), leaking of CSF into the nasopharynx, or CSF fluid collection or drainage at an operative site. To differentiate between mucus and a CSF leak, the drainage can be tested with a glucose indicator strip (Dextrostix). If CSF is present, the indicator has a positive reaction, because CSF contains sugar.

(continued)

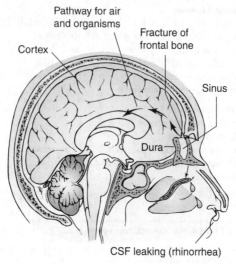

CSF leaking (rhinorrhea)

■ Cerebrospinal fluid leak.

HEMANGIOBLASTOMA *(see Tumors, Neurogenic, p. 62)*

HERNIATION

Herniation is the abnormal protrusion of an organ or other body structure through a defect or natural opening in a covering membrane, muscle, or bone. Neurologically, herniation is divided into three types:

1. Central (transtentorial) herniation is evidenced by compression and downward displacement of the hemispheres, resulting in compression against the tentorium cerebelli. Signs include small pupils (1 to 3 mm) at first, then both pupils dilate. It is usually seen in chronic disorders.
2. Uncal herniation is a displacement of the temporal lobe (uncus) against the brain stem and third cranial nerve. It is found in CVA with ipsilateral pupil dilation. It is also seen in neurologic emergencies, such as epidural hematoma. Patient exhibits a "blown" pupil, because the herniation compresses the cranial nerves.
3. Infratentorial herniation is a compression on the brain stem or cerebellum, either upward against the tentorium cerebelli or downward through the foramen magnum.

(continued)

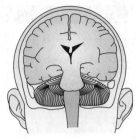
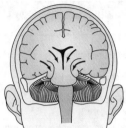
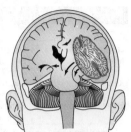

Normal	Central transtentorial herniation	Uncal and transtentorial herniation
	The brain is swollen, the diencephalon is compressed and elongated, and the medial temporal lobes are forced along the brain stem through the tentorial notch.	The cingulate gyrus is herniated under the falx cerebri, the uncus herniates through the tentorial notch, and the brain stem is compressed and shifted laterally and downward.

■ Coronal views of supratentorial and infratentorial compartments. (Reprinted from Arbour, R. [2004]. Intracranial hypertension, *Critical Care Nurse*, 24, [5, 19–32], with permission from Elsevier.)

Types of Herniation*

Central (Transtentorial)		
	Early	**Late**
Pupils	Small, reactive bilaterally	Bilateral fixed, dilated
Level of arousal	Difficulty with concentration; agitated or drowsy	Stupor leads to coma
Motor	Contralateral hemiparesis	Bilateral decortication, decerebration, flaccidity
Respiration	Pauses, central neurogenic hyperventilation	Cheyne-Stokes, ataxia
Extraocular signs	Normal or slightly roving	Dysconjugate gaze, extraocular paralysis
Uncal (Lateral Transtentorial)		
	Early	**Late**
Pupils	Ipsilateral dilated pupil; sluggish nonreactive	Dilated and fixed
Level of arousal	Normal to restless	Stupor may rapidly become coma
Motor	Slight weakness, pronator drift	Decortication, decerebration, flaccidity
Respiration	Normal	Cheyne-Stokes, ataxia, respiratory arrest
Extraocular signs	Ptosis	Extraocular paralysis
Infratentorial		
	Early	**Late**
Pupils	Midposition or small and nonreactive	Bilateral fixed

(*continued*)

Types of Herniation* (Continued)		
	Early	**Late**
Level of arousal	Stupor	Coma
Motor	Hemiparesis, hemiplegia	Decortication, decerebration, flaccidity
Respiration	Variable depending on level of lesion	Respiratory arrest
Extraocular signs	Ophthalmoplegias; early loss of upward gaze	Extraocular paralysis

*An important point to keep in mind when observing a patient with a possible herniation is that there is a predictable order to the development of the signs and symptoms. The neurologic deterioration in both central and uncal herniation proceeds in an orderly scheme (the diencephalon, midbrain, pons, and finally medulla are affected by increasing pressure). Notice that the last stages of central and uncal herniation are the same.

Revised and adapted from Hickey, J. V. (1997). The clinical practice of neurological and neurosurgical nursing (4th ed.). Philadelphia: Lippincott-Raven.

HOMONYMOUS HEMIANOPIA

Homonymous hemianopia is the loss of vision in half the field of each eye (hemi = half; anopia = of each field). It indicates damage to the optic nerve.

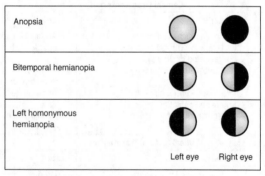

Anopsia		
Bitemporal hemianopia		
Left homonymous hemianopia	Left eye	Right eye

■ Visual field defects. Black area = no vision.

HUNT AND HESS SCALE (see Aneurysms, p. 5)

HYDROCEPHALUS

Hydrocephalus is an abnormal accumulation of CSF in the cranial vault. In infants, the head enlarges. In adults, because the cranium is fixed in size and cannot give, there is no enlargement. The mounting pressure caused by the excess fluid squeezes the brain tissue against the skull, causing tissue atrophy and tissue death, as well as seizures. Hydrocephalus can be surgically corrected by placing a ventroperitoneal (VP) shunt that runs from the brain ventricle, under the skin, downward to the peritoneum for drainage.

INCREASED INTRACRANIAL PRESSURE (see also Cerebral Perfusion Pressure, p. 13; Cushing's Reflex and Cushing's Triad, p. 22; Intracranial Pressure Monitoring, p. 37; Monro-Kellie Hypothesis, p. 43)

When the nondistendable intracranial cavity is filled to capacity with noncompressible contents—that is, CSF, blood, or brain tissue—the result is an increase in intracranial pressure (ICP).

Normal ICP	3 to 15 mm Hg
Severe increase	>20 mm Hg

CONDITIONS CAUSING AN INCREASE IN ICP

Increased brain volume	• Space-occupying lesions such as epidural and subdural hematomas, abscesses, or aneurysms
	• Cerebral edema related to head injuries, cardiopulmonary arrest, and metabolic encephalopathies
Increased blood volume	• Obstruction of venous outflow
	• Hyperemia
	• Hypercapnia

> **REMEMBER:**
>
> *Receptors in the brain constantly analyze blood gases. Therefore, an increase in PCO_2 (hypoventilation) means vasodilation of cerebral vessels and an increase in blood flow to the brain: ICP rises. Conversely, a decrease in PCO_2 (hyperventilation) means vasoconstriction of cerebral vessels and a decrease of blood flow to the brain: ICP decreases.*

	• Disease states associated with increased blood volume
	• Reye's syndrome
Increased CSF	• Increased production of CSF
	• Decreased absorption of CSF
	• Obstruction of CSF flow

FACTORS CONTRIBUTING TO INCREASED ICP

Hypercapnia (PCO_2 >5 mm Hg)	• Sleep, sedation, shallow respirations, coma, neuromuscular impairment, improper mechanical ventilator settings
Hypoxemia (PCO_2 >30 mm Hg)	• Insufficient oxygen concentration in supplemental oxygen therapy; inadequate lung perfusion; inadequate lung ventilation; drug-induced cerebral vasodilation; administration of nicotinic acid, cyclandelate, histamine, and anesthetic agents such as halothane, enflurane, isoflurane, and nitrous oxide
Valsalva's maneuver	• Straining at stool, moving or turning in bed, coughing, sneezing
Body positioning	• Any position that obstructs venous return from the brain, i.e., Trendelenburg's, prone, extreme flexion of hips, neck flexion
Isometric muscle contractions	• Isometric exercises, i.e., pushing against resistance, shivering, decerebration

(continued)

| REM sleep | • Rapid eye movements are associated with cerebral activity; sleep arousal also increases ICP |
| Noxious stimuli | • Visceral discomfort, painful procedures, stimuli associated with assessment, loud noises |

CLASSIC SIGNS AND SYMPTOMS OF INCREASED ICP

Decreased LOC	• Confusion, increasing headache, blurred vision, vomiting
Impaired motor function	• Change in motor ability, change in cranial nerve function (especially oculomotor function)
Alteration in pupil reflex	• Papilledema (edema of the optic disc; a positive sign of increased ICP but not seen in acute intracranial hypertension), sluggish or absent light responses, photophobia
Change in vital signs	• A change in baseline from one assessment to the next may indicate a change in neurologic status

MANAGEMENT OF INCREASED ICP

Management of increased ICP (>15 mm Hg) includes one or several of the following:

• Analgesia/sedation. Anxiety, restlessness, and pain will increase ICP. Morphine sulfate is the preferred analgesic, with hydromorphone as an alternative. Fentanyl is the best choice if the patient is hemodynamically unstable. Midazolam (Versed) and propofol (Diprivan) are preferred for short-term anxiety (<24 hours), and lorazepam (Ativan) is preferred for prolonged anxiety. Haloperidol (Haldol) is typically reserved for delirium.

• Barbiturate coma. Phenobarbital or pentobarbital produce complete unresponsiveness and therefore decreased metabolic demands. *Note:* Patient must be intubated and ventilated with continuous arterial blood pressure monitoring.

• Blood pressure control. Since hypotension is directly related to cerebral ischemia, MAP should be maintained above 90 mm Hg at all times, with cerebral perfusion pressure above 70 mm Hg (treat with fluid bolus and/or vasopressors). Conversely, hypertension shows little effect on ICP or cerebral blood flow.

• Elevate head of bed to 30°. Use of gravity facilitates venous drainage (because brain has no valves) and will concomitantly lower ICP. This measure is contraindicated in hypovolemic states.

• Fluid management. Deliver only hypertonic or isotonic fluids. **No D5W or ½ NS** (fluid would go from blood vessels to brain matter and increase edema).

• Hyperventilate. Lowering $PaCO_2$ causes vasoconstriction (CO_2 is a potent vasodilator) and results in decreased cerebral blood flow, thereby decreasing ICP. Currently this method is used only during an emergent rise in ICP. Typically, CO_2 levels in the low 30 range and higher are acceptable. If the ICP suddenly rises to dangerous levels, aggressive "bagging" is typically done, while other interventions get underway.

• Hypothermia. Early studies showed decreased cerebral edema as a result of moderate hypothermia (core temperature 32° to 33°C), but more recent studies are inconclusive. While still sometimes used, the treatment is falling out of favor.

• Neuromuscular blockade. Used as a chemical restraint to control behavior that contributes to an increase in ICP. Pancuronium is the preferred drug for most critically ill patients, and vecuronium is used for patients with cardiac disease or unstable hemodynamics.

(*continued*)

- Osmotic diuretics. Mannitol, urea, and glycerol are used to decrease interstitial fluid in the brain by drawing water from the extracellular space of edematous brain tissue into the plasma.
- Oxygenation. PaO_2 below 60 mm Hg must be avoided, because adequate cerebral perfusion levels cannot be maintained.
- Seizure control. Prophylaxis for high-risk patients (within 7 days of injury) should be initiated. Dilantin and carbamazepine are effective agents.
- Temperature control. Hyperthermia should be treated aggressively with antipyretic drugs and/or a cooling blanket. For every 1°C rise in body temperature, the cerebral blood flow increases 5% to 6%. (Avoid shivering, however, because this will also increase ICP).

INTRACRANIAL PRESSURE MONITORING
(see also Cerebral Perfusion Pressure, p. 13; Increased Intracranial Pressure, p. 35)

Normal ICP   3 to 15 mm Hg
Severe increase   >20 mm Hg

THE WAVEFORM
The ICP waveform results from transmission of arterial and venous pressure waves through the CSF and brain parenchyma. The normal ICP waveform has an upstroke that corresponds to systole and three small peaks of decreasing amplitude (see figure). The waveform resembles a somewhat dampened arterial waveform.

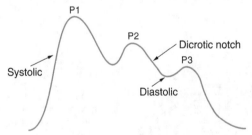

■ Normal intracranial pressure waveform. (Adapted from Hudak, C. M., Gallo, B. M., & Morton, P. G. [1998]. *Critical care nursing* [7th ed.]. Philadelphia: Lippincott-Raven.)

A waves (plateau waves) are seen in the decompensatory stage of increased ICP and are associated with cerebral ischemia. They may last 2 to 20 minutes and occur from a baseline of an already increased ICP (usually >20 mm Hg but may be as high as 40 to 50 mm Hg). Physician should be notified.

B waves (sawtooth waves) occur in multiples and are associated with fluctuations of ICP related to respiratory patterns. They may occur every 30 seconds to 2 minutes with an ICP in the range of 20 to 50 mm Hg. They signify a decreased intracranial compliance and are a precursor of A waves.

C waves (small, rhythmic waves) occur four to eight times per minute. They correlate to normal fluctuations in respiration and blood pressure. They have no clinical significance but may be associated with increased ICP by as much as 20 mm Hg.

(continued)

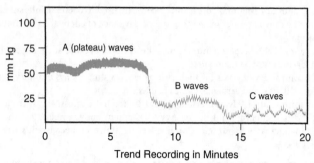

■ Intracranial pressure waves. Composite drawing of A (plateau) waves, B waves, and C waves.

MONITORING DEVICES

Ventriculostomy

The ventriculostomy is considered the "gold standard" for ICP monitoring. Though its accuracy is unquestionable, it is associated with the highest risk of infection and requires that the user have a sound working knowledge of the system. The ventriculostomy is inserted into the anterior horn of the lateral ventricle (sometimes posterior horn), usually in the nondominant hemisphere, and can be incorporated into a hydraulic, fluid-filled, or fiberoptic monitoring system.

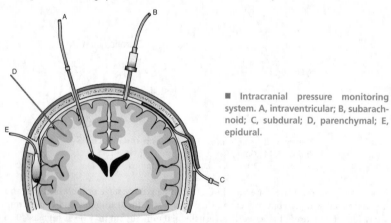

■ Intracranial pressure monitoring system. A, intraventricular; B, subarachnoid; C, subdural; D, parenchymal; E, epidural.

Setup specifics:
- Head of bed should be elevated 20° to 30°.
- If a fluid-filled transduced system, prime line with nonbacteriostatic normal saline. No air bubbles in system.
- Level transducer at the foramen of Monro (halfway between the outer canthus of the eye and the tragus of the ear).
- Remember to relevel with any change in the patient's position.
- Connect to bedside monitor, and zero the monitor (open to air, closed to the patient). Remember to rezero with any change in the patient's position. Check for adequate waveform.

(continued)

- Physician may order the drainage collection chamber to be elevated at a specific level above the patient for CSF drainage.
- This is usually in centimeters H_2O, but it can also be in millimeters Hg. These are different levels, so be sure to be consistent with the order. Alternately, orders may be received to drain a specific amount of CSF, then clamp the ventriculostomy, or to open the ventriculostomy to drainage when a certain ICP level is reached.
- If the patient's ICP exceeds the level at which the bag is positioned, CSF should flow into the bag. Conversely, if the bag is leveled too low, the patient drains CSF that should not be drained. This is dangerous.
- Be sure all tubing is air-bubble–free, and never fast-flush the ventricular catheter.
- To obtain CSF samples, always use the port below the collection chamber, and swab with Betadine only.
- Remember to always close the stopcock to the patient during temporary change of position, e.g., for x-ray films or turning, and remember to always reopen it on completion of task.

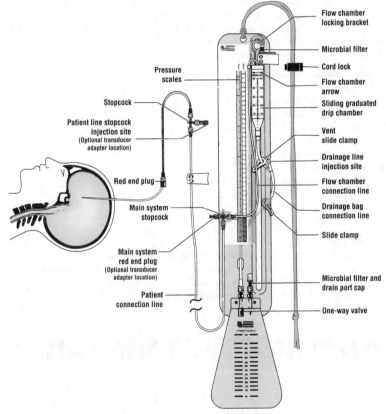

■ Becker external drainage and monitoring system for intracranial pressure monitoring and intermittent cerebrospinal fluid drainage. (Adapted from Medtronic PS Medical, Goleta, CA.)

(continued)

Troubleshooting—fluid-filled system:
- Loss of waveform
    Check stopcock connections.
    Check for air in system.
    Check monitor cable.
    Increase gain or range on monitor.
- False high or low
    Rezero and calibrate.
    Reposition transducer.
    Check system for air bubbles.
- Low ICP
    Check patient for otorrhea and rhinorrhea.

Fiberoptics

The fiberoptic catheter is extremely versatile and can be placed in virtually any intracranial location because the transducer is at the tip of the catheter. Usually, it is incorporated within a subarachnoid bolt or ventriculostomy. The system requires no flush and is calibrated only once immediately before insertion. The problems of a fluid-filled system are eliminated, but the system is difficult to maintain securely fixed to the patient, and the fragile fiberoptic filaments are easily damaged as a result of tension or catheter crimping, all too often rendering the system inoperable.

Troubleshooting—fiberoptic system:
- Loss of waveform
    Check cable connections, reconnecting as needed.
    Increase gain or range.
    Assist physician in repositioning catheter.
- False high or low
    Assist physician in repositioning catheter.
- Monitor reads 888
    Assist physician in repositioning catheter.
- Microprocessor and bedside monitor do not correlate
    Rezero and calibrate.
    Check connections.

Subarachnoid Bolt

No penetration of the brain is necessary for insertion of this device, because it is "screwed" into the subarachnoid space (see figure). The risk of infection is markedly decreased. However, the system affords no way to drain CSF and is unreliable at high ICPs, when the brain tissue herniates up into the monitoring device.

(*continued*)

NOTES

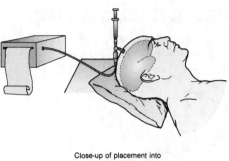

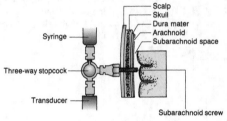

Close-up of placement into
subarachnoid space

Scalp
Skull
Dura mater
Arachnoid
Subarachnoid space

Syringe

Three-way stopcock

Transducer

Subarachnoid screw

■ Subarachnoid bolt.

Troubleshooting—subarachnoid bolt:
- Loss of waveform
    Check stopcock connections.
    Check for air in system.
    Check monitor cable.
    Increase gain or range on monitor.
- False high or low
    Recalibrate.
    Check system for air bubbles.
- Low ICP
    Check patient for otorrhea and rhinorrhea.

INTRATHECAL ANALGESIA

Unlike epidural analgesia (where drugs are injected into a "potential" space), intrathecal analgesia (also known as "spinal analgesia") is injected directly into the subarachnoid space in the spine, where CSF is present. This allows for a rapid onset of pain relief with a very small volume of drug. Typically, opioids are administered intrathecally for the treatment of both acute postoperative pain and various chronic pain syndromes. Cancer pain was the first indication for intrathecal opioid administration, although using it to treat noncancer pain is now more common. The advantages of intrathecal therapy are reduced incidence of adverse reactions and simplified medical regimens. Side effects are much the same as those for epidural analgesia: respiratory depression, itching, constipation, and urinary retention. Long-term complications of intrathecal administration of opioids may include catheter fracture or dislodgement, resulting in abrupt cessation of intrathecal drug therapy and onset of acute opioid withdrawal.

KERNIG'S SIGN *(see also Brudzinski's Sign, p. 12)*

To test for Kernig's sign, flex patient's hip 90° and extend knee. Response is positive if there is pain and/or spasm and indicates a bleed into subarachnoid space. It is also positive in meningitis.

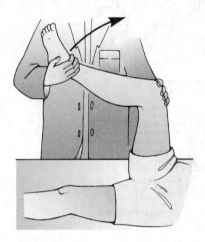

■ Kernig's sign. (From Hickey J. V. [2009]. *Neurological and neurosurgical nursing* [6th ed., p. 667]. Philadelphia: Lippincott Williams & Wilkins.)

KUSSMAUL'S RESPIRATION *(see Respiratory Patterns in Part 3, p. 204)*

LOBE FUNCTIONS *(see Anatomy: Brain Structures and Function, p. 2)*

LUMBAR PUNCTURE *(see also Cerebrospinal Fluid, p. 14; Cerebrospinal Fluid Lab Values in Part 9, p. 343)*

Lumbar puncture is performed below the second lumbar vertebra, so spinal cord won't be hit. It is diagnostic for subarachnoid hemorrhage and meningitis.

Normal lumbar pressures:
with patient side lying 8–180 cm H_2O via ICP monitoring: 4–15 mm Hg

The procedure carries a relative contraindication with increased ICP, since pressure may be released lower in the spinal cord and theoretically cause cerebellar herniation leading to seizures.

LYMPHOMA *(see Tumors, Neurogenic, p. 63)*

MEAN ARTERIAL PRESSURE *(see also Increased Intracranial Pressure, p. 35)*

Normal MAP: 70 to 110 mm Hg

$$\frac{\text{Systolic blood pressure} + (\text{diastolic blood pressure} \times 2)}{3}$$

REMEMBER:

$$\frac{1 + 2}{3}$$

MEDULLOBLASTOMA *(see Tumors, Neurogenic, p. 63)*

MENINGIOMA *(see Tumors, Neurogenic, p. 63)*

MENINGITIS *(see also Brudzinski's Sign, p. 12; Cranial Nerves, p. 19; Kernig's Sign, p. 42; Lumbar Puncture, p. 42)*

Diagnosis of meningitis is related to pathologic organism found in subarachnoid space (meninges) causing disruption of the blood-brain barrier. Exudate forms and collects, resulting in tissue congestion, edema, and increased ICP. Meningitis leads to necrosis of the cortex and nerve damage. Several sources are possible: sinus, midear, skull fracture, drains, and so on. Pay attention to eighth cranial nerve (acoustic) because disease itself can cause deafness. Cause may be bacterial or viral.

The signs and symptoms form a common triad: Stiff neck, fever, and acute onset of altered neurologic status. Signs may also include headache, positive Kernig's and Brudzinski's signs, increased ICP, and petechiae. The two types of meningitis, bacterial and viral, are diagnosed by lumbar puncture, in which the CSF may exhibit the characteristics noted in the table.

Cerebrospinal Fluid in Viral versus Bacterial Meningitis

	Bacterial	Viral
Appearance	Cloudy	Clear, sometimes turbid
Protein	↑↑ (100–500 mg/dL)*	Normal or slightly ↑
Glucose	↓↓ (below 40 mg/dL)*	Relatively normal
WBCs	↑↑ (above 1,000–2,000 mm³ or more)	Mildly elevated (300 mm³)
Type cells	Predominantly neutrophils	Predominantly mononuclear

*REMEMBER: Bacteria like to eat things and viruses don't. Therefore, in bacterial meningitis, the bacteria "gobble up" all the glucose (it's so yummy!), resulting in decreased glucose in the CSF and increased protein, because it's left over.

Bacterial meningitis is treated with large doses of penicillin, and isolation of patient is required. The disease is further broken down into three subtypes:

- *Haemophilus influenzae* (children)   Gram–   *Haemophilus influenzae*
- Meningococcal (young adult)   Gram–   *Neisseria meningitidis*
- Pneumococcal (after 40)   Gram+   *Streptococcus pneumoniae*

Viral meningitis is also known as acute benign lymphocytic meningitis or acute aseptic meningitis. It is related to an enterovirus, but isolation is not necessary. It is usually seen in children, and complete recovery is standard.

MONRO-KELLIE HYPOTHESIS
(see also Increased Intracranial Pressure, p. 35)

The skull is a closed box containing three intracranial volumes:

1. CSF (about 10%)
2. Intravascular blood (about 10%)
3. Brain tissue (about 80%)

An increase in any one of the three, without a decrease in one or both of the others, will result in an increase in ICP.

MOYAMOYA DISEASE

Moyamoya disease is a rare, progressive cerebrovascular disorder, characterized by the spontaneous occlusion of one, more commonly both, internal carotid arteries and the resultant formation of a collateral network called moyamoya vessels (Japanese for "puff of smoke"). The disease primarily affects children in the first decade of their life, though it has been diagnosed in patients from 6 months to 67 years. Females are typically more affected than males. Although the pathophysiology is not fully understood, narrowed main trunks of intracranial arteries and lipid deposits in a thickened intima are common. Similar vessel changes also occur in the heart, kidneys, and other organs. Thus, this is a systemic vascular disease. Researchers suspect a genetic link because of the 9% incidence found in certain Japanese families. A gene for moyamoya has been found on a chromosome, and further study is under way. There is no cure. Pharmacologic therapy for the primary disease is disappointing. Treatment is primarily directed at the complications of the disease: Management of hypertension for intracerebral hemorrhage, and, in cases of severe stroke, consideration of anticoagulant and antiplatelet medications. Surgical treatment involves various methods to revascularize the ischemic brain, or placement of frontal burr holes with opening of the underlying dura and arachnoid. Mortality is in the 30% range.

MULTIPLE SCLEROSIS

Multiple sclerosis is a chronic, progressive demyelinating disease of the nervous system with an overgrowth of glial cells in the white substance of the brain and spinal cord. Early in the disease, the lesions formed by the destruction of the myelin sheath are temporary; later, they are permanent. Some common symptoms are these:
- Blurred vision
- Diplopia
- Nystagmus
- Weakness, tingling of extremity
- Ataxia
- Paralysis (usually of lower extremities)
- Intention tremor

These symptoms often appear gradually, then disappear, only to return later in months or even years. Some patients have severe, long-lasting exacerbations, whereas others experience only occasional, mild symptoms for several years after onset. The course is unknown, and there is no cure.

MUSCULAR DYSTROPHY

Muscular dystrophy is characterized by progressive weakness and finally by atrophy of groups of muscles. It is a general term for a group of inherited diseases involving a defective gene. It develops mostly in children, and in at least half of all cases, there is a history of at least one other family member who had the disease. There are several forms, pseudohypertrophic being one of the most common. It is characterized by enlargement of the calf muscles, accompanied by limitation of muscle function. No effective medical treatment is known. The disease does not have remissions and gets progressively worse. Unfortunately, few affected children live to adulthood, since over time, even the muscles that control breathing get weaker. Patients frequently die from respiratory failure, heart failure, pneumonia, or other medical problems.

MYASTHENIA GRAVIS

Myasthenia gravis is a disease of the neuromuscular junction characterized by abnormal muscle fatigue brought on by activity and improving with rest. The cause is unknown, although a link to autoimmunity is suspected. Sometimes, removal of the thymus is helpful. Diagnosis is based on the Tensilon (edrophonium) test. Tensilon is a rapid-acting anticholinesterase and causes the symptoms of the disease to rapidly and transiently improve.

A myasthenia crisis occurs when there is not enough cholinesterase in the system, or when a tolerance for it has been reached. Anticholinesterase then has no effect on the patient, and the muscle fatigue persists.

A cholinergic crisis occurs when there is too high a level of anticholinesterase in the system. It may cause respiratory paralysis. The condition is reversible with atropine. To identify a cholinergic crisis,

REMEMBER:

- Red as a beet (vasodilation)
- Mad as a hatter (neurologic changes)
- Hotter than hell (core temperature rises)
- Dry as a bone (saliva decreases, no sweating)

Normal:

Nerve impulse → ACh liberated → depolarization → muscle contracts

(a neurotransmitter)

Abnormal:

Nerve impulse → ACH liberated *but*

Cholinesterase destroys ACh → muscle weakness

Rx: Anticholinesterase (neostigmine, Mestinon) to destroy antibodies.

■ Myasthenia gravis diagram.

NERVE STIMULATOR *(see Peripheral Nerve Stimulator, p. 47)*

NEURINOMA *(see Tumors, Neurogenic, p. 61)*

NEUROFIBROMATOSIS

Neurofibromatosis is a genetic disorder of the nervous system, also known as von Recklinghausen's disease, that causes tumors to form on the nerves anywhere in the body at any time. Type 1 is carried on chromosome 17, and Type 2 is carried on chromosome 22. The effects of the disease are unpredictable and have varying manifestations and degrees of severity. There is no known cure for either form, and no treatment other than the surgical removal of tumors, which may sometimes grow back.

NEUROGENIC HYPERVENTILATION
(see Respiratory Patterns in Part 3, p. 203)

NEUROGENIC PULMONARY EDEMA
(see Pulmonary Edema in Part 3, p. 198)

NEUROGENIC SHOCK *(see Shock, Neurogenic, p. 52)*

NEURONS

Neurons are composed of a cell body and two types of processes: axons and dendrites. An axon is a single extension carrying impulses away from the cell body. Dendrites (meaning "treelike") are processes carrying impulses toward the cell body. There is only one axon, but several dendrites. A myelin sheath (made by Schwann cells) surrounds some axons. The nodes of Ranvier are areas along the axon not covered by myelin. They increase the speed of conduction. Synaptic knobs are the end portions where acetylcholine and epinephrine are stored.

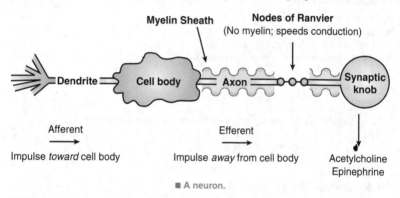

■ A neuron.

FUNCTION

Upper motor neurons conduct impulses from the motor area of the cerebral cortex to the brain stem or spinal cord. They are responsible for voluntary movement of specific body parts.

Lower motor neurons conduct impulses from the brain stem or spinal cord to specific muscle groups. Their function is to "relay" commands from the upper motor neurons to effect voluntary muscle movement. If either of these two neuron pathways is injured, the patient will exhibit specific symptoms, as illustrated in the table.

Symptoms of Upper Motor Neuron/Lower Motor Neuron Damage	
Upper Motor Neurons	**Lower Motor Neurons**
Loss of voluntary muscle control No inhibition of lower motor neurons, resulting in • Preservation of reflexes • Spastic muscles • Increased muscle tone • Little or no atrophy	Loss of voluntary muscle control Inhibition of lower motor neurons, resulting in • Absent or decreased reflexes • Flaccid paralysis of muscles • Decreased muscle tone • Significant atrophy

REMEMBER: Injury to the upper motor neurons (upper = <u>superior</u>) results in <u>spasticity</u>
Injury to the lower motor neurons (lower = <u>floor level</u>) results in <u>flaccidity</u>

NEUROTRANSMITTERS *(see also Myasthenia Gravis, p. 45)*

Acetylcholine is the major transmitter at the neuromuscular junction. Other neurotransmitters are norepinephrine, dopamine, and serotonin.

NUCHAL RIGIDITY *(see also Brudzinski's Sign, p. 12)*

Nuchal rigidity occurs in meningeal irritation and produces pain and stiffness when the patient attempts to flex the head to the chest.

OCULOCEPHALIC REFLEX *(see Doll's Eyes, p. 23)*

OCULOVESTIBULAR REFLEX *(see Caloric Test, p. 12)*

OLIGODENDROGLIOMA *(see Tumors, Neurogenic, p. 63)*

OPISTHOTONOS

Extension of the body with the neck and back arched is opisthotonos. It is seen in patients with tetany or with damage to the brain stem.

PARKINSON'S DISEASE *(see also Stereotactic Surgery, p. 56)*

Parkinson's disease belongs to a group of conditions known as motor system disorders and is related to a deficiency of dopamine in the basal ganglia. It is characterized by four primary symptoms: tremors ("pill rolling"); rigidity of movement; slow motion and shuffling gait; and postural instability. The progression of the disease varies from person to person. Since dopamine itself does not cross the blood-brain barrier, L-dopa, a precursor of dopamine, is given as a replacement. Stereotactic surgery is sometimes helpful.

PERIPHERAL NERVE STIMULATOR

When administering neuromuscular blocking agents, a peripheral nerve stimulator is used to monitor the level of blockade. Electric stimulation is applied to the ulnar nerve, the facial nerve, or the posterior tibial nerve, with the ulnar nerve being the preferred site.

1. Place electrodes along ulnar nerve, 3 to 5 cm apart.
2. Apply alligator clips to electrodes (polarity is insignificant).
3. Establish a baseline before beginning therapy by setting the output dial on the stimulator to 4.
4. Press TOF (train of four) to elicit four mild electric stimuli. If four twitches are not seen, increase the current by one until four twitches are observed. Be sure to wait 15 seconds between stimuli to allow for nerve repolarization. The level at which four twitches are seen is the stimulation threshold.
5. Commence therapy (pancuronium usually preferred; vecuronium for patients with cardiac disease or hemodynamic instability).

As the depth of the blockade increases, the number of twitches on the TOF will decrease (see table). A TOF is generally assessed every hour, but frequency depends on whether the drug is being titrated or an infusion is being maintained.

(continued)

Twitch Responses for Degrees of Blockade

Train of Four Twitch Response	Approximate Degree of Blockade (%)
4/4	0–75
3/4	75–80
2/4	80–90
1/4	90
0/4	100

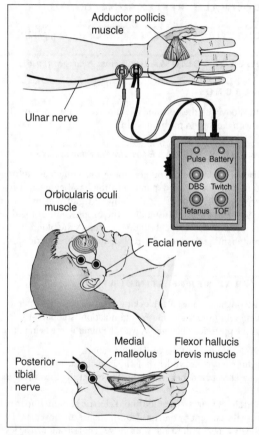

■ Nerve stimulator. (Courtesy of Neuro Technology, Inc., Houston, TX.)

PINEAL REGION TUMORS (see Tumors, Neurogenic, p. 63)

PITUITARY ADENOMA (see Tumors, Neurogenic, p. 63)

PLASMAPHERESIS

Plasmapheresis is removal of one or more components of blood after the blood is separated into component parts. It is used in myasthenia gravis or Guillain-Barre syndrome to remove autoantibodies, as well as in other immune-related disorders such as multiple myeloma, lupus, and rheumatoid arthritis, or the palliative treatment of disseminated intravascular coagulation (DIC).

Access is established via a large-bore, double-lumen central venous line or a large antecubital vein, and the patient is connected to an extracorporeal circuit. The "old" plasma is removed from whole blood by flow through a cell separator, where it is centrifuged down (or passed through a microporous membrane filter) and exchanged for "new" plasma in the form of replacement fluid. (In an alternative method, the plasma is separated out, filtered to remove the disease mediator, then returned to the patient.) In both methods, because the extracorporeal circuit contains 150 to 400 mL of blood during the procedure, the patient needs to be able to tolerate the low volume.

PONS

The pons consists of fibers and nuclei situated at the base of the brain that receive impulses from the cerebral cortex. A lesion in the pons is accompanied by pinpoint pupils and apneustic breathing.

POSTURING *(see Decerebrate, p. 22; Decorticate, p. 22; Opisthotonos, p. 47)*

PUPIL GAUGE

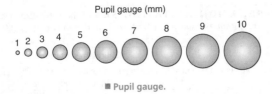

Pupil gauge (mm)

■ Pupil gauge.

RACCOON EYES *(see Basilar Skull Fracture, p. 8)*

RAMSEY SCALE *(see also Bispectral Index Monitoring, p. 9; Riker Sedation-Agitation Scale, p. 50; Moderate Sedation in Part 8, p. 323)*

	Level	Clinical Description
Desired level during moderate sedation	1	Awake, anxious, bordering agitation/restlessness
	2	Awake, cooperative, accepting ventilation, oriented, tranquil
	3	Awake, responds only to verbal commands
	4	Asleep but responds briskly to loud auditory or light tactile stimuli
	5	Asleep, sluggish response to loud auditory or light tactile stimuli but retains brisk response to painful stimulus
	6	Asleep, no response to any stimulation

RASS SCALE (*see Richmond Agitation Sedation Scale, p. 50*)

RETICULAR ACTIVATING SYSTEM

The reticular activating system is essential for arousal from sleep, alert wakefulness, focusing of attention, and perceptual association. Destructive lesions of upper pons and midbrain produce coma.

RICHMOND AGITATION SEDATION SCALE (RASS)
(*see also Ramsey Scale, p. 49*)

Score	Term	Description
+4	Combative	Overly combative, violent, immediate danger to staff
+3	Very agitated	Pulls or removes tubes or catheters; aggressive
+2	Agitated	Frequent nonpurposeful movement, fights ventilator
+1	Restless	Anxious, but movement not aggressive
0	Alert, calm	
−1	Drowsy	Awakens to voice (eye opening/contact) >10 seconds
−2	Light sedation	Briefly awakens to voice (eye opening/contact) <10 seconds
−3	Moderate sedation	Movement or eye opening to voice (but no eye contact)
−4	Deep sedation	No response to voice, but movement or eye opening to physical stimulation
−5	Unarousable	No response to voice or physical stimulation

RIKER SEDATION-AGITATION SCALE (*see also Bispectral Index Monitoring p. 9; Ramsey Scale, p. 49; Moderate Sedation in Part 8, p. 323*)

	Level	Clinical Presentation
7	Dangerous agitation	Pulling at ET tube, trying to remove catheters, climbing over bed rail, striking out at staff, thrashing side to side
6	Very agitated	Does not calm despite frequent verbal reminding of limits, biting ET tube, requires physical restraints
5	Agitated	Anxious or mildly agitated, attempting to sit up but calms down to verbal instructions
4	Calm	Cooperative, awakens easily, follows commands
3	Sedated	Difficult to arouse, awakens to verbal stimuli or gentle shaking but drifts off again. Follows simple commands
2	Very sedated	Arouses to physical stimuli but does not communicate or follow commands. May move spontaneously
1	Unarousable	Minimal or no response to noxious stimuli, does not communicate or follow any commands

RINNE TEST (*see also Caloric Test, p. 12; Weber's Test, p. 66*)

The Rinne test is used to diagnose middle ear disease by testing the eighth cranial nerve. Place vibrating tuning fork on mastoid bone. When sound is no longer heard, fork is

(*continued*)

placed in front of the ear, where sound is normally louder (conduction through bone vs. through air).

ROMBERG'S TEST

Patient is asked to stand with legs together, arms out, and eyes closed. Position is to be maintained for 20 to 30 seconds. A minimal sway is acceptable, but if the patient exhibits a major sway or falls, this signifies a positive result, indicative of cerebellar dysfunction.

SCHWANNOMA *(see Tumors, Neurogenic, p. 61)*

SEIZURES *(see also Electroencephalogram Monitoring, p. 24)*

A seizure is an electric discharge in the neurons of the cerebral cortex and possibly neurons of the brain stem. Definitive diagnosis is determined by EEG monitoring. The causes or precipitating factors are many, including genes, cerebral tumors, metabolic disorders, AVMs of the brain, trauma, infections, and cerebral vascular disease, to name a few.

Treatment involves first preventing injury during seizure activity and protecting the airway. Improved control of seizure activity by monitoring and maintaining therapeutic drug levels must follow. (See also Therapeutic Drug Levels in Part 9.)

GENERALIZED SEIZURE

The manifestations of this type of seizure are seen bilaterally and in both hemispheres.

- Absence (petit mal). Sudden loss of awareness. Mostly in children, sometimes as many as 300 in 24 hours.
- Generalized motor (grand mal). Tonic movement (abrupt increase in muscle tone) and clonic movement (jerky, rhythmic movement) to both sides of body.
- Myoclonic. Sudden, brief muscular contractions that may occur singly or repetitively; usually involves arms.
- Akinetic. Sudden, brief loss of muscle tone; "drop attacks."

PARTIAL SEIZURE

Initial neuronal discharge is limited to one focal site or one cerebral hemisphere. Clinical symptoms usually begin on one side of body. Partial seizures may progress into generalized seizures.

- Simple partial. No impaired level of consciousness
- Complex partial. Impaired level of consciousness. Inability to respond to external stimuli. No memory of event. Repeat of inappropriate acts called automatisms, such as smacking of lips, chewing movements.

STATUS EPILEPTICUS

Most clinicians agree that SE is defined as either a continuous seizure lasting more than 5 minutes; or two or more sequential seizures, where there is no recovery of consciousness in between. SE is a medical emergency and is associated with significant morbidity and mortality (20%). Prolonged, uncontrolled seizure activity may lead to cardiorespiratory problems, hyperthermia, and ultimately metabolic imbalances that result in irreversible brain death. The most common cause of SE is abrupt withdrawal from anti-epileptic drugs, or noncompliance with them, although other causes such as withdrawal from alcohol, sedative, or other drugs have been cited. Clinically, SE patients can present with convulsive or nonconvulsive seizure activity (in which case, an EEG is required to detect the presence of seizure activity). Treatment is focused on maintaining an airway and controlling the seizure activity promptly.

(continued)

STATUS EPILEPTICUS ALGORITHM

INITIALLY

Lorazepam (Ativan) 0.1 mg/kg IV given at 2 mg/min
This may control the immediate seizure activity but will not provide long term protection against recurrence.

⇩

IF SEIZURES DO NOT TERMINATE

Phenytoin (Dilantin) 20 mg/kg IV at 50 mg/min
or
Fosphenytoin 20 mg/kg PE IV at 150 mg/min
The use of Fosphenytoin is gaining popularity due to the fact that it can be mixed in D5W or 0.9 NS, no IV filter is required, and it has fewer reported infusion site reactions.

⇩

IF SEIZURES DO NOT TERMINATE

Additional Phenytoin (Dilantin) 5-10 mg/kg IV
Or
Additional Fosphenytoin 5-10 mg/kg PE IV

⇩   ⇩

IF SEIZURES DO NOT TERMINATE AND HAVE CONTINUED LONGER THAN 90 MINUTES; OR IF THE PATIENT HAS SEVERE SYSTEMIC PROBLEMS; OR IS IN ICU

IF THE PATIENT DOES NOT FIT CRITERIA LISTED ON LEFT, AND SEIZURES DO NOT TERMINATE

Proceed to anesthesia with midazolam or propofol

Phenobarbital 20 mg/kg IV at 50-75 mg/min

IF SEIZURES CONTINUE

Additional Phenobarbital 5-10 mg/kg IV

IF SEIZURES CONTINUE

Proceed to anesthesia with midazolam or propofol

SHOCK, NEUROGENIC *(see also Shock Parameters in Part 2, p. 147)*

It is characterized by severe autonomic dysfunction resulting in hypotension, bradycardia, peripheral vasodilation, and hypothermia (body heat is lost due to passively dilated vascular bed). Initially, neurogenic shock may mimic hypovolemic shock; however, the compensatory tachycardia will not occur. In neurogenic shock, bradycardia is generally due to the unopposed vagal tone. Neurogenic shock tends to occur more commonly in

(continued)

spinal cord injuries above the level of T6. It may last from several days to several months. In the acute phase, administration of pressor agents may be required to support blood pressure and heart rate.

SIADH (see Syndrome of Inappropriate Antidiuretic Hormone in Part 6, p. 273)

SKULL FRACTURE (see Basilar Skull Fracture, p. 8)

SPINAL CORD (see also Lumbar Puncture, p. 42; Spinal Injury, p. 55; Vertebrae, p. 65)

The spinal cord extends from the foramen magnum to the second lumbar vertebra. The anterior gray column (anterior horn) contains efferent or motor fibers. The posterior gray column (posterior horn) contains cell bodies of the afferent or sensory fibers. The lateral column (prominent in upper cervical, thoracic, and midsacral regions) contains preganglionic fibers of the autonomic nervous system. The white matter, arranged into three longitudinal columns called anterior, lateral, and posterior funiculi, contains mostly myelinated axons. The funiculi also contain tracts that are functionally distinct (i.e., have the same or similar origin, course, and termination) and are classified as ascending or descending.

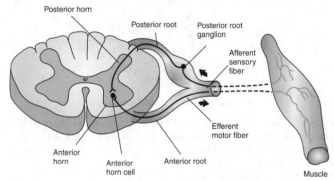

■ Cross-section of the spinal cord.

The major ascending tracts of the spinal cord (afferent, sensory, posterior) (see figure) are pathways to the brain for impulses entering the cord via the dorsal root of the spinal nerves.

- Fasciculus gracilis and fasciculus cuneatus convey sensations of position, movement, touch, and pressure.
- Lateral spinothalamic tract conveys sensations of pain and temperature.
- Ventral spinothalamic tract transmits stimuli of touch and pressure.
- Dorsal spinocerebellar tract conveys sensory impulses from muscles and muscle tendons to cerebellum.
- Ventral spinocerebellar tract is the same as dorsal spinocerebellar tract.
- Spinotectal tract pathway correlates with pathway of spinal cord.

(continued)

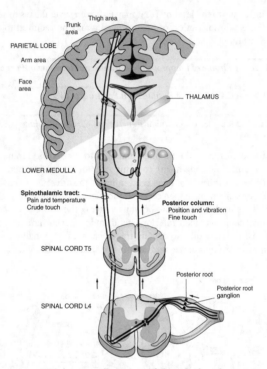

Thigh area

Trunk
area

PARIETAL LOBE

Arm area

Face
area

THALAMUS

LOWER MEDULLA

Spinothalamic tract:
Pain and temperature
Crude touch

Posterior column:
Position and vibration
Fine touch

SPINAL CORD T5

Posterior root

Posterior root
ganglion

SPINAL CORD L4

■ Major ascending tracts of the spinal cord.

The major descending tracts of the spinal cord (efferent, motor, anterior) (see figure) transmit impulses from the brain to the motor neurons of the spinal cord.

- Corticospinal (pyramidal) tract is the major pathway from the cortex to the peripheral motor nerves for voluntary movement.
- Tectospinal tract mediates optic and auditory reflexes.
- Rubrospinal tract conveys impulses from the cerebellum to the anterior column motor cells.

(*continued*)

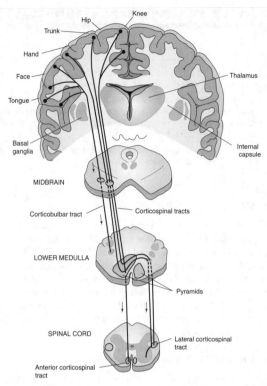

■ Major descending tracts of the spinal cord.

SPINAL INJURY *(see also Brown-Sequard Syndrome, p. 11; Lumbar Puncture, p. 42; Spinal Cord, p. 53; Vertebrae, p. 65)*

The degree and location of injury to the spinal cord determine the extent of the disability (see table p. 56). If the injury is high in the cervical region, respiratory failure and death follow paralysis of the diaphragm.

REMEMBER:

C1, C2, a pine box for you;
C3, 4, 5 keep the diaphragm alive;
S3, S4 keep caca off the floor.

Midcervical injuries result in breathing only by diaphragmatic movement, because the muscles of the upper thorax are paralyzed. Thoracic vertebrae are seldom injured because they are protected by the rib cage. The fifth and sixth cervical vertebrae and the first and fifth lumbar vertebrae are especially vulnerable, and injury to the cord at these levels is frequent. The severity of injury to the cord also determines how much function is lost. When the cord is completely severed, function is lost permanently below the level of the injury. If the damage to the cord is partial, some function may be maintained or, at times, even regained.

(continued)

Location of Spinal Cord Injury and Related Disability	
Injury to	**Findings**
C1, C2, C3	Usually fatal
C4	Quadriplegia, respiration difficulty
C5–C8	Variable function of neck, shoulder, and arm muscles
T1–T11	Paraplegia. Respiration is a concern because upper thoracic region innervates intercostal muscles. Loss of vasomotor tone, vagal responses. Inability to regulate heart rate. Loss of autonomic nerve impulses. Occasionally, leg braces can be used when injury is to lower thoracic spine.
T12–13	Paraplegia. Mixed picture of motor and sensory loss, bowel and bladder dysfunction. Probable wheelchair; leg braces necessary.

SPINAL SHOCK

Spinal shock is a temporary reflex depression of spinal cord function below the level of injury with associated loss of sensorimotor function. This is frequently the first picture of a patient with spinal cord injury. The cord is "jolted" so that nothing works. *Below* the level of the injury, the patient is areflexic with flaccid paralysis, has loss of pain and sensation, has bowel and bladder dysfunction, and is anhydrous. The duration can be days, weeks, or months. Interventions include close monitoring of the respiratory status. Blood pressure may drop, and if it does, there is probably damage to the thoracic area or above. Bradycardia (vagus nerve involvement) as well as decreased temperature and decreased potassium levels may also be seen.

STATUS EPILEPTICUS *(see Seizures, p. 51)*

STEREOGNOSIS

Stereognosis is tactile discrimination, or recognizing the form and size of objects by touch. It is determined by parietal lobe function.

STEREOTACTIC SURGERY

Stereotactic surgery (stereo = three-dimensional; tactic = to touch) is based on atlases of three-dimensional coordinates compiled from dissections. Current techniques would be more appropriately termed "image-guided stereotactic surgery," because a computed tomographic (CT) scan, magnetic resonance imaging (MRI), or occasionally an angiogram is performed with a compatible device affixed to the patient's head, allowing the target to be precisely localized.

Many different frames have been developed, the most common of which are the Leksell, Todd-Wells, Brown-Robert-Wells, and Guiot. A set of guides, oriented to the same coordinate system, is used to direct biopsy needles to the target location. This method is useful for biopsy or for aspiration of small, deeply situated tumors or abscesses. The combination of stereotactics with craniotomy provides for a more direct localization and obviates the need for ventriculography.

(continued)

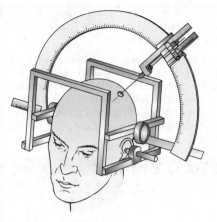

■ Stereotactic frame. (Reprinted with permission from the CIBA Collection of Medical Illustrations [1991]. *Neurology and neurosurgery* [Vol. I, Part II.]. New York: Churchill Livingstone.)

Brown-Robert-Wells (BRW) system:

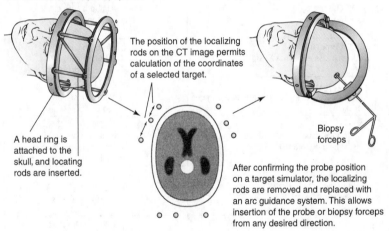

The position of the localizing rods on the CT image permits calculation of the coordinates of a selected target.

A head ring is attached to the skull, and locating rods are inserted.

Biopsy forceps

After confirming the probe position on a target simulator, the localizing rods are removed and replaced with an arc guidance system. This allows insertion of the probe or biopsy forceps from any desired direction.

■ Stereotactic procedure. (Adapted from Lindsey, K., Bone, I., & Callender, R. [1991]. *Neurology and neurosurgery illustrated* [2nd ed.]. New York: Churchill Livingstone.)

STROKE *(see also Alteplase in Part 8, p. 298)*

A life-threatening event in which the brain's vital supply of O_2 is disrupted, affecting senses, speech, behavior, thought patterns, and memory. About 10% of strokes are preceded by TIAs occurring days, weeks, or months before a major stroke. Strokes fall into two major categories:

1. Ischemic (80% to 85%), due to interruption or blockage of blood flow to brain and including thrombotic, embolic, lacunar, and dissecting events.

(continued)

2. Hemorrhagic (15% to 20%), due to rupture of a blood vessel, characterized by bleeding within or surrounding brain, and often a result of intracerebral or subarachnoid hemorrhage. Typically, these patients exhibit rapid deterioration.

If a CT scan is negative for bleeding or edema, and the exact time of onset of symptoms can be identified, the patient may be a candidate for fibrinolytic therapy. Following a stroke, the blood pressure may fluctuate dramatically, often requiring treatment with labetalol or nipride.

The National Institutes of Health Stroke Scale (NIHSS) was developed as a tool to measure the neurologic deficits most often seen with an acute stroke. It shows good correlation with 3-month outcomes and a direct relationship between a score of ≥15 and the presence of an arterial clot in ischemic stroke.

National Institutes of Health Stroke Scale		
Category	**Description**	**Score**
1a. Level of Consciousness	Alert	0
	Drowsy	1
	Stuporous	2
	Coma	3
1b. LOC Questions (Month, age)	Answers both correctly	0
	Answers one correctly	1
	Incorrect	2
1c. LOC Commands (Open, close eyes, make fist, let go)	Obeys both correctly	0
	Obeys one correctly	1
	Incorrect	2
2. Best Gaze (Eyes open, patient follows examiner's finger or face)	Normal	0
	Partial Gaze Palsy	1
	Forced Deviation	2
3. Visual (Introduce visual stimulus/threat to patient's visual field quadrants)	No Visual Loss	0
	Partial Hemianopsia	1
	Complete Hemianopsia	2
	Bilateral Hemianopsia	3
4. Facial Palsy (Show teeth, raise eyebrows, and squeeze eyes shut)	Normal	0
	Minor	1
	Partial	2
	Complete	3
5. Motor Arm-Left/Right (Elevate extremity to 90° and score drift/movement)	No Drift	0
	Drift	1
	Can't Resist Gravity	2
	No Effort Against Gravity	3
	No Movement	4
	Amputation, Joint Fusion (explain)	9
6. Motor Leg-Left/Right (Elevate extremity to 30° and score drift/movement)	No Drift	0
	Drift	1
	Can't Resist Gravity	2
	No Effort Against Gravity	3
	No Movement	4
	Amputation, Joint Fusion (explain)	9
7. Limb Ataxia (Finger to nose, heel down shin)	Absent	0
	Present in one limb	1
	Present in two limbs	2
	Amputation, Joint Fusion	9

(continued)

National Institutes of Health Stroke Scale (*Continued*)		
Category	**Description**	**Score**
8. Sensory (Pinprick to face, arm, trunk, and leg compare side to side)	Normal Partial Loss Severe Loss	0 1 2
9. Best Language (Name items, describe a picture, and read sentences)	No Aphasia Mild to Moderate Aphasia Severe Aphasia Mute	0 1 2 3
10. Dysarthria (Evaluate speech clarity by patient repeating listed words)	Normal Articulation Mild to Moderate Dysarthria Near to Unintelligible or Worse Intubated or Other Physical Barrier	0 1 2 9
11. Extinction and Inattention (Use information from prior testing to identify neglect or double simultaneous testing)	No Neglect Partial Neglect Complete Neglect	0 1 2

Another stroke scale, the Cincinnati Prehospital Stroke Scale (CPSS), is a three-item scale based on a simplification of the NIHSS. If any one of the three parameters is abnormal, there is a 72% probability that the patient is positive for a stroke. The scale has a high sensitivity and specificity in identifying patients with stroke who are candidates for thrombolysis.

Cincinnati Prehospital Stroke Scale		
	Normal	**Abnormal**
Facial Droop	Both sides of face move equally	One side of face does not move at all
Arm Drift	Both arms move equally or not at all	One arm drifts compared with the other
Speech	Patient uses correct words with no slurring	Slurred or inappropriate words or mute

Another popular scale used to measure overall functional disability and handicap following stroke is the Modified Rankin Scale. A score of ≤1 is considered favorable.

Modified Rankin Scale

This simplified scale ranks patients according to six classifications:

0 = No symptoms at all.
1 = No significant disability. Patient is able to carry out all previous activities.
2 = Slight disability. Patient is unable to carry out all previous activities but is able to attend to bodily needs without assistance.
3 = Moderate disability. Patient requires some help for bodily needs and to walk.
4 = Moderate severe disability. Patient requires some assistance for bodily needs and is unable to walk without assistance or physical device.
5 = Severe disability. Patient is unable to attend to bodily needs and/or unable to walk without assistance.

SUBARACHNOID BOLT *(see Intracranial Pressure monitoring, p. 37)*

SUBARACHNOID HEMORRHAGE *(see also Aneurysms, p. 5; Arteriovenous Malformation, p. 7; Transcranial Doppler Studies, p. 60; Vasospasm, p. 64)*

Subarachnoid hemorrhage (SAH) is caused by the rupture of an aneurysm, trauma, tumor, or arteriovenous malformation. The patient presents with a classic triad of symptoms and signs: (1) sudden explosive headache, (2) decreased level of consciousness, and (3) nuchal rigidity. In addition, SAH is well known to cause EKG changes in the ST segment and the T wave, with a prominent U wave.

Vasospasm risk: 40% to 60% incidence, with 20% to 30% of patients showing symptoms. It can begin anytime, most likely 5 to 7 days postbleed (not postoperative), and usually resolves by day 21. It is diagnosed by transcranial Doppler studies and/or arteriogram.

Rebleed risk: A rebleed is possible 7 to 10 days after the initial bleed, with peak incidence on days 4 through 8. This is the greatest cause of death.

SUBDURAL HEMATOMA

Subdural hematoma is usually caused by a venous bleed causing blood to accumulate between the dura mater and arachnoid layers. It is often related to trauma. Patient will appear sleepy with a decreased level of consciousness, similar to a TIA. The pupil on the side of the lesion is usually dilated. The onset of the symptoms is slow: For an acute bleed, 24 to 72 hours is common; for a subacute bleed, 48 to 72 hours. A chronic, slow bleed can take from several weeks to as long as 6 months after injury to manifest symptoms. Diagnosis is confirmed by CT scan.

SYNDROME OF INAPPROPRIATE ANTIDIURETIC HORMONE *(see Part 6, p. 273)*

TENTORIUM CEREBELLI

A tentorium is a fold made by dura mater between the occipital lobe and cerebellum. It is used as a line of demarcation.

TRAIN OF FOUR *(see Peripheral Nerve Stimulator, p. 47)*

TRANSCRANIAL DOPPLER STUDIES *(see also Ultrasound in Part 10, p. 367)*

Utilizing an ultrasound beam directed into a column of blood, this study is a noninvasive way to assess the velocity of red blood cells, thus yielding information about cerebral blood flow. It is quick, easy to administer, and easily repeatable.

In neuro patients, it is frequently used to assess for vasospasm (patients with subarachnoid hemorrhage have up to a 70% chance of being positive, usually between day 2 and 17). It is common practice to monitor serial TCDs in order to track increasing velocity trends.

Normal velocities:
- MCA 50 to 60 cm/sec
- AC 30 to 40 cm/sec

(continued)

Criteria:

- 120 cm/sec bears watching
- 140 to 170 cm/sec = mild to moderate vasospasm
- 170 to 250 cm/sec = moderate to severe vasospasm
- >250 cm/sec = trouble (angioplasty?)

TROUSSEAU'S SIGN *(see also Chvostek's Sign, p. 16)*

Apply sphygmomanometer cuff to upper arm, and inflate until radial pulse is obliterated. Keep inflated for about 3 minutes. A positive sign is evidenced by spasm of the lower arm and hand muscles (carpal spasm), indicating hypocalcemia. If there is no spasm, the sign is negative.

TUMORS, NEUROGENIC *(see also Anatomy: Brain Structures and Function, p. 2; Tumors, Grading/Staging in Part 11, p.391)*

The names given to brain tumors can be confusing because there are different types of classification systems. Most institutions, however, follow the World Health Organization (WHO) system, which is based on a tumor's biologic behavior and cells of origin. The following are the most common brain and spinal tumors, listed alphabetically.

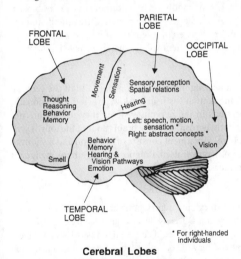

■ Cerebral function and associated anatomical areas. (Reproduced with permission from the American Brain Tumor Association, Des Plaines, IL.)

Cerebral Lobes

ACOUSTIC NEUROMA (SCHWANNOMA, NEURINOMA)

A benign tumor of the eighth cranial nerve (hearing) located in the posterior fossa, acoustic neuroma commonly occurs in adults, usually in the middle years. Symptoms are loss of hearing of one ear, buzzing or ringing in the ear (tinnitus), and occasionally some dizziness. If the tumor also affects the adjacent seventh cranial nerve (facial nerve), some facial paralysis, difficulty in swallowing, loss of sensation in the face, impaired eye movement, and unsteadiness may occur. In most cases, this tumor can be completely removed by surgery and has an excellent prognosis. After surgery, there may be permanent or temporary damage to the facial nerve, resulting in some facial paralysis.

(continued)

ASTROCYTOMA

Astrocytoma is a tumor arising from the astrocyte cells (support cells) and named for its starlike appearance. This tumor is the most common CNS tumor, constituting about 50% of all brain and spinal cord tumors. The lower grades (Grade I and II astrocytomas) are noninfiltrating, slow growing, and often successfully treated with surgery alone. Radiation may be used in addition to surgery for any leftover tumor. They have a better prognosis (6 to 7 years) than the higher grades. Grade III tumors (anaplastic astrocytomas) and Grade IV tumors (glioblastoma multiforme) are malignant tumors (see also Glioblastoma). Usual treatment is partial or complete removal by surgery, followed by radiation therapy. The tumors tend to recur frequently and infiltrate surrounding tissue.

CHORDOMA

An extremely rare (2%) tumor that occurs at the base of the skull or end of the spine, chordoma is a benign extradural tumor, but frequently invades adjacent bone. Treatment is surgery, followed by radiation. The prognosis is generally poor.

CRANIOPHARYNGIOMA

Craniopharyngioma is a benign congenital tumor, cystic in nature, representing 2% to 3% of all primary brain tumors and 5% to 13% of childhood brain tumors. It usually appears in the sellar region, near the pituitary gland. Surgery is the preferred treatment, and the prognosis is excellent if the tumor can be removed in its entirety. Radiation therapy may be administered if excision is incomplete. The patient will frequently receive DDAVP.

EPENDYMOMA

Ependymoma is a childhood tumor appearing in the posterior fossa and in the cerebral hemisphere. It may be benign or malignant and is usually slow growing. Occasionally, these tumors may seed to other locations in the nervous system. They usually are not totally removable by surgery because of their position in the brain (floor of the fourth ventricle or deep in the cerebral hemisphere). Treatment consists of radiation and a shunt to relieve the increased ICP. Often, chemotherapy is used. Prognosis: 1 month for malignant tumors and 7 to 8 years for benign tumors.

GLIOBLASTOMA

Glioblastoma is a Grade IV malignant astrocytoma, representing about 30% of all primary brain tumors and about 50% of the astrocytomas. Because it can double its size every 10 to 11 days and contains a mixture of cells, it is one of the most difficult brain tumors to treat. Whereas one cell type is responsive to treatment and may die off, other types are waiting to take over. Radiation therapy is almost always used after surgery, followed by aggressive chemotherapy. Prognosis is generally poor: 10 weeks with surgery alone and 10 months with radiation alone.

GLIOMA

Glioma is a general "family" name for a variety of different types of tumor of the glial (supportive) tissue of the brain (see Astrocytoma, Oligodendroglioma, and Glioblastoma).

HEMANGIOBLASTOMA

Hemangioblastoma is a benign tumorlike mass that arises from blood vessels, often cystic in nature, representing about 2% of all primary brain tumors. Most commonly found in the cerebellum, it is slow growing and does not metastasize. Surgery is the treatment of

(continued)

choice unless the tumor is attached to the brain stem, in which case radiation is preferred. The prognosis is excellent.

LYMPHOMA

Lymphoma is a malignant tumor common in people with impaired immune function. The most common site is the cerebral hemispheres, and multiple tumors may be present. Metastasis is common. Radiation is the standard therapy (because this tumor infiltrates large areas, the entire brain may be radiated). Depending on the exact location, size, and number of tumors, sometimes surgery alone may be performed, or chemotherapy in combination with radiation. The overall prognosis is poor, with an average survival of 2 years.

MEDULLOBLASTOMA

A rapidly growing, malignant tumor of the cerebellum, occurring mainly in children, medulloblastoma is an invasive tumor, frequently metastatic via the spinal fluid. Surgical removal followed by radiation of the tumor area and the entire brain and spinal cord is the treatment of choice. The tumor is very radiosensitive and is often cured by this treatment alone. Recurrent tumors may be treated with chemotherapy.

MENINGIOMA

Meningioma is a benign, slow-growing tumor that arises from the meninges of the brain and spinal cord, representing about 15% to 20% of all primary brain tumors. If the tumor is accessible, the standard treatment is surgery. Radiation may be used if the tumor is not entirely resected and may prolong life for many years. With total tumor removal the prognosis for long life is excellent.

OLIGODENDROGLIOMA

As with astrocytomas, these are tumors of the supportive (glial) tissue of the brain. They most frequently occur in middle-aged individuals and are usually located in the cerebral hemispheres. They are generally slow growing and benign, although malignant forms are possible. Often they are present for many years before diagnosis and permit survival for years afterward. Treatment consists of surgical removal of as much of the tumor as possible, followed by a course of radiation. Recurrence is not unusual.

PINEAL REGION TUMORS

Tumors in this region are most commonly germ cell tumors, which arise from developmental abnormalities, or tumors that come from the pineal gland itself. Hydrocephalus is a common result, along with brain stem and cerebellum compression. The tumors can be either malignant or benign. The usual treatment is radiation because the surgical approach is very difficult. A shunt procedure is frequently done at the same time to relieve the increased intracranial pressure. The response is often curative. However, surgery remains a viable option, with the extent of the surgical removal being a significant factor in the outcome.

PITUITARY ADENOMA

Tumors of the pituitary gland commonly occur in young or middle-aged adults. Treatment typically consists of surgical removal using a transsphenoidal approach and is often curative. Other treatment may include various forms of radiation or drug therapy.

UNCAL HERNIATION *(see Herniation, p. 32)*

VASOSPASM

Vasospasm is a sustained constriction or narrowing of a cerebral artery or arteries subsequent to a subarachnoid bleed. The spasms cause ischemia and decreased cerebral blood flow, and they play a major part in determining the patient's overall outcome. They occur in 40% to 60% of all patients with SAH, with 20% to 30% showing symptoms, which vary from mild to severe. Diagnosis is by transcranial Doppler studies or angiogram. It has been shown that an internal carotid aneurysm has a greater propensity to produce vasospasm than a middle cerebral aneurysm. Also of note is that a decreased sodium level increases the chance of spasm, because less sodium creates less fluid as it takes H_2O with it. Research to date has failed to provide evidence of the reason for the spasms, and it remains unclear whether the vasospasm is a normal or abnormal contraction, whether it is a failure of arterial smooth muscle cells to relax, or whether it represents a thickening in the vessel wall.

Peak incidence: Day 5 to 7 postbleed (not postsurgery) but can occur from day 1 to 21.

Treatment

Angioplasty	An attempt to improve blood flow by dilating vessels interfering with circulation via a balloon-tip.
Calcium channel blockers	Nimotop (nimodipine) has been shown to have a special affinity for cerebral vessels. Although it does not appear to affect the severity of spasms, it has demonstrated an improved patient outcome overall.
Hemodilution	Allows easier blood flow past site of constriction. Give fluids to reduce hematocrit to approximately 30%.
Hypervolemia	Crystalloids, colloids (albumin, Plasmanate). Keep CVP up to 10 mm Hg; PCWP 16 to 18.
Hypertension	Dopamine, dobutamine, and/or norepinephrine (Levophed). Keep SBP 160 to 220.
Papaverine	A smooth muscle relaxant; possibly works by blocking calcium channels. Injected during angioplasty.

Known as "Triple H" Therapy

VENTRICULOSTOMY *(see Intracranial Pressure Monitoring, p. 37)*

VERTEBRAE *(see also Lumbar Puncture, p. 42; Spinal Cord, p. 53; Spinal Injury, p. 55)*

Referred to as 26 in number (not 33), vertebrae are named and numbered from above downward:

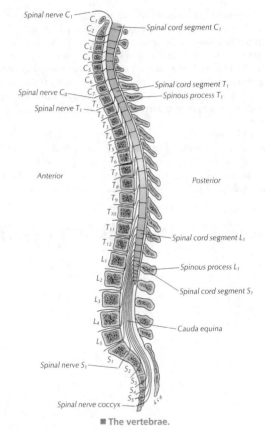

■ The vertebrae.

Vertebrae (number of each type):
- 7 cervical
- 12 thoracic
- 5 lumbar
- 1 sacral (5 sacral fused by adulthood to form 1)
- 1 coccygeal (4 coccygeal united firmly to form 1)

WEBER'S TEST *(see also Caloric Test, p. 12; Rinne Test, p. 50)*

This is an acoustic test for the eighth cranial nerve. A vibrating tuning fork is placed on middle of patient's forehead. Hearing sound equally in both ears is a normal finding. If sound balance is skewed, impaired function of the cochlear nerve is suspected.

WEST NILE VIRUS

This virus was recognized as a cause of human meningitis and encephalitis during an outbreak in 1957. It is transmitted by infectious mosquitoes (the vectors) and birds (the reservoir hosts), but is known to be transmitted human-to-human as well, via blood transfusions, organ transplant, breast milk, and intrauterine transmission. The incubation period is 2 to 14 days (longer if the patient is immunosuppressed), with 80% of those infected showing no symptoms at any time during their life. Conversely, however, exposure may manifest itself as West Nile fever, in which mild flu-like symptoms such as headache, a maculopapular rash on the trunk of the body, swollen lymph glands, and eye pain are prevalent.

The more serious form, West Nile encephalitis, presents with the extreme symptoms of altered mental status, progressing to confusion, coma, and often death. Neurologic deficits include limb paralysis and cranial nerve palsies. Diagnosis is determined from history, CSF analysis (lumbar puncture), CT scan, MRI scan, EEG and EMG testing, IgM antibody capture, and direct ELISA testing. Medical and nursing care is supportive.

NOTES

PART 2

Cardiovascular System

ABLATION *(see also Electrophysiology Studies, p. 106; Wolff-Parkinson-White Syndrome, p. 165)*

Based on results of electrophysiology studies, ablation therapy may be used to eliminate an accessory pathway in the electrical system of the heart. When this circuit is eliminated, fast heart rates should not occur. For this procedure, a specially designed catheter is positioned next to the extra pathway. A form of energy (radio frequency waves) is then delivered into the catheter, heating the heart tissue under the catheter tip and causing the normal cells to no longer function, thus resulting in elimination of the pathway. Much of the success of this approach depends on the pathway location. If the path is on the left side of the heart, the success rate is 90% to 95%. If the pathway is in the center or on the right side of the heart, the success rate is 85% to 90%. In approximately 5% to 10% of patients, even though the extra pathway appears to have been successfully eliminated, the pathway function may return later, requiring a repeat procedure.

ACTION POTENTIAL

Heart muscle cells and nerve cells share many things in common, one of which is the fact that they are both capable of rapidly reversing their resting membrane potential from negative to slightly positive values. This is known as the "action potential" and is brought on by a change in membrane permeability by certain ions. The cardiac action potential, which is associated with contraction, has five distinct phases (numbered 0–4) as described below.

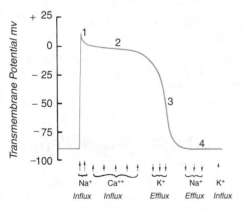

■ Action potential of human ventricular myocardium together with probable electrolyte movements. (Schlant, R. C., & Alexander, R. W. [1994]. *Hurst's the heart* [8th ed.]. New York: McGraw-Hill.)

Phase 0:   Rapid depolarization (sodium in)

On depolarization, the cell becomes permeable to sodium through "fast" channels, and sodium, previously outside the cell, rushes inside. This causes the initial rapid upstroke of

(continued)

the curve and a reversal of potential (resting cell was negative on the inside and becomes positive on the inside when depolarized).

Phase 1:   Initial repolarization (sodium stops, chloride in)

The brief, rapid start of repolarization is believed to be due to the inactivation of the inbound sodium as well as a secondary influx of chloride.

Phase 2:   Repolarization plateau (calcium in, potassium out)

The repolarization slows as a result of a complex interaction between a slow influx of calcium entering the cell and a slow exiting of potassium. Phases 1 and 2 are periods of absolute refractoriness.

Phase 3:   Repolarization Continues (calcium stops, potassium out)

The influx of calcium ceases, whereas the outward flow of potassium continues. Phase 3 is a period of relative refractoriness.

Phase 4:   Resting (sodium/potassium pump)

Most cardiac cells are -70 to -90 mV at rest. The net negative electrical charge is restored by a sodium/potassium exchange across the membrane. The slow diastolic depolarization is caused by a time-dependent fall in outbound potassium. This, combined with an increase in the sodium influx, causes the threshold to be reached.

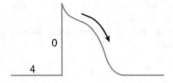

■ Action potential memory aid. Remember, once you hit 40, it's downhill!

ACUTE CORONARY SYNDROME

Acute coronary syndrome is an umbrella term used to cover a group of three clinical entities:

1. Unstable angina (USA)
2. Acute non-ST segment elevation myocardial infarction (N-STEMI)
3. Acute ST segment elevation myocardial infarction (STEMI)

The initial diagnosis of ACS is based on the patient's clinical history (including risk factors), on clinical presentation, and changes on serial ECG tracings. The following table summarizes the similarities and differences of each diagnosis.

(continued)

Acute Coronary Syndrome

	Cause	Signs Symptoms	Diagnostic Findings	LV Function	Complications
USA	Thrombus partially or intermittently occludes CA	• Pain with or without radiation • Occurs at rest with exertion • Limits activity	• ST segment depression or T wave inversion • Cardiac markers not ↑	• Return to normal	• Few initially but potential for recurrence
N-STEMI	Thrombus partially or intermittently occludes CA	• Longer in duration and more severe than USA	• ST segment depression or T wave inversion • Cardiac markers ↑	• Moderate damage	• Few initially but high potential for recurrence
STEMI	• Thrombus fully occludes CA	• Longer in duration and more severe than USA	• ST elevation or new LBBB. • Cardiac markers ↑↑ • Injury	• Major damage	• High potential for an incident

	Treatment
USA	O_2 NTG/MSO_4 to control pain Beta-blockers, ACE inhibitors, statins, glycoprotein IIb/IIIa inhibitors, antiplatelet therapy (ASA, plavix) unless contraindicated, heparin
N-STEMI	O_2 NTG/MSO_4 to control pain Beta-blockers, ACE inhibitors, statins, glycoprotein IIb/IIIa inhibitors, antiplatelet therapy (ASA, plavix) unless contraindicated, heparin, cardiac cath, possible PCTA
STEMI	O_2 NTG/MSO_4 to control pain Beta-blockers, ACE inhibitors, statins, glycoprotein IIb/IIIa inhibitors, antiplatelet therapy (ASA, plavix) unless contraindicated, heparin PCTA within 90 minutes of medical evaluation Fibrinolytic therapy within 30 minutes of medical examination

AFTERLOAD *(see Swan-Ganz: Hemodynamic Algorithm, p. 154)*

AICD *(see Automatic Implantable Cardiac Defibrillators, p. 79)*

ALLEN'S TEST

Allen's test is a quick bedside procedure performed specifically to assess ulnar arterial circulation to the hand and evaluate the patency of the ulnar artery prior to radial arterial puncture. Elevate patient's hand with fist clenched while both radial and ulnar arteries are compressed to occlude arterial blood flow. Pressure is then released over only the ulnar artery. Color should return to the hand within 6 seconds, indicating a patent ulnar artery and adequate collateral blood flow to the hand.

(continued)

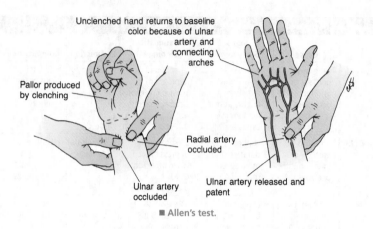

Unclenched hand returns to baseline color because of ulnar artery and connecting arches

Pallor produced by clenching

Radial artery occluded

Ulnar artery occluded

Ulnar artery released and patent

■ Allen's test.

ANEURYSM: AORTIC

An aortic aneurysm is an abnormal dilation of a weakened aorta arterial wall that expands the diameter of the vessel >1½ times normal. (Normal aorta diameter range = 1.4–3 cm.)

Development: At first, pressure increases from the aneurysm cause the aorta lumen to widen and blood flow to slow. An aneurysm typically expands on an average of 0.3 to 0.4 cm per year, with larger aneurysms expanding faster. As the growth progresses, hemodynamic compromise ensues, creating pulsatile stresses on the weakened wall and resulting in the aorta becoming bowed and torturous. Without surgical intervention, the aneurysm may ultimately rupture or tear suddenly and cause possible death.

Sites: The abdominal aorta is the most common site for aortic aneurysms, with 80% developing below the bifurcation of the renal arteries.

Signs/Symptoms: Most aneurysms do not cause any symptoms and are usually discovered incidentally. Unfortunately, asymptomatic aneurysms have a higher risk for rupture. When symptoms do occur, they typically include flank pain (because of the pressure placed on other organs by the expanding size of the aneurysm) or back pain (between the shoulder blades and chest), bradycardia, different pressures in the right and left arms, bruit, jugular venous distention, and unequal carotid and radial pulses. An aneurysm must be at least 5 cm in diameter to be detected on a routine physical exam, and is definitively diagnosed by ultrasound, MRI, or CT.

Treatment: Elective surgical repair is considered for aneurysms that exceed 5.5 cm in diameter, or when small aneurysms increase 0.5 cm within a 6-month period.

Postoperative care focuses on strict blood pressure control in the first 24 to 48 hours to prevent bleeding, tearing of suture lines, and formation of a pseudoaneurysm.

Dissection: This occurs when there is a progressive tear in the aorta, allowing blood to collect and form a hematoma between the intimal and medial layers of the aortic wall.

(*continued*)

Dissections are classified according to location and severity and defined by two systems; see table below.

Aortic Aneurysm Dissection Classifications		
System	**Type**	**Involves**
Daily System	A	Ascending aorta
	B	Descending aorta
DeBakey System	I	Ascending aorta, extending beyond aortic arch
	II	Ascending aorta, extending from the aortic valve to the innominate artery
	III (a)	Descending aorta, extending from the aortic arch to the level of the diaphragm
	III (b)	Descending aorta, extending from the aortic arch to below the level of the diaphragm

Treatment of dissection is based on the extent and location of the dissecting segment. Daily Type A and DeBakey Type I or II are treated as surgical emergencies, and the dissecting segment is replaced with a synthetic graft or endovascular placement of a stent. Daily Type B and DeBakey Type III are generally treated medically unless hemorrhage is suspected, although grafting is an option.

ANGIOGRAPHY, CORONARY *(see also Closure Devices, p. 86; Stents, p. 149)*

Coronary angiography, also called an angiogram, a heart catheterization, or a ventriculogram, is the main diagnostic test used to pinpoint where obstructions are in the coronary arteries and to determine their severity. Conscious sedation is administered, and access is accomplished via the femoral artery. A catheter is then threaded through the entry site, up the artery, through the aorta, and into the openings of the left and right coronary arteries. Contrast dye is injected, and under x-ray, the coronary arteries are viewed in motion, making it possible to visualize plaques. After visualizing the coronary arteries (sometimes before then), another catheter is threaded into the heart's left ventricle, which allows visualization of the wall motion, wall thickness, chamber size, and determination of ejection fraction. (This is known as a ventriculogram.) Throughout the procedure, heart pressures are monitored to determine if any pressure gradients exist. Because there are no nerve endings in the arteries, the patient is unaware that the test is being done (except for a warm sensation following injection of the contrast dye). (*See Schematics on next page.*)

(continued)

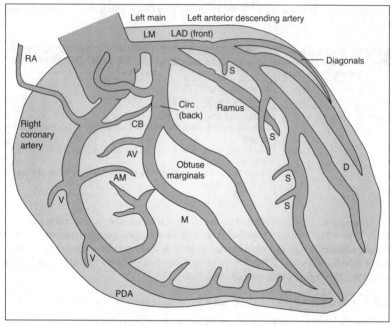

■ RIGHT DOMINANT Cardiac Catheterization Schematic Report.

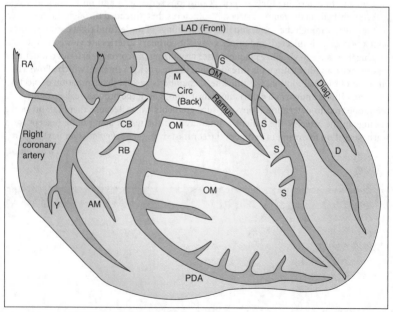

■ LEFT DOMINANT Cardiac Catheterization Schematic Report.

ANGIOPLASTY (see also Atherectomy, p. 78; Closure Devices, p. 86; Stents, p. 149)

Coronary angioplasty is accomplished using a balloon-tipped catheter inserted through the femoral or brachial artery (and threaded to the coronary artery) to widen a vessel that is narrowed due to stenosis or occlusion. Also known as percutaneous transluminal coronary angioplasty (PTCA), if successful, can alleviate myocardial ischemia, relieve angina, and prevent myocardial necrosis. The indications for PTCA have expanded with the advent of improved equipment and techniques; however, the procedure is generally reserved for patients with at least a 50% narrowing of vessels. There are a number of different balloons that can be used; a discussion of the most common follows.

SALINE BALLOON

Typically, a coaxial catheter system with an outer diameter of 6 to 10 F is introduced via the cephalic or femoral vein into the coronary artery tree. The tips of the guiding catheters have curves that are preshaped for selective access to either the right or the left coronary artery and are carefully advanced into the area of coronary stenosis. A balloon attached to the catheter is then inflated with saline solution, increasing the luminal diameter and improving blood flow through the dilated segment. Exact placement of the dilation balloon within the stenosis is facilitated by fluoroscopy. The most common complication of the procedure is peripheral arterial injury at the site of the catheter insertion, leading to thromboembolism, hematoma, arterial perforation, pseudoaneurysm, or arteriovenous fistula. Other complications include stroke, myocardial infarction (MI), and arrhythmias. However, even though this is an invasive procedure, morbidity is minimal, and clinical success ranges from 80% to 95%. Unfortunately, long-term restenosis of the dilated artery occurs in 30% of patients within 3 months.

CUTTING BALLOON

Another option when performing coronary angioplasty is the use of a cutting balloon, where three or four microsurgical blades are mounted longitudinally on the balloon's outer surface. The balloon is positioned across the lesion and is inflated. Tiny cuts are made within the surface of the plaque, and the balloon is deflated, rotated, and then inflated again. The process is repeated several times. It is believed that the cuts in the plaque allow the balloon to enlarge the narrowed lumen using less pressure (and thus lessening the chance of restenosis). This technique is most often used for "old" plaque, which may be resistant to traditional angioplasty, or for restenosis.

CRYOPLASTY

More recently, a technique called cryoplasty has evolved. In effect, it is angioplasty on ice. The procedure is performed much the same way as the traditional angioplasty, but when the balloon is inflated, nitrous oxide is used instead of saline. The nitrous cools to a temperature of $-10°C$, freezing the plaque and inducing a process called apoptosis (programmed cell death). This newer technique appears to be less traumatic to blood vessels and boasts a lower rate of restenosis.

ANKLE-BRACHIAL INDEX

The ankle-brachial index is a noninvasive examination that provides baseline data regarding circulation in the lower limbs. A blood pressure cuff is put around the ankle above the malleolus. When the dorsalis pedis pulse has been located via Doppler, the cuff is inflated

(continued)

in the usual manner until the Doppler signal is no longer heard. As the cuff is slowly deflated, the systolic pressure is recorded when the signal returns. The same procedure is done by using a Doppler on the posterior tibial pulse. The higher pressure of the two pressures is used for the calculation of the index. The brachial systolic pressure is then measured in the same manner and is divided into the ankle systolic pressure. The lower of the two numbers (right vs. left) results in the overall ABI.

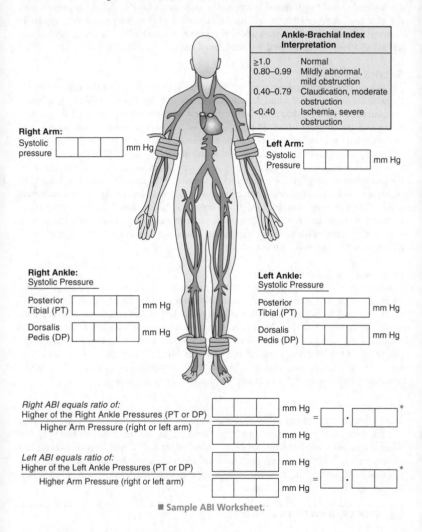

Ankle-Brachial Index Interpretation	
≥1.0	Normal
0.80–0.99	Mildly abnormal, mild obstruction
0.40–0.79	Claudication, moderate obstruction
<0.40	Ischemia, severe obstruction

Right Arm:
Systolic pressure ☐☐☐ mm Hg

Left Arm:
Systolic Pressure ☐☐☐ mm Hg

Right Ankle:
Systolic Pressure
Posterior Tibial (PT) ☐☐☐ mm Hg
Dorsalis Pedis (DP) ☐☐☐ mm Hg

Left Ankle:
Systolic Pressure
Posterior Tibial (PT) ☐☐☐ mm Hg
Dorsalis Pedis (DP) ☐☐☐ mm Hg

Right ABI equals ratio of:
Higher of the Right Ankle Pressures (PT or DP) ☐☐☐ mm Hg
Higher Arm Pressure (right or left arm) ☐☐☐ mm Hg
= ☐ . ☐☐ *

Left ABI equals ratio of:
Higher of the Left Ankle Pressures (PT or DP) ☐☐☐ mm Hg
Higher Arm Pressure (right or left arm) ☐☐☐ mm Hg
= ☐ . ☐☐ *

■ Sample ABI Worksheet.

ANNULOPLASTY RING

An annulus is a ring of tissue around the opening of a valve. When the annulus is dilated, it allows blood to leak back through the valve after it has closed. Most commonly used on the mitral valve, the implantation of an annuloplasty ring (either rigid or flexible) will bring the annulus back to a more normal position, facilitate the meeting of the valve leaflets, and aid in eliminating the regurgitant blood flow.

AORTIC ANEURYSM *(see Aneurysm: Aortic, p. 70)*

AORTIC REGURGITATION/INSUFFICIENCY

Aortic regurgitation/insufficiency is a condition in which there is a weakening or ballooning of the aortic heart valve, causing the valve to fail to close tightly, leading to backflow of blood into the ventricle. This reduces the amount of blood available to perfuse the coronary artery and leads to myocardial ischemia. Over time, it also causes dilatation and hypertrophy of left ventricle.

Causes:
- Most commonly caused by rheumatic fever (fibrous infiltrates on the valve cusps, which causes malalignment)
- Endocarditis (tissue destruction of leaflets, leading to cusp perforation or prolapse)
- Myxomatous changes (enlarged, thickened, floppy, gelatinous leaflets and elongated chordae tendineae)
- Aortic root disease (aortic annulus becomes so large that the valve cusps no longer approximate)
- Congenital abnormalities

Assessment:
- Murmur (louder and longer as severity increases)
- Widening pulse pressure (may be greater than 60 mm Hg)
- Decreased diastolic pressures
- PMI may be displaced laterally
- Quincke's sign (pulsatile flushing/blanching of nail bed when pressure applied)
- DeMusset's sign (bobbing of head with each pulse)
- Corrigan's or Waterhammer pulse (sharp systolic upstroke and diastolic collapse of pulse)

Diagnosis:
- 2-D echo (shows changes in the valve, left ventricular end-diastolic volume, ejection fraction, and mass)
- Transesophageal echo (TEE, shows images in both ascending and descending aorta)
- EKG (left axis deviation, patterns of left ventricular strain, i.e., Q waves in I, AVL, V_3–V_6)
- CXR (shows left ventricular enlargement, signs of CHF)
- Cardiac catheterization (visualizes extent of disease)

Management:
- ACE inhibitors (reduces afterload)
- Vasodilators (reduces afterload)
- Nifedipine (reduces left ventricular size and mass)
- Antibiotic prophylaxis
- Surgery (aortic valve replacement)

AORTIC STENOSIS

Aortic stenosis is a narrowing or constriction of the opening of the aortic valve, which results in a decrease in the outflow of blood from the left ventricle to the aorta. This causes a pressure overload in the left ventricle, an increase in left ventricular systolic pressure, and hypertrophy. As the left ventricular pressure continues to increase, the pulmonary system becomes congested, and the right side of the heart begins to fail. Stenosis reduces stroke volume, and without a compensatory increase in heart rate, cardiac output falls and perfusion of the coronary arteries is reduced.

Causes:
- Age-related degenerative calcific changes
- Rheumatic fever (scars the valve, causing fibrosis, calcification, and fusion of the leaflets)
- Congenital abnormalities

Assessment:
- Midsystolic murmur (rough, low pitched, loudest at second right intercostal space, radiating up neck)
- Low systolic blood pressure with a normal diastolic pressure; pulse pressure may be narrowed
- Indicators of left ventricular failure (increased wedge pressure)

Diagnosis:
- 2-D echo (defines extent of leaflet thickening, determines left ventricular function and hypertrophy, measures aortic valve pressure gradient, determines left atrial enlargement)
- EKG (QRS amplitude changes associated with hypertrophy, ST/T wave changes due to left ventricular strain, possible LBB, left axis deviation, atrial fibrillation in late stages)
- CXR (shows left ventricular enlargement, rounding at apex and slight backward displacement of the heart)
- Cardiac catheterization (visualizes extent of disease)
  Calcification of aortic valve area:

Normal	3.0 to 3.5 cm^2
Mild AS	1.0 to 1.5 cm^2
Moderate	0.85 to 1.0 cm^2
Severe AS	Less than 0.85 cm^2

Management:
- No preventative measures; surgical replacement only effective for long-term treatment
- Mild stenosis, echocardiography every 2 years
- **REMEMBER:** Use meds cautiously! Medications can lower preload, and the left ventricle is very dependent on preload for adequate functioning. If preload is too low, cardiac output will be too low, and there will not be enough pressure generated to open the noncompliant valve.

APHERESIS

Apheresis is a process using the Liposorber system, indicated for use in removing LDL cholesterol from the plasma of the following high-risk patient populations for whom diet has been ineffective and maximum drug therapy has either been ineffective or not tolerated:
- Patients with LDL-C >300 mg/dL
- Patients with LDL-C >200 mg/dL and documented coronary heart disease

(continued)

The patient's blood is withdrawn via a venous access and is pumped to a plasma separator, where it is separated and pumped into one of the two LDL absorption columns. As the plasma passes through the column, LDL, Lp(a), and VLDL are selectively absorbed by dextran sulfate cellulose beads within the column. There is minimal effect on other plasma components such as HDL and albumin. The LDL-depleted plasma leaves the column and is recombined with the blood cells exiting the separator, all of which are returned to the patient via a second venous access. When the first column has completed absorbing the LDL, the computer-regulated machine automatically switches the plasma flow to the second column. The plasma remaining in the first column is returned to the patient. The column is then regenerated, eluting the LDL, Lp(a), and VLDL to the waste lines. After elution, the column is reprimed completely and is ready for the next cycle of absorption, allowing continuous treatment. A typical treatment takes about 2 to 4 hours to complete and may be repeated every 2 to 3 weeks.

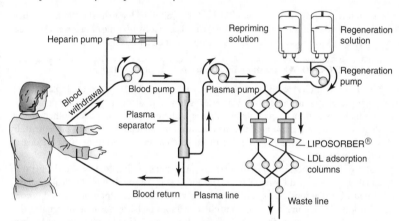

■ Liposorber schematic used with permission of Kaneka Pharma America LLC.

ARTERIAL PRESSURE *(see Intra-arterial Pressure, p. 123)*

ASHMAN'S PHENOMENON

Ashman's theory states that aberrant conduction is more likely to complicate atrial fibrillation when a longer cycle is succeeded by a shorter one.

■ Ashman's phenomenon: atrial fibrillation with long-short-long cycle.

The phenomenon may also occur when sinus bradycardia is complicated by a premature atrial contraction (PAC). The cycle of sinus bradycardia is long, but PAC

(continued)

shortens cycle and is conducted aberrantly (usually in right bundle branch [RBB] pattern, rsR′):

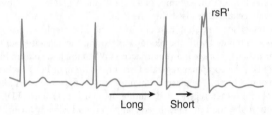

rsR'

Long   Short

■ Ashman's phenomenon: sinus bradycardia with premature atrial contraction.

Therefore, according to Ashman, the beat that follows a long/short cycle favors aberrancy. This, however, is not a hard-and-fast rule, because by the rule of bigeminy, a longer cycle also tends to produce a ventricular ectopic beat equally as many times.

ATHERECTOMY *(see also Angioplasty, p. 73; Stents, p. 149)*

Atherectomy is indicated in conditions not well treated by standard angioplasty, such as when the plaque in the coronary arteries is too large or the plaque is hardened to a degree that it is no longer possible to flatten it. Atherectomy creates a smoother surface by debulking the vessel and is sometimes followed by angioplasty or stent placement. In theory, the process permits a more controlled vascular injury and minimizes the degree of arterial stretch.

- **Rotational atherectomy** (Rotablator) uses a catheter with a high-speed drill (up to 200,000 rpm) to grind away plaque. The abrasive tip of the drill is elliptical in shape, coated with diamond chips, and comes in a variety of sizes. Rotational speed is controlled by air pressure, which is controlled by a foot pedal. Atherosclerotic material is shredded into millions of tiny particles (much smaller than red blood cells) and is then washed away in the bloodstream by passing through the capillaries. This process is most useful for treating plaque that has hardened with calcium.

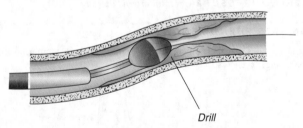

Drill

■ Rotational atherectomy.

- **Directional atherectomy** uses a catheter with a small cutting device to actually "shave off" tiny pieces of plaque. The tiny plaques are then stored in a collection chamber attached to the catheter and, at the completion of the procedure, are removed from the body when the catheter is withdrawn. This process is most useful for treating atherosclerotic deposits that are bulky, not hardened with calcium, and limited to one side of the arterial wall.

(continued)

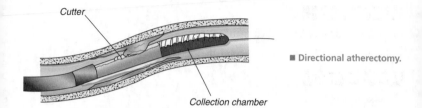

Cutter

■ Directional atherectomy.

Collection chamber

Potential complications in both procedures include perforation of the coronary artery, abrupt closure, embolization distal to the lesion site, and myocardial infarction. The rate of restenosis and other complications is comparable to that of angioplasty.

AUTOMATIC IMPLANTABLE CARDIAC DEFIBRILLATORS

An automatic implantable cardiac defibrillator is a device implanted transvenously with local anesthetic, using a simple surgical procedure (the patient is usually able to be discharged with 24 hours) to treat ventricular arrhythmias with pacing and shock therapy. Current versions also have the capability to treat and suppress atrial arrhythmias, resynchronize the ventricles to manage heart failure symptoms, or pace the heart with all the features of a dual-chamber pacemaker. Originally indicated for patients who have survived two cardiac arrests, the devices have recently been shown to improve survival in all patients with prior myocardial infarction and an ejection fraction of 30% or less (identifying them as high risk for sudden death).

AXIS DEVIATION

The axis is the mean direction (vector) in which electrical activity spreads across the heart. The strength of the vector is indicated by recording a small deflection for a weak vector and a large deflection for a strong vector.

Normal axis is described by some authors to be in the narrow bounds of $+30°$ to $+60°$ and by others to be between $0°$ and $+90°$. Using the range from $-30°$ to $+110°$ allows easier definition of hemiblock.

QUICK METHOD FOR DETERMINING AXIS

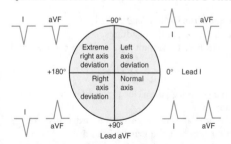

■ Determining electrical axis. (Adapted from Morton, P. G., & Fontaine, D. K. [2009]. *Critical care nursing* [9th ed.]. Philadelphia: Lippincott Williams & Wilkins.)

1. Examine deflections in leads I and aVF.
2. If they point toward each other on the 12-lead electrocardiogram (EKG) (lead I negative, aVF positive), the deviation is to the right.
3. If they point away from each other on the 12-lead EKG (lead I positive, aVF negative), the deviation is to the left.

(*continued*)

REMEMBER:

The axis is "right together" or "left apart."

4. If leads I and aVF both deviate upward, the axis is normal.

REMEMBER:

It's good to be up!

5. If leads I and aVF both deviate downward, the axis is in "no man's land," or indeterminate (usually because of a junctional rhythm).

MORE EXACT, HEXAXIAL METHOD FOR DETERMINING AXIS

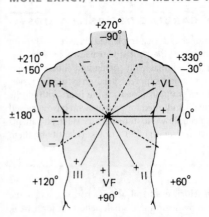

■ Hexaxial figure to pinpoint axis. (Goldman, M. J. [1996]. *Principles of clinical electrocardiography* [12th ed.]. Los Altos, CA: Lange Medical Publications.)

1. Find the most equiphasic lead (lead that equals zero when the values of the positive and negative deflections are added) using leads I, II, III, aVR, aVL, and aVF (no V leads!).
2. Use the hexaxial figure to determine which lead is perpendicular to the equiphasic one.
3. Check to see whether the QRS of this lead is a negative or positive deflection. This gives the direction of the vector.

If there is no equiphasic deflection present in the six limb leads:
- Look at leads I and aVF to place the axis in one of the quadrants.
- Determine which of the other two leads in that quadrant has the largest complex, and place the axis closest to that vector.

Hints:
- V tach commonly has an axis in no man's land, giving a clue to the differential diagnosis between ventricular ectopy and aberrance.
- Axis shifts to the left with age. An axis of −30° is not necessarily a cardiac disorder.
- ALL complexes in the V lead deflecting either up or down are definitive of V-tach.
- Axis deviates **toward** bundle branch block (RBBB = R axis deviation).
- Axis deviates away from MI.

Left axis deviation caused by:
- Advanced age, obesity, pregnancy
- Left ventricular hypertrophy

(*continued*)

- Inferior MI
- Wolff-Parkinson-White (WPW) syndrome
- Ascites, tumors
- Hypertension
- Ischemic heart disease

Right axis deviation caused by:
- Youth, tall, and thin body form
- Right ventricular hypertrophy
- Chronic obstructive pulmonary disease (COPD), pulmonary emboli, lateral myocardial infarct
- Dextrocardia
- Right bundle branch block

BNP *(see Heart Failure, p. 110; see also BNP in Part 9, p. 341)*

BODY MASS INDEX *(see Bariatrics in Part 4, p. 217)*

BRACHYTHERAPY, VASCULAR

Many technologies are currently under investigation for the treatment and prevention of restenosis following angioplasty and stenting, but the most promising appears to be brachytherapy. This technique, approved by the FDA in 2002, delivers either beta or gamma radiation to the blocked site (via a catheter, postangioplasty) utilizing a miniaturized x-ray emitter. Once delivered, the radiation "beads" remain in place from 3 to 20 minutes before being withdrawn. No radioactive material is left in the body. The radiation is not felt, and the normal healing process is unaffected. The procedure works on the principle that the radiation interacts with vessel walls, destroying their capability for cell division and regrowth.

BRUGADA SYNDROME

Brugada syndrome is a condition associated with sudden cardiac death, idiopathic ventricular fibrillation, or self-terminating polymorphic ventricular tachycardia in an otherwise structurally normal heart. Characterized by a right bundle branch block pattern and ST segment elevations in leads V_1 to V_3, the syndrome is seen more frequently in males than in females and primarily in a mean age group of 35 to 40 years. It is consistent with a chromosomal mutation and predisposes individuals to a lifetime risk of sudden cardiac death. There is no effective pharmacologic treatment, and genetic counseling is advised.

CABG *(see Cardiac Surgery, p. 82)*

CARDIAC INDEX *(see also Swan-Ganz: Hemodynamic Normals, p. 157)*

Cardiac index = cardiac output ÷ body surface area   Normal: 2.5 to 4.5 L/min/m²

CARDIAC MARKERS *(see Cardiac Markers in Part 9, p. 342)*

CARDIAC OUTPUT *(see also Swan-Ganz: Hemodynamic Normals, p. 156)*

Cardiac output = stroke volume × heart rate   Normal: 4 to 8 L/min

CARDIAC SURGERY

CABG (CORONARY ARTERY BYPASS GRAFT)

Developed in 1954, CABG is a procedure used to reroute or bypass blood around blocked coronary arteries and to improve blood supply to the myocardium. Cardioplegic solution is used to cause intentional cardiac arrest and to provide a bloodless operating field and a motionless heart. The solution helps to protect the heart from ischemia by providing a substrate for ongoing cellular metabolism during the time on the bypass pump. The body is cooled to reduce metabolic demand.

OpCAB (OFF-PUMP CORONARY ARTERY BYPASS)

The heart continues to beat through OpCAB. No cannulation is needed, and the body is not cooled. A specialized stabilizer is used, resulting in suction to minimize heart movement only at the site of anastomosis. Shunts are placed in the coronary vessel to be anastomosed and to continue blood flow through the vessel until the anastomosis is complete. The shunt is removed just prior to securing the suture. A mister is utilized to keep the site free of blood for better visualization for the surgeon.

MIDCAB (MINIMALLY INVASIVE DIRECT CORONARY ARTERY BYPASS)

MIDCAB is similar to OpCAB, except this procedure is done with a short incision in the left chest cavity, rather than a sternotomy. The left anterior descending artery and the internal mammary artery are sutured together in the front of the heart.

Comparing Types of CABG

Features	On-pump CABG	OPCAB	MIDCAB
Access site	Breastbone severed for heart access	Breastbone severed for heart access	Incision made between ribs for anterior heart access, no bones cut
Indications	Suitable for multivessel disease, any coronary artery	Suitable for multivessel disease, any coronary artery	Used only for one-vessel diseases in anterior portions of heart, such as left anterior descending artery, or some portions of the right coronary and circumflex arteries
Graft types	Combination of artery and vein grafts	Combination of artery and vein grafts	Arterial grafts (better long-term results)
Complications	Highest risk of postoperative complications	Reduced blood usage, fewer rhythm problems, less kidney dysfunction than on-pump CABG	Reduces blood usage, fewest complications, fastest recovery
Intubation	Up to 24 hours	Up to 24 hours	Usually 2 to 4 hours
Incisions	Leg incisions for vein grafting, possibly arm incisions for radial artery grafting	Leg incisions for vein grafting, possibly arm incisions for radial artery grafting	No leg incisions, possibly arm incision for radial artery grafting
Heart and lung function	Heart and lung circulation bypassed mechanically, affecting blood cells	Drugs and special equipment used to slow heart and immobilize it; cardiopulmonary and systemic circulation still function	Drugs used to slow heart; cardiopulmonary and systemic circulation still function

From Visual Nursing: A Guide to Diseases, Skills, and Treatment. *Lippincott, Williams & Wilkins, 2008.*

(*continued*)

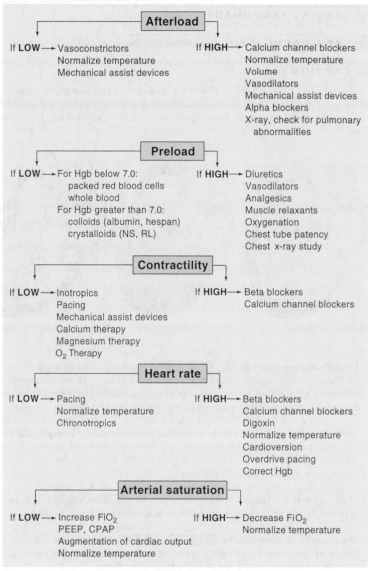

Afterload

If **LOW** → Vasoconstrictors
Normalize temperature
Mechanical assist devices

If **HIGH** → Calcium channel blockers
Normalize temperature
Volume
Vasodilators
Mechanical assist devices
Alpha blockers
X-ray, check for pulmonary
abnormalities

Preload

If **LOW** → For Hgb below 7.0:
packed red blood cells
whole blood
For Hgb greater than 7.0:
colloids (albumin, hespan)
crystalloids (NS, RL)

If **HIGH** → Diuretics
Vasodilators
Analgesics
Muscle relaxants
Oxygenation
Chest tube patency
Chest x-ray study

Contractility

If **LOW** → Inotropics
Pacing
Mechanical assist devices
Calcium therapy
Magnesium therapy
O_2 Therapy

If **HIGH** → Beta blockers
Calcium channel blockers

Heart rate

If **LOW** → Pacing
Normalize temperature
Chronotropics

If **HIGH** → Beta blockers
Calcium channel blockers
Digoxin
Normalize temperature
Cardioversion
Overdrive pacing
Correct Hgb

Arterial saturation

If **LOW** → Increase FiO_2
PEEP, CPAP
Augmentation of cardiac output
Normalize temperature

If **HIGH** → Decrease FiO_2
Normalize temperature

■ Postcardiac surgery algorithm.

CARDIAC TAMPONADE *(see Tamponade, p. 159)*

CARDIOGENIC SHOCK *(see Shock, Cardiogenic, p. 146)*

CARDIOMYOPATHY

Cardiomyopathy is an irreversible primary disease of the heart muscle, most commonly affecting the myocardial layer but occasionally affecting the endocardial, subendocardial, and/or pericardial layers of the heart. Cardiomyopathies are divided into the following three types:

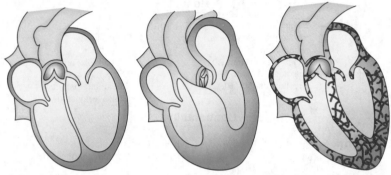

■ Dilated cardiomyopathy.   ■ Hypertrophic cardiomyopathy.   ■ Restrictive cardiomyopathy.

- **Dilated cardiomyopathy** *REMEMBER:* Heart thins and enlarges. Most cases of dilated cardiomyopathy are idiopathic (no exact cause is known), although viral infections, myocarditis, heredity, and use of toxic substances have been linked to the disease. It is characterized by damaged heart muscle, which causes an increase in size of the right and left ventricles. (A damaged heart muscle cannot pump enough blood to meet the demands of the body, so the heart compensates by enlarging the size of the ventricles.) The larger chambers temporarily move more blood, but eventually, the stretched out walls become weak. Inadequate cardiac output results, and ultimately, mitral and tricuspid insufficiency occurs.

  If the cause can be determined, management is focused on treating the cause. Otherwise, treatment is directed toward maximizing heart function (digoxin, dobutamine, vasodilators, heparin, diuretics, etc.). Fifty percent of all deaths occur suddenly and are usually caused by ventricular arrhythmias and, secondarily, clots.

- **Hypertrophic cardiomyopathy** *REMEMBER:* Heart muscle thickens. Also known as idiopathic hypertrophic subaortic stenosis (IHSS), hypertrophic cardiomyopathy occurs without any systemic precipitating factors. The cause is thought to be genetic, with as high as 60% to 80% of the cases being inherited through autosomal dominant transmission. It is characterized by thickened walls of the left ventricle and septum. The thicker muscle walls cause the chambers to hold less blood, and the heart muscle remains stiff in diastole. The primary goals of treatment center on decreasing the risk of sudden cardiac death and treating symptoms of angina, fatigue, dyspnea, and syncope.

(continued)

• **Restrictive cardiomyopathy** *REMEMBER:* Heart muscle becomes hard and stiff. This type of cardiomyopathy is rare in the United States and is seen mostly in Africa. It is frequently idiopathic, sometimes genetically linked, and is often seen in amyloidosis, sarcoidosis, endomyocardial fibrosis, and other infiltrative diseases. Clinically, it presents like congestive heart failure, but the heart is small or only slightly enlarged. Systemic and pulmonary venous pressures are high, with peripheral edema and possible ascites. Atrial fibrillation is common. There is no known treatment, so therapy is supportive and includes diuretics, steroids, anticoagulants, inotropic agents, oxygen, and fluid restriction.

CARDIOVERSION, SYNCHRONIZED *(see also Defibrillation, p. 92)*

Electrical cardioversion (also known as direct current, or DC cardioversion) is the delivery of a synchronized electrical shock through the chest wall to the heart via conducting pads. Its purpose is to suddenly and simultaneously interrupt the abnormal electrical circuit(s) in the heart, and restore a normal electrical rhythm. Most cardioversions (synchronized shocks) are performed to treat rhythms such as atrial fibrillation, atrial flutter, ventricular tachycardia with a pulse, or any other perfusing rhythm that is undesirable due to complications or symptoms.

Cardioversion differs from defibrillation in that the shock is *synchronized,* meaning it is timed to deliver current during the safest point of the cardiac cycle (the R wave phase). A defibrillator placed in the synchronized mode will actually *delay* delivery of the shock, waiting instead until it senses an R wave before firing. This avoids the delivery of energy during the electrically vulnerable downslope of the T wave, and prevents possible R on T phenomenon, where a perfusing rhythm can deteriorate to a chaotic, pulseless one.

REMEMBER:

Most defibrillators have a safety feature designed to automatically reset the defibrillator *back* to the NON-synchronized (defibrillation) mode after each shock. If repeated synchronized shocks are required, the user must remember to key in the synchronous setting *each time*.

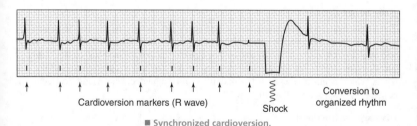

Cardioversion markers (R wave)　　　Shock　　　Conversion to organized rhythm

■ Synchronized cardioversion.

CENTRAL VENOUS PRESSURE *(see Swan Ganz: Hemodynamic Normals, p. 155)*

CLOSURE DEVICES

Closure devices assist in achieving hemostasis postfemoral artery puncture and have proven to be an efficient alternative/adjunct to manual compression. They can be divided into four categories:

- Passive devices **REMEMBER:** "push"
    Delivers compression via a device, or requires manual compression in addition to a surface pad.
    Example: (devices): FemoStop, C Clamp, Safe Guard, Hemoband
        (surface pads): Syvek, Chito-Seal, Clo-Sur, D-Stat Dry,
    Safe Seal, V+ Pad, Neptune Pad
- Sealing devices **REMEMBER:** "pull"
    A mechanical seal is activated by sandwiching the arteriotomy between a suture anchor and a collagen sponge.   Example: AngioSeal, VasoSeal, Duett Pro, Boomerang
- Suturing devices **REMEMBER:** "stitch"
    Delivers an intravascular suture.   Example: Perclose, SuperStitch, X-Press, VasoLock
- Stapling devices **REMEMBER:** "click"
    Delivers a metal clip on surface of the procedure site.   Example: Star Close, AngioLink

The number of devices available on the market is numerous and continues to expand. A short discussion of only the more "classic" models follows. In general, the principles for all devices in the same category are similar, and some universal rules apply:

REMEMBER:

1. If a patient has an arterial and a venous sheath, both lines should NOT be pulled at once. Hemostasis of one line should be achieved before pulling the other, to aid in the prevention of AV fistula formation.
2. While parameters for safe removal are institution specific, in general, the ACT should be <170 seconds, the INR >1.5, and the platelets >50,000.

ANGIO-SEAL
The Angio-Seal device is composed of a small collagen sponge and an absorbable anchor, connected by an absorbable suture. It stops bleeding from the puncture site by "sandwiching" the puncture between the anchor (inside the artery) and the collagen sponge (outside the artery). Bleeding is also stopped by the clot-inducing properties of the collagen, which is effective even if the patient is anticoagulated. The Angio-Seal device is completely absorbed in 60 to 90 days.

Discharge instructions:
- Patient may not take a tub bath, swim, or soak in a hot tub until puncture site healed.
- Patient may shower after 24 hours.
- Wash site with soap and water and cover with a bandage for at least 3 days.
- There may be a small olive pit-size knot over the puncture site for 5 to 7 days.
- Angio-Seal is MRI compatible.
- Patient needs to keep a wallet card for 90 days, then it can be discarded. (Repuncture of the same artery within 90 days is not recommended.)

(continued)

D-STAT DRY

D-Stat Dry is a dry hemostatic bandage, packaged as a pad to be applied to surface bleeding from vascular sites. Utilizing the power of thrombin, D-Stat works on the clotting cascade by activating clotting factors V, VIII, and XIII while stimulating platelet aggregation and cleaving endogenous fibrinogen to fibrin. Apply shiny side down.

DUETT PRO

The Duett Pro catheter is designed to be inserted at the completion of the procedure through the sheath already in place. A small balloon at the end of the catheter is inflated and pulled back against the artery. Then, the liquid procoagulant (a gluelike substance) is delivered on top of the puncture site to permanently seal it. The Duett Pro catheter and sheath are removed, and after a few minutes of light pressure, the site is sealed.

Discharge instructions:

- In most cases, sitting up in bed and moving the leg is allowed 1 hour after the procedure.
- Ambulation is dependent on type of catheterization procedure and the amount of anticoagulant given.
- Patient may not take a tub bath, swim, or soak in a hot tub until the puncture site is healed.
- Patient may shower normally.
- Use routine puncture site care; keep clean and dry.
- Activity may be used as tolerated, avoid heavy lifting or straining (more than 10 lb) for several days.

FEMOSTOP

FemoStop is a femoral compression system, consisting of an arch with a sterile pneumatic pressure dome, a belt, and a reusable pump with a manometer. The pressure dome is placed over the vessel puncture site in the groin. The belt is placed around the patient. The dome applies a mechanical pressure over the vessel puncture site to induce hemostasis. The pressure of the dome is controlled by the reusable pump and the manometer. The arch and the belt provide counterpressure for the dome.

HEMOBAND (RADIAL ARTERY STASIS)

HemoBand is an adjustable, single-use band with a molded V-shaped pressure pad to allow graft flow while controlling bleeding after sheath withdrawal (used also for removal of dialysis catheters). The band is placed into position. One person draws blood from the sheath during removal (to remove clot debris), and as the sheath exits the site, the artery is permitted to spurt slightly. Digital pressure is applied above and below the site. A sterile 4 × 4 is placed over the site so that pressure is applied over the skin entry site and the actual arteriotomy site. If the radial artery is not compressed this way, retrograde flow from the ulnar artery will occur. The band is tightened until bleeding is stopped. The ulnar pulse has to be intact so that the distal wrist and the hand continue to be perfused. The band is released two "clicks" every 15 to 20 minutes over the next 2 hours. Pulses are often checked throughout the procedure. The patient is positioned in bed with the arm draped across a pillow on the upper abdominal area.

PERCLOSE

Perclose is a suture-mediated closure (SMC) device that involves a suture and knotting technique to directly close the arterial puncture. The sutures are cut below the level of the skin. Primary healing is not dependent upon clot formation, and this device can be used with anticoagulated patients.

(continued)

Discharge instructions:
- In most cases, sitting up in bed is allowed immediately postprocedure, and depending on the type of catheterization, the patient may be allowed bathroom privileges.
- Patient may not take a tub bath, swim, or soak in a hot tub until the puncture site is healed.
- There may be formation of a small lump (1.5–2.5 cm), which may last up to 6 weeks.
- Use routine puncture site care; keep clean and dry.
- If steri strips are in place, allow them to remain until they fall off on their own.
- Patient needs to permanently retain wallet card.

STARCLOSE

The StarClose system utilizes a tiny circumferential flexible clip, which, when placed on the surface of the femoral artery, causes the artery to be closed securely in a matter of seconds following a catheterization. The clip is designed for delivery "through the sheath"—a feature intended to avoid contact with the skin and thus decreasing the rate of infection. The device requires only four clicks to achieve a secure closure, leaving nothing inside the artery itself but achieving stasis entirely from outside the vessel. The clip is made of nitinol, a nickel-titanium composite that "remembers" its shape once released from the StarClose device. While oozing from the site is usually minimal, if oozing increases, D-Stat should never be used to obtain stasis.

Discharge instructions:
- The patient may sit up at a 45° angle and move freely in bed immediately postprocedure as long as any subcutaneous ooze is minimal. Ambulation is allowed as directed by the physician.
- Use routine site care; keep clean and dry.
- Patient may shower the day after the procedure, but no tub bath or swimming for at least 5 days or until the site is healed.
- Normal activity may be resumed in 2 days, but discomfort should be the guide.

SYVEK PATCH

The SyvekPatch is made from a polymer that is isolated from microalga. Its mechanism of action is local vasoconstriction and clot formation to achieve a hemostatic effect. In addition to an adjunct to manual pressure sheath removal, it can also be used to achieve hemostasis on groin "oozes." The patch is external and does not leave foreign matter in the subcutaneous tissue.

Discharge instructions:
- Remove the dressing and SyvekPatch 24 hours after application by soaking the patch with water (may be done in the shower). Gently peel off the patch.
- Use routine site care; wash site with soap and water, and cover with a bandage for 1 day.
- Patient may not take a tub bath, swim, or soak in a hot tub until the site is healed.

V + PAD

The V+Pad is a small three-layer woven gauze pad covered with a D-glucosamine–enriched coating, which, when applied to the angiography site, works to accelerate platelet aggregation and enhance platelet plug formation. The pad promotes the body's natural thrombin to convert fibrinogen to fibrin and results in a "mesh" forming around the platelet plug. More platelets continue to be trapped, and ultimately a clot is formed. Post hemostasis,

(continued)

the V+Pad remains in place and is covered with a Tegaderm dressing. Patients are usually ambulatory 90 minutes post hemostasis and are able to be discharged home with instructions to remove the V+Pad within 24 hours by soaking with water and gently peeling away from the skin.

VASOSEAL

VasoSeal is a closure device that enhances the body's natural method of achieving hemostasis by delivering collagen extravascularly to the surface of the femoral artery. The collagen (Type I, produced from bovine tendons) attracts and activates platelets in the arterial puncture, forming a coagulum at the surface of the artery and resulting in a seal at the puncture site. The collagen reabsorbs over a 6-week period.

Discharge instructions:
- Decreased bedrest time and greater flexibility of movement (head of bed may be elevated).
- There may be a knot under the skin at the groin site for 5 to 7 days.
- Use routine site care; keep clean and dry.
- Patient may not take a tub a bath, swim, or soak in a hot tub until the site is healed.

COARCTATION OF THE AORTA

Aortic constriction, usually distal to the left subclavian artery, stresses the left ventricle and causes an increase in afterload.

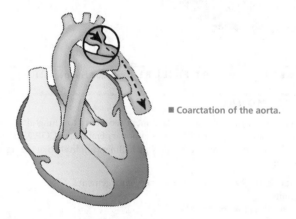

■ Coarctation of the aorta.

Signs/symptoms:
- Headaches, dizziness, syncope (exercise intolerance)
- Cold legs and feet, with leg pain or cramps after exertion
- Shortness of breath, nosebleeds
- Chest pain or palpitations
- Blood pressure noted higher in arms than in legs (related to upper extremity hypertension). Femoral pulse may be noted weak, or even absent.

Treatment: Usually corrected by surgery or by nonsurgical balloon dilation.

(*continued*)

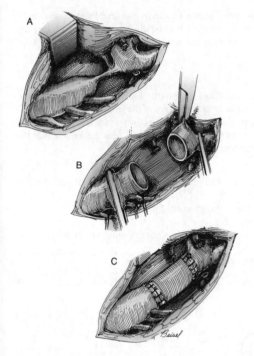

■ Surgical repair of coarctation of the aorta using a tubular graft prosthesis. A, The coarctation is exposed through a left lateral thoracotomy incision. B, Clamps are applied to the aorta above and below the area of coarctation and the coarcted segment is excised. C, A tubular prosthetic graft is placed to bridge the defect and sutured to the aorta in end-to-end fashion. (Waldhausen, J. A., Pierce, W. S., & Campbell, D. B. [Eds.]. [1996] *Surgery of the chest* [6th ed.]. St. Louis: Mosby, Inc. Reprinted with permission.)

CONGESTIVE HEART FAILURE *(see Heart Failure, p. 110)*

COR PULMONALE

Cor pulmonale is a right ventricular enlargement secondary to a lung disorder that produces pulmonary artery hypertension (i.e., pulmonary embolism, COPD, loss of lung tissue related to surgery or trauma). The following hallmarks indicate that the right ventricle is feeling strain:

1. Chest x-ray shows RV and pulmonary artery enlargement.
2. EKG exhibits:
   - Right axis deviation (by >30%)
   - Inverted, diphasic, or flattened T waves in leads V_1 to V_3
   - ST depression in leads II, III, and aVF
   - P waves are tall and peaked (>2.5 mm) in leads II, III, and aVF
   - P waves are inverted in lead aVL
   - P waves in V_1 to V_3 are sharp and pointed
   - Low-voltage QRS is common

CORONARY ANGIOGRAPHY *(see Angiography, p. 71)*

CORONARY ARTERIES

Right coronary artery (RCA) perfuses:
- SA node in 60% of population
- AV node in 80% to 90% of population
- Bundle of HIS
- Part of left bundle branch
- Posterior third of septum
- Right atrium and ventricle
- Inferior wall of left ventricle

Left anterior descending (LAD) artery perfuses: (Branches are "diagonals"):
- Anterior wall of left ventricle
- Two thirds of septum
- Right bundle branch
- Part of left bundle branch
- SA node in 40% of population

Left circumflex artery (LCA) perfuses: (Branches are "obtuse marginals"):
- Part of the left bundle branch
- Lateral wall of left atrium and ventricle

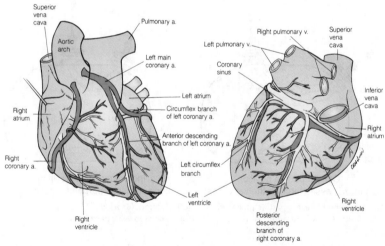

■ Coronary circulation: Coronary arteries and some coronary sinus veins.

CORONARY ARTERY BYPASS GRAFT *(see Cardiac Surgery, p. 82)*

CORONARY STENTS *(see Stents, p. 149)*

CRYOPLASTY *(see Angioplasty, p. 73)*

CVP *(see Swan-Ganz: Hemodynamic Normals, p. 155)*

DEFIBRILLATION

Defibrillation is the discharge of energy (joules) in the form of a nonsynchronized shock, generally delivered to the heart via transthoracic paddles or pads for the purpose of reestablishing normal electric conduction in the presence of VF or pulseless V-tach.

DEFIBRILLATOR HINTS

Energy stored in the defibrillator is constant, so the only variance to the delivered current results from the operator and the impedance of the individual patient's chest. To minimize this variance:

- Use the hands-free adhesive defibrillation pads (always preferred) rather than the hands-on paddles. The hands-free pads provide the lowest resistance and greatest amount of safety.
- If paddles are required, 25 lb of pressure per paddle must be applied.
- Use the proper pad (paddle) placement so the heart (primarily the ventricles) is in the path of the current.
- Placing the defibrillation pad over a medication patch can decrease the effectiveness of the electrical therapy. **REMEMBER:** Remove any transdermal medication patches from the patient's chest before defibrillating.

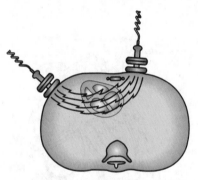 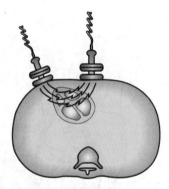

Correct paddle position   Incorrect paddle position
(current passes through the ventricles)   (current misses part of the ventricles)

■ Correct and incorrect paddle placement for defibrillation. (Crockett, P. [1991]. *Defib: What you should know.* Redmond, WA: Physio-Control. Reprinted with permission.)

The sternum/apex position is most frequently used, with sternum pad on upper right side of chest to right of sternum, below clavicle, and apex pad on lower left side of chest over cardiac apex, to left of nipple in midaxillary line.

DEFIBRILLATION OF A PATIENT WITH AN IMPLANTED PACEMAKER

Place the pads as far away from pulse generator as possible. Standard anterior/lateral placement is most convenient, but it delivers defibrillation energy in the same direction as the pacemaker's sensing vector and may damage the pacemaker. Place pads in the anterior/posterior position so that energy is delivered perpendicular to sensing vector.

(continued)

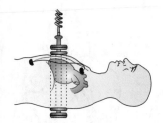

■ Anterior/posterior paddle placement for patient with an implanted pacemaker. (Crockett, P. [1991]. *Defib: What you should know.* Redmond, WA: Physio-Control. Reprinted with permission.)

DEFIBRILLATION OF A PATIENT WITH AN IMPLANTED DEFIBRILLATOR

If an unconscious patient receives shocks from an implanted defibrillator but V-tach or ventricular fibrillation (V-fib) persists, external countershock should be delivered. It is possible that the limited energy output of the implant is insufficient to defibrillate the heart. If initial attempts at external defibrillation are unsuccessful, change the placement of the pad electrodes. For example, if the sternum/apex position fails, try the anterior/posterior position.

MONOPHASIC VERSUS BIPHASIC DEFIBRILLATION

Defibrillators are classified according to two types of waveforms: monophasic and biphasic. Monophasic defibrillators were introduced first, and although they are no longer being manufactured, many remain in use today. They deliver current in one direction only. Biphasic defibrillators deliver two-way current. During the first phase of the shock, the current flows in one direction. During the second phase, the current reverses, and travels backwards.

DEFIBRILLATION ENERGY LEVELS

Research indicates that lower-energy biphasic defibrillation has equivalent or higher success for termination of VF than does monophasic defibrillation which delivers escalating energy (200–300–360 J) with successive shocks. Although the optimal energy for biphasic waveform defibrillation has not been conclusively determined, shocks with relatively low energy (<200 J) have been shown to terminate VF with equivalent or higher success rates than do monophasic shocks of equivalent or higher energy.

DOR PROCEDURE *(see also Ventricular Restoration, p. 164)*

The Dor procedure, also known as left ventricular reconstructive surgery, or EVCPP (endoventricular circular patch plasty), is a surgical approach that is sometimes used after an aneurysm forms following a heart attack. By restoring the normal elliptical geometry of the left ventricle, the ability of the ventricle to contract is improved, resulting in improved heart function.

The heart is placed on heart-lung bypass, and a small incision is made into the left ventricle to find the exact location of the scarred tissue. Two or more rows of circular stitches are then placed around the border of the dead tissue to separate it from healthy muscle tissue and then are pulled together like a purse string to permanently separate the dead tissue from the rest of the heart. (Sometimes an area of scar tissue is removed first before the stitches are pulled together, of if there is a lot of dead tissue to remove and the stitches are not enough to isolate the area, a patch must be placed.) Lastly, the outside of the ventricle is closed and reinforced with another row of stitches. Often, other surgeries, such as CABG or valve surgery, are often done at the same time.

(continued)

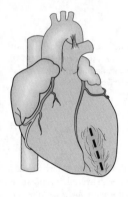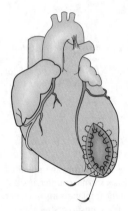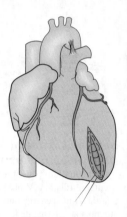

| Incision line through dead scarred tissue | Purse-string stitches around the dead tissue | Pulling of purse string and closing of left ventricle |

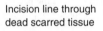

■ Dor procedure. (Adapted with permission, Cleveland Clinic Center for Medical Art and Photography © 2004–2010. All Rights Reserved.)

DRESSLER'S SYNDROME

A pronounced form of pericarditis that develops in some patients weeks or months after an MI, characterized by pleuritic chest pain, fever, pericardial friction rub, and mild to moderate pleural effusion, Dressler's syndrome is rarely serious, although it often recurs several times before finally resolving spontaneously.

ECMO *(see Extracorporeal Life Support, p. 108)*

EDEMA GRADING SCALE *(see also Third Spacing in Part 7, p. 293)*

Pitting >1 inch = 4+
Pitting ½ to 1 inch = 3+
Pitting ¼ to ½ inch = 2+
Pitting <¼ inch = 1+

EECP *(see Enhanced External Counterpulsation, p. 107)*

EINTHOVEN'S TRIANGLE *(see EKG Lead Placement, p. 101)*

EJECTION FRACTION

First-pass angiocardiography is used to show end-diastolic and end-systolic images, shunts, and details of heart wall motion. From these values, an ejection fraction (EF) can be determined, indicating the percentage of ventricular chamber emptying. It is determined by this formula:

$$EF = \frac{EDV - ESV}{EDV} \times 100$$

Normal ejection fraction is 60% to 65% ($\pm$8%); lower values indicate ventricular dysfunction, whereas an ejection fraction of <35% indicates serious ventricular problems.

EKG: FUSION BEATS

Fusion beats occur when two opposing electrical currents meet and collide within the same chamber at the same time. The ensuing EKG complex is often narrower and of lesser amplitude than an ectopic beat alone.

REMEMBER:

With a fusion beat: The P to P is regular, the R to R is regular, and the P *does* bear a relationship to the QRS (the PR interval may be shorter than that of the sinus rhythm, but never by more than 0.06).

(continued)

NOTES

EKG: INTERPRETATION PARAMETERS *(see also Myocardial Infarction: EKG Patterns, p. 131)*

EKG Interpretation Parameters

Rhythm	P Wave	PR Interval	QRS Rate and Rhythm	Comment
Sinus	Before each QRS	0.12–0.20	60–100; regular	
Sinus arrhythmia	Before each QRS	0.12–0.20	60–100; phasic variation with respiration	
Sinus bradycardia	Before each QRS	0.12–0.20	<60; regular	Not often below 40
Sinus tachycardia	Before each QRS	0.12–0.20	>100; regular, but may vary a little	Usually 100–160; may be higher in children
Sinus arrest		Pause does not march out		R to R regular except for missed beat
Sinus block		Pause marches out		2nd or 3rd degree may follow
Wandering pacemaker	Morphology changes; may be hard to see	Varies as site changes		R to R varies as site changes
Premature atrial contraction (PAC)	Premature P may have different configuration; P may be buried in T	May be <0.12 or >0.20	QRS may be normal or widened; irregular	No compensatory pause, **usually;** frequent PACs can lead to A fib
Premature atrial tachycardia (PAT)	Before each QRS; may be buried in preceding wave or T fused P & T	May be <0.12 or >0.20	160–250; absolutely regular, **usually**	QRS normal, **usually;** abrupt onset and termination; carotid pressure may terminate attack
Atrial flutter	Atrial rate is 200–300; Ventricular rate varies; Sawtooth pattern	Constant or variable	75–300, depending on amount of AV block; regular or irregular	Carotid pressure produces temporary slowing, if any; Watch for emboli
Atrial fibrillation (A fib)	Atrial rate 300 or more; Ventricular rate varies; Irregular, undulant baseline ("F" waves)	Variable; R → R never march out; exception: CHB	50–250, depending on degree of AV block; irregular	"F" waves may be shown better in V_2 than lead II; Watch for emboli

EKG Interpretation Parameters (*Continued*)

Rhythm	P Wave	PR Interval	QRS Rate and Rhythm	Comment
PJC			Single premature beat interrupts rhythm; slight delay before next	
Junctional	Before, after, or in QRS Often inverted	Usually <0.12	40–100	
Premature ventricular contraction (PVC)	None preceding the premature QRS		Usually normal, can occur at any rate	Compensatory pause, **usually;** QRS configuration different, >0.12, **usually**
Ventricular tachycardia (V tach)	Usually not seen; if present, not related to QRS	Variable	100–220, **usually** regular or nearly regular	QRS broad, different, >0.10, **usually** Can be with or without pulse
Ventricular fibrillation (V fib)	None		No well-defined QRS complexes	No palpable pulse and no audible tones
1st-degree AV block	Before each QRS	0.21 or more	Regular	May be a warning that 2nd- or 3rd-degree block will follow
2nd-degree AV block (Type 1, Mobitz 1, or Wenckebach)	Before each QRS except for blocked P	Lengthens until one beat is dropped; first of the PR series is usually >0.20 seconds	Normal	"Group beating" is obvious; usually a transient rhythm
2nd-degree AV block (Type II or Mobitz II)	Before each QRS except for blocked P	Normal or prolonged but constant	Normal if block is at bundle of HIS, wide if at the level of the bundle branches	Is often irreversible and progresses into 3rd degree; may need pacemaker; **REMEMBER:** "Out of the blue, Mobitz II drops a Q (wave)"
3rd-degree AV block (complete heart block)	Occurs regularly but without relationship to QRS	Variable	Below 60, **usually;** regular, **usually**	Spells of syncope common (Adams-Stokes attacks); pace-maker is in the ventricles (idioventricular rhythm)

EKG LEAD PLACEMENT *(see also ST Segment Monitoring, p. 148)*

Depending on the monitoring system, the number of EKG electrodes (wires) positioned on the patient will differ. **But remember**: One electrode (wire) cannot be a "lead." Leads are *pictures*, so this means that a *group* of electrodes is required to capture a specific view. (For example, to obtain a 12-lead EKG, there are six "chest" electrodes, and four "limb" electrodes. This is only 10 wires, but the different combinations of the wires yield 12 different views.)

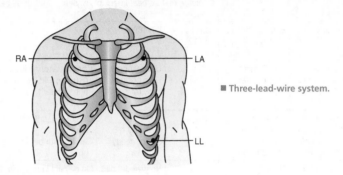

■ Three-lead-wire system.

THREE-LEAD SYSTEM

A three-lead system can only give you a choice of limb leads: I, II, III, aVR, aVL, and aVF.

Position:

RA (white) Below right clavicle, 2nd ICS, MCL

REMEMBER: White is right

LA (black) Below left clavicle, 2nd ICS, MCL
LL (red) Left lower rib cage, 8th ICS, MCL

Chest leads are unavailable with a three-lead system; however, *changing the lead selector on the monitor to lead III* and *repositioning an electrode* can facilitate a *modified* chest lead (MCL) tracing. To monitor modified chest leads: LL (red) must move to the appropriate chest lead position, either:

MCL_1 = 4th ICS, right sternal boarder or
MCL_6 = 5th ICS, L midaxillary line to heart

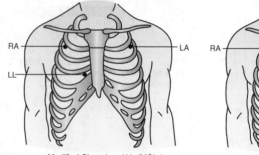

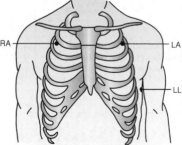

Modified Chest Lead V_1 (MCL_1) Modified Chest Lead V_6 (MCL_6)

■ Modified chest leads. *(continued)*

FIVE-LEAD SYSTEM

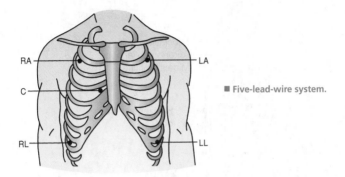

■ Five-lead-wire system.

A five-lead system allows monitoring in the limb leads: I, II, III, aVR, aVL, and aVF and by using the lead select on the monitor, a chest lead can be obtained as well.

Position:

RA (white)	Below right clavicle, 2nd ICS, MCL
RL (green)	Right lower rib cage, 8th ICS, MCL
LA (black)	Below left clavicle, 2nd ICS, MCL
LL (red)	Left lower rib cage, 8th ICS, MCL
CHEST (brown)	Any V lead position, usually V_1

> **REMEMBER:**

Clouds over grass, smoke over fire.

   (White electrode above green electrode; Black electrode above red electrode)

(*continued*)

NOTES

TWELVE-LEAD SYSTEM

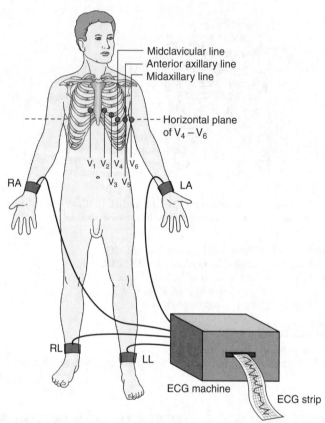

Midclavicular line
Anterior axillary line
Midaxillary line

Horizontal plane of $V_4 - V_6$

V_1 V_2 V_4 V_6
V_3 V_5

RA

LA

RL

LL

ECG machine

ECG strip

■ Electrode placement for limb leads and precordial leads. (From Morton, P. G., & Fontaine, D. [2009]. *Critical care nursing: A holistic approach* [9th ed.]. Philadelphia: Lippincott Williams & Wilkins.)

The 12-lead EKG views six limb leads in the *frontal plane* of the body, and six chest leads in the *horizontal plane*.

Position:

RA (white)	Anywhere on right arm (below shoulder)
LA (black)	Anywhere on left arm (below shoulder)
LL (red)	Anywhere on left leg (below inguinal fold anterior; below gluteal fold posterior)
RL (green)	Anywhere on right leg (below inguinal fold anterior; below gluteal fold posterior)
V_1 (brown)	4th ICS, right sternal boarder
V_2 (brown)	4th ICS, left sternal boarder

(continued)

V$_3$ (brown)	Halfway between V$_2$ and V$_4$
V$_4$ (brown)	5th ICS, left MCL
V$_5$ (brown)	5th ICS, left anterior axillary line
V$_6$ (brown)	5th ICS, left midaxillary line

REMEMBER:

When you think of how the **LIMB** leads "look" at the heart, imagine looking at the face of a clock:

Lead I	views the heart from	3 o'clock
Lead II	views the heart from	5 o'clock
Lead III	views the heart from	7 o'clock
aVR	views the heart from	10 o'clock
aVL	views the heart from	2 o'clock
aVF	views the heart from	6 o'clock

REMEMBER:

When you think of how the **CHEST** leads "look" at the heart, imagine a vector projecting through the AV node toward the patient's back. V$_1$ to V$_6$ are like the spokes of a wheel, with the center being the heart.

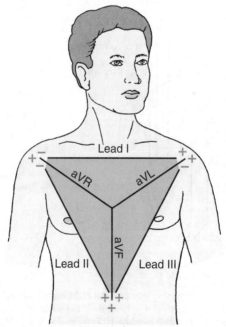

■ EKG planes. (From Morton, P. G., & Fotaine, D. [2009] *Critical care nursing: A holistic approach* [9th ed.]. Philadelphia: Lippincott Williams & Wilkins.)

(*continued*)

Limb leads give information on a vertical plane: right, left, inferior, superior | Chest leads give information on a horizontal plane: right, left, anterior, posterior

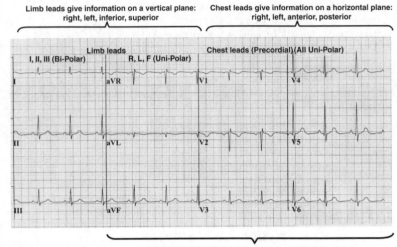

REMEMBER: All Uni-Polar leads have a "V" in their name.
■ Normal 12-lead EKG configuration.

RIGHT CHEST LEADS

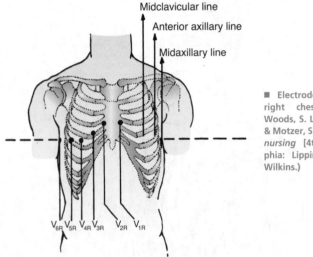

Midclavicular line
Anterior axillary line
Midaxillary line

■ Electrode placement for right chest leads. (From Woods, S. L., Froelicher, E. S., & Motzer, S. U. [1999]. *Cardiac nursing* [4th ed.]. Philadelphia: Lippincott Williams & Wilkins.)

In the case of right ventricular hypertrophy and right ventricular infarct, often times it is helpful to look further "around" the heart than the standard V_1 to V_6 leads. This is when the use of right chest leads is employed. Designated as V_1R to V_6R, they are a "mirror image" of the standard (left) chest leads, and yield information related to right-sided anomalies. The tracings of V_4R, V_5R, and V_6R will look similar to that of the standard V_1 but will be smaller. V_4R is the lead most indicative of right-sided involvement.

(*continued*)

Position:

V_1R (brown)	(Standard V_2 lead) 4th ICS, left sternal boarder
V_2R (brown)	(Standard V_1 lead) 4th ICS, right sternal boarder
V_3R (brown)	Halfway between V_2R and V_4R
V_4R (brown)	5th ICS, right MCL
V_5R (brown)	5th ICS, right anterior axillary line
V_6R (brown)	4th ICS right midaxillary line

LEFT POSTERIOR CHEST LEADS

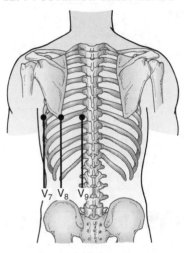

■ Electrode placement for left posterior leads. (From Woods, S. L., Froelicher, E. S., & Motzer, S. U. [1999]. *Cardiac nursing* [4th ed.]. Philadelphia: Lippincott Williams & Wilkins.)

Only rarely used, left posterior chest leads can diagnose a posterior infarct in a patient with a suspected MI, but a nondiagnostic standard 12 lead. Placement of left posterior chest leads allows direct visualization of the posterior surface of the heart.

REMEMBER:

All leads will print out as a straight line, except those labeled V_4, V_5, and V_6 (since these are the only three lead wires connected). They must be relabeled V_7, V_8, and V_9, respectively. However, some EKG machines won't operate unless *all* electrodes are connected. In that case, the limb leads as well as V_1, V_2, and V_3 would need to be applied, but will be nondiagnostic.

Position:

V_7 (brown)	5th ICS (at level of V_4), left posterior axillary line
V_8 (brown)	5th ICS (at level of V_4) left midscapular line
V_9 (brown)	5th ICS (at level of V_4) immediately to left of spine

FIFTEEN- OR EIGHTEEN-LEAD SYSTEM

Nonstandard EKG tracings may lead to the increased detection of infarctions of the right ventricle and posterior wall. Right chest leads V_4R, V_5R, and V_6R and left posterior chest leads V_7, V_8, and V_9 when combined with a standard 12-lead EKG, can produce either a 15- or 18-lead EKG. (See previous discussion of right chest leads, and left posterior chest leads). Some 12-lead EKG recorders actually have the capacity to record three extra leads

(continued)

simultaneously with the 12 standard leads, but this is not essential. A 15- or 18-lead EKG can be obtained by first running a standard 12-lead EKG, then adding electrodes in the specified locations, and running the "12 lead" a second time. **REMEMBER:** The "new" leads will need to be relabeled (for right chest or left posterior leads) when the EKG is run a second time, as the machine does not know where the electrodes are located.

Lead Placement for 12-Lead EKG		
Lead	**Direction of Electrical Potential**	**View of Heart**
Standard Limb Leads (Bipolar) (Einthoven's Triangle)		
I	Between L arm (+) and R arm (−)	Lateral wall LV
II	Between L leg (+) and R arm (−)	Inferior wall LV
III	Between L leg (+) and L arm (−)	Inferior wall LV
Augmented Limb Leads (Unipolar)		
aVR	R arm to heart	No specific view; superior aspect LV
aVL	L arm to heart	Lateral wall; superior aspect LV
Avf	L foot to heart	Inferior wall LV
Precordial or Chest Leads (Unipolar)		
V_1	4th ICS; right sternal border to heart	Anteroseptal wall LV
V_2	4th ICS; left sternal border to heart	Anteroseptal wall LV
V_3	Halfway between V_2 and V_4 to heart	Anterior wall LV
V_4	5th ICS; left midclavicular line to heart	Anterior wall LV
V_5	5th ICS; left anterior axillary line to heart	Lateral wall LV
V_6	5th ICS; left midaxillary line to heart	Lateral wall LV

Which Lead Is Best?	
To See	**Lead**
PACs Abnormal sinus rhythm Most heart blocks	Any lead that displays clear P waves and QRS complexes
Atrial fibrillation	Recognizable in most leads by the irregular R-R intervals
Differentiate wide QRS rhythms	V_1 and V_6 (or their bipolar equivalents, MCL_1 and MCL_6)
Arrhythmias in general (Inadequate for ischemia)	II, V_1
Ischemia, infarcts*	III, V_3
ST segment changes of the right coronary artery*	III, aVF, sometimes II useful (standard 12 lead)
Occlusion or reocclusion of the LAD*	V_2, V_3, sometimes V_1, V_4 useful (standard 12 lead)
ST segment changes of circumflex*	A variety of leads depending on myocardial zone affected: V_5, V_6 for lateral III, aVF, II for interior V_1, V_2, V_3 for posterior
Unsure about where occlusion exists*	III, aVF most reliable for showing ST deviation with involvement of all three major coronary arteries

ST elevation should not be more than 1 mm in standard leads or more than 2 mm in precordial leads. Presence of ST depression of 1 to 2 mm or more for a duration of 0.08 seconds may indicate ischemia.

(*continued*)

Normal 12-Lead EKG Waveforms

Lead	P Wave	Q Wave	R Wave	S Wave	T Wave	ST Segment
I	Upright	Small	Largest wave of complex	Small (less than R or none)	Upright	May vary from +1 to −0.5 mm
II	Upright	Small or none	Large (vertical heart)	Small (less than R or none)	Upright	May vary from +1 to −0.5 mm
III	Upright, diphasic, or inverted	Usually small or none (for large Q to be diagnostic, a Q must also be present in a VF)	None to large	None to large (horizontal heart)	Upright, diphasic, or inverted	May vary from +1 to −0.5 mm
aVR	Inverted	Small, none, or large	Small or none	Large (may be QS complex)	Inverted	May vary from +1 to −0.5 mm
aVL	Upright, diphasic, or inverted	Small, none, or large (to be diagnostic, Q must also be present in one or precordial leads)	Small, none, or large (horizontal heart)	None to large (vertical heart)	Upright, diphasic, or inverted	May vary from +1 to −0.5 mm
aVF	Upright	Small or none	Small, none, or large (vertical heart)	None to large (horizontal heart)	Upright, diphasic, or inverted	May vary from +1 to −0.5 mm
V_1	Upright, diphasic, or inverted	None or QS complex	Less than S wave or none	Large (may be QS)	Upright, diphasic, or inverted	May vary from 0 to +3 mm
V_2	Upright	None (rare QS)	Less than S wave, or none (larger than V_1)	Large (may be QS)	Upright	May vary from 0 to +3 mm
V_3	Upright	Small or none	Less, greater, or equal to five wave (larger than V_2)	Large (greater, less, or equal to R wave)	Upright	May vary from 0 to +3 mm
V_4	Upright	Small or none	Greater than S (larger than V_3)	Smaller than R; (smaller than V_3)	Upright	May vary from +1 to −0.5 mm
V_5	Upright	Small	Larger than R in V_4; less than 26 mm	Smaller than S in V_4	Upright	May vary from +1 to −0.5 mm
V_6	Upright	Small	Large; less than 26 mm	Smaller than S in V_5	Upright	May vary from +1 to −0.5 mm

U waves may follow T waves, particularly in leads V_2 to V_4; are upright; and are of lower amplitude than T waves. (Adapted from Goldschlager, N., & Goldman, M. J. [1989]. Principles of clinical electrocardiograph [13th ed.]. Norwalk, CT: Appleton & Lange. With permission.)

ELECTROPHYSIOLOGY STUDIES *(see also Ablation, p. 67)*

Electrophysiology studies (EPS) are performed in a specialized lab to determine an arrhythmia diagnosis or an EP mechanism of a known arrhythmia. They provide a valuable adjunct to the traditional 12-lead EKG, Holter monitor, and stress test. Preparation for an EPS is similar to that for cardiac catheterization. The patient is given nothing by mouth and is sedated during the procedure. A peripheral IV is necessary to administer medication, and systemic anticoagulation may be used. During the procedure, transvenous intracardiac catheters are placed (with the aid of fluoroscopy) into various locations of the heart. These catheters allow recording of intracardiac action potentials and programmed electrical stimulation (PES). Lethal dysrhythmias may be induced; therefore, the procedure is performed in an environment where resuscitative equipment is readily available. Complications are rare but include hematoma, pneumothorax, deep vein thrombosis, stroke, and sudden death.

ENDOCARDITIS

The entire inner surface of the heart, the four heart valves and the four heart chambers, is lined with a thin membrane called the endocardium. Endocarditis is a term used to describe inflammation and/or infection of the endocardial tissue, or inner lining. The most common causative organisms of endocarditis are *Streptococcus viridans* and *Staphylococcus aureus*. Bacteria "set up housekeeping" on heart valve(s) and throw septic emboli. The mitral valve is most commonly affected; the aortic valve is second. Causes are related to:

- Rheumatic heart disease
- Open-heart, genitourinary, or gynecologic surgery
- Congenital heart defects
- Dental procedures
- Abscess
- Drug abuse
- Body piercing

Assessment reveals clubbing of fingers, splinter hemorrhages of nails, petechiae, Roth's spots (white spots on retina), and Janeway lesions (painless lesions on palms, soles).

Long-term intravenous antibiotics are required to eradicate the bacteria from the heart chambers and the vegetations on the valves. The chosen drug must be specific for the organism causing the condition, which is determined by blood culture and sensitivity tests. Treatment for up to 6 weeks is not uncommon.

ENDOTHELIAL FUNCTION TESTING

Recently developed, this noninvasive finger device is used to measure the health of endothelial cells by measuring blood flow. It promises to be a highly predictive tool for a heart attack or stroke in patients who are considered low to moderate risk.

The test, which takes about 15 minutes, consists of digital recording equipment and two finger probes that look like large thimbles. The patient is fitted with one probe on each index finger, and hooked up to a machine that will measure the blood flow. A standard blood pressure cuff is placed on one arm; the arm without the cuff is the control. A reading of the fingers' blood flow rate begins. The blood pressure cuff is inflated for a few minutes, then deflated, and the normal blood flow response that occurs when occlusion is released is documented. Three readings are taken. A low blood flow response correlates with endothelial dysfunction and impaired vascular health, and serves as a biomarker for future events.

ENHANCED EXTERNAL COUNTERPULSATION (EECP)

A noninvasive treatment of angina, usually reserved for patients who have either failed or are not candidates for bypass or angioplasty. Typically done on an outpatient basis, patients are treated 1 hour daily for up to 7 weeks. An EKG monitor is placed on the patient, and three pneumatic inflatable cuffs are wrapped around the calf, the thigh, and the buttock. Using the EKG signal, these cuffs sequentially inflate (calf, thigh, buttock) to gently compress blood vessels and force blood back to the heart. Then all three simultaneously deflate. Studies indicate that this treatment may stimulate the formation of collaterals (small branches of blood vessels), and thereby create a natural bypass around blocked arteries.

ENZYMES, CARDIAC *(see Cardiac Markers in Part 9, p. 342)*

ERB'S POINT *(see Heart Sounds: Landmarks, p. 111)*

ESOPHAGEAL DOPPLER MONITORING
(see also Ultrasound in Part 10, p. 367)

Using Doppler ultrasound technology, EDM provides noninvasive beat-to-beat information on how well the heart is functioning, how effectively patient fluid levels are being maintained, and the impact of therapeutic interventions. The technology uses a thin silicone probe, about 6 mm in diameter. The flexible, patient-specific probe is inserted into the esophagus of an intubated and sedated patient and positioned alongside the descending aorta. The other end of the probe is connected to the monitoring system, and the ultrasound signal is transformed into meaningful cardiac function information (see figure).

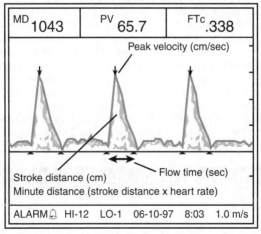

■ EDM waveform. (Courtesy of Deltex Medical, Inc. Irving, TX.)

(continued)

EDM waveform interpretation:

The base of the waveform is used as in index to *preload* and is displayed as FTc (systolic flow time in seconds, corrected for heart rate).

The waveform height is used as an index to *contractility* and appears as PV (peak velocity) in cm/sec.

Concurrent shifts in FTc and PV are used as an index to afterload (see table).

Waveform Interpretation		
PV	**FTc**	**Possible Indication**
Decreased	Decreased	Increased afterload
Decreased	Normal	Decreased contractility
Normal	Decreased	Decreased preload
Increased	Increased	Hyperdynamic, vasodilation, sepsis

MD (minute distance) is a cardiac output parameter. It is the distance (cm) moved by the column of blood through the aorta in 1 minute:

MD <800 cm = low flow state
MD >1,200 cm = high flow state

EXTRACORPOREAL LIFE SUPPORT

Extracorporeal life support (ECLS) is a broad term that includes many methods of mechanical cardiopulmonary support. When it is used for respiratory support with extrathoracic cannulation, it is known as extracorporeal membrane oxygenation (ECMO). The term ECMO is often used interchangeably with ECLS to denote prolonged extracorporeal circulation with mechanical devices. When the heart/lung machine is used in the operating room in venoarterial mode, the technique is known as cardiopulmonary bypass (CBG). Generally, all these devices include a venous cannula used to drain blood from the right side of the heart to a circuit. As blood is pumped through the circuit it is oxygenated, filtered, cooled, or warmed, and returned by means of an arterial cannula to the systemic circulation. Some form of anticoagulation (usually heparin) is used, and therefore, bleeding is always a potential problem. Blood pumps alone can be used as left ventricular assist devices (LVADs), right ventricular assist devices (RVADs), or biventricular assist devices (BiVADs). VADs, however, differ from ECLS in that the patient's pulmonary vasculature is not bypassed. (Blood is oxygenated by the patient, not the device.) Another difference is that the VADs are designed for long-term use, whereas CBG is used only for the duration of the operation, usually 6 to 8 hours.

NOTES

FEMORAL BYPASS SURGERY

Femoral bypass surgery is an option when an arterial blockage(s) is causing significant symptomatic distal tissue ischemia. The procedure causes the surgical redirection of blood flow, via a transplanted healthy blood vessel or man-made graft, to bypass the blocked artery. One end of the vein, or man-made graft, is attached above the blockage, with the other end attached below the blockage, rerouting blood flow and restoring distal circulation.

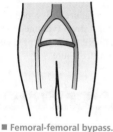

Femoral-femoral bypass: Performed in poor-risk patients with unilateral claudication or ischemia. Performed only if donor artery has no marked proximal stenosis.

■ Femoral-femoral bypass.

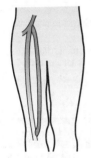

Femoral-popliteal bypass: Remains the standard operation for relieving ischemic symptoms secondary to femoral-popliteal occlusive disease. Patients with this disease usually have involvement of distal popliteal artery and its tibial branches as well.

■ Femoral-popliteal bypass.

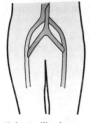

Aorto-iliac bypass: Limb-threatening ischemia is not usually seen with aorto-iliac occlusions unless femoral-popliteal disease is also present. In aorto-iliac occlusive disease, the distal aorta, including the iliac arteries, is affected.

■ Aorto-iliac bypass.

FIBRINOLYTIC THERAPY (see *Thrombolytic Therapy, p. 161*)

FUSION BEATS (see *EKG: Fusion Beats, p. 95*)

HEART FAILURE (see also *BNP, in Part 9, p. 341*)

Heart failure is a complex clinical syndrome characterized by dyspnea and fatigue, secondary to structural and functional changes in the heart. It can stem from any cardiac disorder where the left ventricle either fills inadequately (diastolic dysfunction) or ejects insufficiently (systolic dysfunction). It is the most common diagnosis of hospitalized patients older than 65 years.

B-type natriuretic peptide (BNP) is a great predictor of heart failure. It is a peptide released from granules in the ventricles in response to ventricular stress (volume overload, pressure overload). At a blood concentration of 80 pg/mL, BNP accurately predicts heart failure, while lower concentrations are highly negative for heart failure.

New York Heart Association Functional Classification System	
Class I	**Symptoms cause little or no limitations** of physical activity.
Class II	Symptoms cause **slight limitations** of physical activity. Comfortable at rest, but ordinary activities result in fatigue, palpitations, and/or dyspnea.
Class III	Symptoms cause **marked limitations** of physical activity. Comfortable at rest, but even slight activity causes marked fatigue, palpitations, and/or dyspnea.
Class IV	**Inability to engage in any physical activity without symptoms.** Unable to carry out ADLs without discomfort. Symptoms of fatigue, palpitations, and/or dyspnea present even at rest.

American College of Cardiology (ACC) and American Heart Association (AHA) Classification of Chronic Heart Failure		
Stage A	High risk for developing heart failure	HTN, DM, CAD, family history of cardiomyopathy
Stage B	Asymptomatic heart failure	Previous MI, LV dysfunction, valvular heart disease
Stage C	Symptomatic heart failure	Structural heart disease, dyspnea, and fatigue, impaired exercise intolerance
Stage D heart failure	Refractory end-stage medical therapy	Marked symptoms at rest despite maximum

Opportunities to improve outcomes:
- Digoxin (decrease HR, increase contractility)
- Diuretics (decrease preload)
- ACE inhibitor (decrease preload and afterload) PLUS beta-blocker
- Natrecor (recombinant human BNP) (reduces wedge pressure)

HEART SOUNDS: LANDMARKS

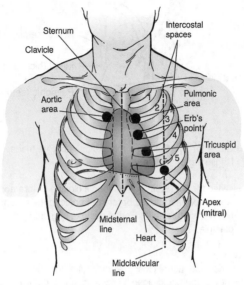

■ Heart sound landmarks. (Adapted from Porth, C. M.
[1994]. *Pathophysiology: Concepts of altered health states*
[4th ed.]. Philadelphia: J.B. Lippincott.)

A logical, systematic approach to auscultation is recommended by listening to the follow-ing areas in this order:

1. Aortic area (loud S_2 here) R sternal boarder, 2nd ICS.
2. Pulmonic area (split S_2 best heard here) L sternal boarder, 3rd ICS
3. Tricuspid area (soft S_1, not always audible here) lower L sternal boarder, 4th ICS
4. Mitral area (loud S_1, and S_3 and S_4 if present, heard here) 5th ICS, L midclavicular line

REMEMBER:

Aortic, pulmonic, tricuspid, mitral:
- **A**ll **p**hysicians **t**ake **m**oney; or
- **A**pple **p**ie **t**astes **m**mmmmmmmm; or
- Aortic on the right, pulmonic on the left,
    Tricuspid neath the sternum.
    Mitral at the apex beat, and this is how we learn 'em!

NOTES

HEART SOUNDS: NORMAL

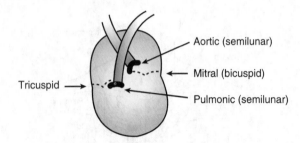

Aortic (semilunar)

Mitral (bicuspid)

Tricuspid →

Pulmonic (semilunar)

- - - - = Close for S_1. (Split S_1 = mitral closes before tricuspid.) Beginning of systole.

▬▬ = Close for S_2. (Split S_2 = pulmonic closing before aortic. Aortic *normally* closes before pulmonic, but ear cannot distinguish this split.) End of systole, beginning of diastole.

Sequence:
S_1 = Tricuspid, mitral close. (Aortic, pulmonic open.)
S_2 = Aortic, pulmonic close. (Tricuspid, mitral open.)

■ Normal sequence of heart sounds.

S_1 (LUB)

S_1 coincides with the R wave. Beginning of systole. Mitral and tricuspid valves close. Loudest at apex.

- Loud S_1 = short PR interval (may be due to structure of AV valve, i.e., mitral stenosis)
- Increased atrial pressures = valve remains open during diastole. May also be due to left-to-right shunting, fever, anemia, or hyperthyroid condition.
- S_1 louder after exercise
- Soft S_1 = decreased strength of contraction (due to infarct, CHF)
- If S_1 is of varied intensity (loud-soft-loud), it may be due to atrial fibrillation or AV block.

S_2 (DUB)

S_2 sound occurs when the aortic and pulmonic valves close.

        ↓   ↓
    Loudest   Slight delay

NOTES

HEART SOUNDS: ABNORMAL

S₃ (LUB-DUP-TA)

S_3 (ventricular gallop) occurs when the mitral and tricuspid valves open and there is an inrush of blood from the atria.

Sounds like KEN—<u>TUC</u>—KY (accent on second syllable)

$$\downarrow \qquad \downarrow \qquad \downarrow$$
$$S_1 \qquad S_2 \qquad S_3$$

- Occurs on inspiration. Best if heard at beginning of expiration. Easier to auscultate if patient holds breath.
- Must use bell at lower left sternal border (left ventricular area)
- S_3 can be felt; it is palpable.
- Heard in 85% of 10- to 25-year-olds and is normal. Not often heard in children younger than 10 years.
- Abnormal finding after 30 years of age. First subtle sign of cardiac failure, because it indicates an increase in preload (LVEDP). Can be auscultated, and S_3 is heard before rales.
- If S_3 persists despite diuretics and digoxin, prognosis is poor.
- S_3 is associated with increase in pressure and blood volume during diastole; therefore, it may be heard in patient with left ventricular failure. May also be present with left-to-right shunt or mitral/tricuspid regurgitation.

S₄ (TA-LUB-DUP)

S_4 (atrial gallop) occurs when the atria contract. An inrush of blood to the ventricles sets up vibrations indicating an increased resistance to filling.

Sounds like <u>TEN</u>—NES—SEE (accent on first syllable)

$$\downarrow \qquad \downarrow \qquad \downarrow$$
$$S_4 \qquad S_1 \qquad S_2$$

- Normal in infants and children
- Abnormal in adults, but common in elderly
- Usually occurs with angina; may occur with MI
- Must use bell. Best heard at apex or left lateral sternal border. Easier to auscultate if patient holds breath.
- Indicates cardiac pathologic condition but is not always diagnostic of a specific dysfunction
- May be due to impairment of ability of ventricle to distend (e.g., after MI) or to increased ventricular pressure (aortic stenosis or hypertension)

Guidelines to help differentiate a left-sided gallop from a right-sided gallop:
- Left-sided gallop sounds are best heard in the apical area, whereas right-sided sounds are best heard at the lower left sternal border.
- The history and the suspected underlying cause of the gallop give clues to whether it is caused by the right or the left side.
- Start at the apex and inch your way to the lower left sternal border. A left-sided gallop fades as you near the sternal border. If the gallop is from the right side, it becomes louder as you near the lower left sternal border area.
- Right-sided gallops are often heard best at the end of inspiration.
- Left-sided gallops are often heard best during expiration.

(continued)

SPLIT S₁ (T-LUB-DUB)

Split S_1 occurs when the mitral valve closes before the tricuspid.

- Occurs with right bundle branch block and premature ventricular contractions (PVCs)
- Heard best at the fourth left intercostal space (right ventricular area), lower left sternal border
- Heard on expiration

SPLIT S₂ (LUB-T-DUB)

Split S_2 is physiologic. The aortic valve normally closes before the pulmonic, but the ear usually cannot distinguish the split.

- Heard only during inspiration at pulmonic area and Erb's point (second or third left intercostal space, adjacent to the sternum)
- After the age of 50 years, split is not usually heard (aortic component is delayed, and valves close closer in time).
- Fixed split occurs on inspiration and expiration. May occur with right bundle branch block (due to much blood backing into the right ventricle, i.e., ventricular septal defect, pulmonic insufficiency).
- Reverse split is due to a delay in aortic valve closure. It is caused by blood overload in the left ventricle resulting from aortic stenosis, left bundle branch block, or ischemia in the left ventricle. It is heard on expiration (as aortic and pulmonic valves fuse on inspiration).

Guidelines to help differentiate a split S₂ from an S₃:

- When listening for an S_3, be sure to use bell.
- Have patient lie in the left lateral position.
- If a split S_2 is suspected, press down firmly on the bell. If it is a low-frequency gallop sound, it usually disappears. But if it is a split S_2, the sound can still be heard.
- If a split S_2 is suspected, inch your way up from the apex to the base (to the pulmonic and aortic area); a split S_2 increases in intensity, and an S_3 fades away.
- An S_3 is low pitched, so if two high-pitched sounds are heard, it is a split S_2.

Guidelines to help differentiate a split S₁ from an S₄:

- When listening for an S_4, be sure to use bell.
- Have patient lie in the left lateral position.
- If a split S_1 is suspected, press down firmly on the bell. If it is a low-frequency gallop sound, it usually disappears. If it is a split S_1, the sound can still be heard.
- If a split S_1 is suspected, feel for the apical pulse. If the sound occurs before the apical pulse, it is an S_4. If it occurs with the apical pulse, it is a split S_1.
- If you hear three sounds where an S_1 should be, it is probably a split S_1 with an S_4.

MURMURS

Murmurs are technically not heart sounds but are related to a pathologic event. They may be due to

- Increased velocity of blood flow (i.e., anemia, hyperthyroid condition)
- Narrowing of vessel (plaque, tumor)
- Blood flowing forward to dilated area of blood vessel (aneurysm)
- Blood flowing forward through abnormal valve (aortic, mitral stenosis)
- Blood flowing through a defect (intraventricular)

(continued)

Systolic Murmurs

Systolic murmurs are heard between S_1 and S_2. The sound is produced when the ventricle contracts. They are related to mitral tricuspid insufficiency (regurgitation) or aortic pulmonic stenosis.

Diastolic Murmurs

Diastolic murmurs are heard between S_2 and S_1. The sound is produced when the ventricle fills. They are related to mitral tricuspid stenosis or aortic pulmonic insufficiency (regurgitation).

REMEMBER:

This chart to help differentiate systolic and diastolic murmurs:

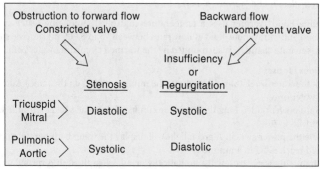

■ **Differentiating systolic from diastolic murmurs.**

Murmur Grades

Two systems are used in general for grading the intensity of murmurs: One based on four and the other on six intensities. The four-grade system is simpler and is usually adequate:

Grade 1	Faintest murmur you can hear
Grade 2	Soft
Grade 3	Loud
Grade 4	Very loud

The six-grade system is more complex but more definitive:

Grade 1	Faintest murmur you can hear; often not heard at first
Grade 2	Faint, but heard without difficulty
Grade 3	Soft, but louder than Grade 2
Grade 4	Loud, but softer than Grade 5
Grade 5	Loud, but not heard if stethoscope is lifted just off chest
Grade 6	Maximum loudness; heard even if stethoscope is lifted from chest

When using either of these grading systems, you must identify which criteria you are using to identify the murmur. That is, Grade 2/4 murmur indicates a Grade 2 murmur on a scale of 4, and Grade 4/6 murmur indicates a Grade 4 murmur on a scale of 6.

If deep inspiration changes the intensity of a murmur, this should be noted. Erb's point (third intercostal space, left sternal border) is usually referred to for murmurs during auscultation.

(continued)

PERICARDIAL FRICTION RUB

Approximately the fourth day after an acute MI, a pericardial friction rub will develop in about 7% of patients. The rub may be transient, sometimes lasting only a few hours. It is a harsh, grating sound, heard in both systole and diastole, and is caused by abrasion of the pericardial surfaces during the cardiac cycle. It can be easily confused with a murmur, so care must be taken during auscultation. Rubs are characteristic of pericarditis, which occurs in more than 15% of the patients with an acute MI. The sound is best heard on exhalation, with the patient sitting upright and leaning forward. Rubs can be present with or without a pericardial effusion.

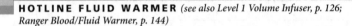

HEMODYNAMICS *(see Swan-Ganz, p. 155)*

HOTLINE FLUID WARMER *(see also Level 1 Volume Infuser, p. 126; Ranger Blood/Fluid Warmer, p. 144)*

The Hotline Fluid Warmer uses a temperature-controlled circulating water system to warm blood and intravenous fluid at flow rates between 75 to 5,000 mL/hr. The sterile IV pathway (separate channel) is surrounded by the warmed circulating water path.

Instructions for use:
1. Check the water level. (Should be above the minimum level on the tank.) Add distilled water only.
2. Plug into power outlet. Plug the twin tube connector into the socket (Hotline warming set REF L-70).
3. Activate the power switch. A green light will display the water bath temperature. (Should reach 37°C in 4 minutes.)
4. The circulating water bath will automatically prime when the unit is turned on.
5. Connect the IV administration set to the Hotline IV set.
6. Fully prime the IV administration set and the Hotline set, and connect to the patient's IV access site without trapping any air.

After use:
1. Turn off the power switch, and remove the Hotline set and dispose of properly.
2. Clean all surface with mild detergent.

HYPOTHERMIA

In patients who have been successfully resuscitated after cardiac arrest due to ventricular fibrillation, therapeutic mild hypothermia has been shown to increase the rate of a favorable neurologic outcome and reduced mortality. Protocols are institution specific but generally require that cooling (via the use of an external cooling blanket) begin within 1 to 2 hours of CPR, to maintain the patient at a temperature of 33°C for no less than 12 hours and no longer than 24 hours. Shivering, which is counterproductive because it increases body temperature, should be controlled by sedation and neuromuscular blockade. Hyperkalemia and hyperglycemia are possibilities, and the patient should be closely monitored. At the end of the cooling period, the patient is passively rewarmed. The lowered temperature is thought to reduce intracranial pressure, reduce heart rate, and reduce the brain's demand for oxygen, with the end result being a better chance of recovering with neurologic function intact.

HYPOVOLEMIC SHOCK *(see Shock, Hypovolemic, p. 146)*

IMPEDANCE CARDIOGRAPHY *(see Noninvasive Cardiac Output Monitoring, p. 133)*

INTRA-AORTIC BALLOON COUNTERPULSATION

Useful in cardiogenic shock, MI, and postoperative support to
- Increase cardiac output
- Decrease myocardial O_2 consumption
- Increase aortic pressure
- Decrease afterload (SVR)

Contraindications:
- Incompetent aortic valve
- Chronic end-stage heart disease
- Peripheral vascular disease
- Dissecting aortic or thoracic aneurysm
- Irreversible brain damage

BALLOON SIZING CRITERIA
- 50 mL—approximate height >6 feet
- **40 mL—approximate height 5′4″ to 6′** (most common)
- 34 mL—approximate height 5′ to 5′4″
- 25 mL—approximate height <5′

PLACEMENT
On x-ray film, tip of intra-aortic balloon (IAB) should be at the second or third intercostal space, 1 to 2 cm from the left subclavian, and above the renal arteries.

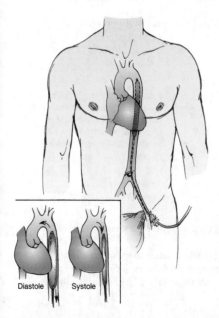

■ Intra-aortic balloon placement.

Diastole   Systole

(continued)

TRIGGERS

In the newest DataScope IABP model, the CS100, the most appropriate trigger source is automatically selected when the pump is place in **Auto mode.**

In DataScope System 98, any of three signals—(1) EKG, (2) arterial wave, or (3) intrinsic (internal) pump rate—can trigger the pump, but the *preferred signal* is the EKG, which triggers the R wave. The pump is initially set to inflate the balloon in the middle of the T wave (diastole) and deflate just before the QRS complex (systole). An appropriately sized EKG signal must be transmitted to the intra-aortic balloon pump (IABP) to initiate pumping.

The *arterial waveform can be used as an alternative to EKG triggering* if an inconsistent EKG trigger occurs. During arterial triggering, the pump is activated by the upstroke of the arterial wave; thus, a steep upstroke is necessary, and the pulse pressure must be at least 20 mm Hg.

TIMING

The balloon should be set to inflate at the dicrotic notch (beginning of diastole when the aortic valve closes). The U shape of the patient's unassisted beat should change to a V shape when the balloon is properly set. The balloon should be set to deflate at the end of diastole, during isovolumetric contraction, just before the opening of the aortic valve.

REMEMBER:

These five key points to setting IABP timing:

1. Inflation at dicrotic notch
2. Crisp V shape on inflation
3. Peak diastolic pressure (PDP) greater than peak systolic pressure (PSP) optimal
4. Balloon aortic end-diastolic pressure (BAEDP) less than patient's aortic end-diastolic pressure (PAEDP) (by 5–15 mm Hg)
5. Assisted peak systolic pressure (APSP) less than peak systolic pressure

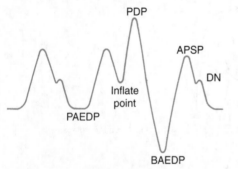

■ Correct intra-aortic balloon pump timing. (Adapted from Hudak, C. M., Gallo, B. M., & Morton, P. B. [1998]. *Critical care nursing* [7th ed.]. Philadelphia: Lippincott-Raven.)

The first three key points refer to inflation:

1. The inflation point should be at or slightly above (within 2 mm) the level of the dicrotic notch (DN).
2. The shape should be a crisp V, showing timely inflation to maximize effect.
3. The peak diastolic pressure reflects augmentation from the balloon due to a displacement of blood volume within the aorta. Ideally, it should be greater than the peak systolic pressure.

(continued)

The last two key points refer to deflation:

4. The balloon-assisted end-diastolic pressure should be 5 to 15 mm lower than the patient's own end-diastolic pressure, producing a lower pressure for the subsequent ventricular systole.

5. Compare systolic pressures. Systolic pressure after an augmented beat (APSP) should be decreased from the patient's own systolic pressure, reflecting the effect of unloading.

REMEMBER:

The IABP must be set on a 1:2 augmentation to assess timing. 1:1 or 1:3 augmentation can be initiated per order after timing has been optimized.

TIMING DURING ARRHYTHMIAS (DATASCOPE)

Atrial Fibrillation

- *System 98.* Inflate and deflate should be adjusted to position the inflation markers of the arterial waveform to correspond with diastole. Moving the deflate slide control all the way to the right will result in automatic R-wave deflation and allow the balloon to stay inflated as long as possible.
- *Model CS 100.* In the **Auto** mode, there are no special pump considerations.

Ectopics

- *System 98* and *Model CS 100* will both automatically deflate when an ectopic beat is sensed and will then inflate during diastole of the ectopic. To ensure reliable triggering, select the lead that minimizes the amplitude differences between the normal QRS and the ectopic.

Cardiac Arrest/Defibrillation

- When defibrillating, the system is completely isolated from the patient. However, the operator should stand clear of the system during defibrillation.
- *System 98.* If possible, use the **ECG** or **Pressure** trigger during CPR. The system will synchronize the trigger to the rate and rhythm of chest compressions. If the **ECG** or **Pressure** trigger cannot be utilized, the **Internal** trigger may be used to allow balloon movement.
- *Model CS 100.* The signal will be automatically selected. If neither the **ECG** nor the **Pressure** signals produce adequate trigger reliability to allow for **Auto** operation, select the **Semi Auto** mode, and set the trigger source to **Internal.**

TIMING ERRORS (ANY MODEL)

Early inflation (inflation of the IAB before aortic valve closure) causes potential premature closure of the aortic valve. This can also cause a potential increase in LVEDV and LVEDP as well as an increase in the pulmonary capillary wedge pressure (PCWP). It increases the stress on the left ventricular wall, resulting in an increased afterload and an increased $M\dot{V}O_2$ demand. The waveform will show inflation before the dicrotic notch, and diastolic augmentation will fade onto systole (see figure below).

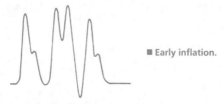

■ Early inflation.

(continued)

Late inflation (marked inflation of the IAB after closure of the aortic valve) results in suboptimal coronary artery perfusion. The waveform shows inflation late after the dicrotic notch and an absence of a sharp V form (see figure).

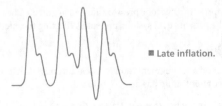

■ Late inflation.

Early deflation (premature deflation of the IAB during the diastolic phase) not only causes suboptimal coronary artery perfusion but also sets up a potential for retrograde coronary and carotid blood flow, resulting in angina (and increased $M\dot{V}O_2$ demand). The waveform will show a sharp drop after diastolic augmentation, and assisted aortic end-diastolic pressure may be equal to or greater than the patient's own aortic end-diastolic pressure (see figure). Assisted systolic pressure may also rise.

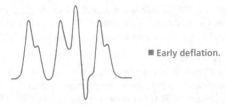

■ Early deflation.

Late deflation (premature deflation of the IAB late in the diastolic phase, as the aortic valve is beginning to open) negates the opportunity for any afterload reduction. The $M\dot{V}O_2$ consumption increases because the left ventricle ejects against a greater resistance, and there is a prolonged isovolumetric contraction phase. In fact, the late deflation of the IAB may impede left ventricular ejection and may actually increase afterload. The waveform will show the assisted aortic end-diastolic pressure and the patient's own aortic end-diastolic pressure as equal (see figure). The rate of rise of the assisted systole is prolonged, and diastolic augmentation may appear widened.

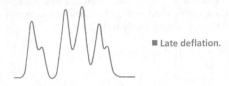

■ Late deflation.

(*continued*)

REMEMBER:

The worst timing errors are **early inflation** and **late deflation,** because both increase the afterload (whereas late inflation or early deflation only reduces coronary artery filling). Keep good etiquette in mind; **do not come to the party too early, or stay too late!**

TIMING APPROPRIATE BUT AUGMENTATION DECREASED

Problem related to balloon itself:
- Sheath not unfolded
- Position too low or size is wrong
- Kink in balloon
- Leak in balloon

Hemodynamic problem:
- Tachycardia
- Low stroke volume (hypovolemia)
- Low ejection fraction (try inotropes)
- MAP 40 to 50 (patient cold?)
- SVR too high (above 1,500) or too low (below 900)

BALLOON PRESSURE WAVEFORM

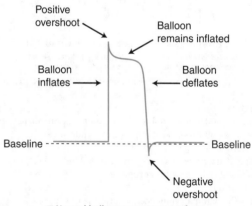

■ Normal balloon pressure waveform.

REMEMBER:

Waveform should look like a church pew. The peak tells how long the balloon is inflated, and should exhibit a positive initial overshoot.

(continued)

Variations in balloon pressure waveforms can be due to a number of conditions:

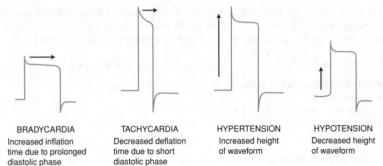

BRADYCARDIA	TACHYCARDIA	HYPERTENSION	HYPOTENSION
Increased inflation time due to prolonged diastolic phase	Decreased deflation time due to short diastolic phase	Increased height of waveform	Decreased height of waveform

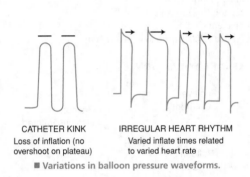

CATHETER KINK	IRREGULAR HEART RHYTHM
Loss of inflation (no overshoot on plateau)	Varied inflate times related to varied heart rate

■ Variations in balloon pressure waveforms.

COMPLICATIONS

- Balloon rupture (Blood seen in tubing. STOP pumping immediately.)
- Lower limb ischemia (14%–45%), compartment syndrome
- Extensive dissection (aorta or iliac artery)
- Occlusion of renal artery (with subsequent renal failure)
- Balloon entrapment (with or without rupture)
- Mesenteric infarction
- Vascular injury (hematoma, lymphedema, false aneurysm, etc.)
- Cerebral embolism during insertion
- Local wound infection

SUGGESTED IABP WEANING CRITERIA

- Cardiac index >2 L/min/m^2
- PCWP <18 to 20 mm Hg
- SBP >100 mm Hg
- Urine output >30 mL/hr
- Absence of crackles, no S$_3$
- Improved mentation
- Absence of life-threatening dysrhythmias
- Absence of ischemia on EKG
- Heart rate <100 beats/min

INTRA-ARTERIAL PRESSURE *(see also Phlebostatic Axis, p. 141)*

Intra-arterial pressure monitoring measures the amount of force exerted by circulating blood over a specific area, also known as arterial tension. It provides a constant beat-to-beat measurement of the systolic, diastolic, and mean arterial blood pressures. The pressure readings are obtained via an arterial cannula connected to pressure tubing, a transducer (connected to an electronic monitor) and a pressurized flush bag. The transducer is an external, disposable, fluid-air interface, which detects changes of pressure within the artery. The transducer interprets the intra-arterial fluctuations and relays the readings and waveform to the bedside monitor.

Four characteristics are inherent to an adequate arterial pressure line tracing:

1. Initial sharp rise
2. Rounded tip
3. Dicrotic notch
4. Tapering off of downstroke after dicrotic notch

The dicrotic notch is the first notch above diastole. If there is a "fling" or "whip" in the catheter, a false dicrotic notch may be produced, resulting in erroneously high readings.

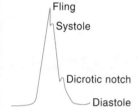

■ Arterial line catheter "fling." (DeGroot, K. [1986]. Monitoring intra-arterial pressure. *Critical Care Nurse, 6* [1]. Reprinted with permission.)

Hypovolemia results in an undulating baseline with respirations, and therefore a lowered dicrotic notch (caused by delay in closing of the aortic valve, resulting from prolonged filling time).

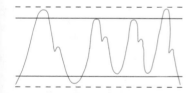

■ Arterial line tracing in a patient with hypovolemia. (DeGroot, K., & Damato, M. [1986]. Monitoring intra-arterial pressure. *Critical Care Nurse, 6* [1]. Reprinted with permission.)

Disparity between arterial line pressure and radial artery cuff pressure is frequently seen in the ICU, leaving the caretaker wondering which to believe. First, remember that the two are not the same. Cuff pressure measurement is based on flow-induced oscillations in the arterial wall. Arterial line pressure is based on exactly that—pressure. Thus, the decision which to use needs to be based on two factors:

1. Clinical status of the patient. The arterial line may be more accurate in shock or low-flow states. Frequent PACs or PVCs (beat-to-beat variability of >15%) can skew cuff pressures. Hypertension and atherosclerosis place unusual demands on the invasive monitoring system, causing a possible overshoot and resultant false high.

(continued)

2. Technical aspects that affect the validity and reliability of each measurement (i.e., dynamic response, correct referencing to the phlebostatic axis, cuff size). If using cuff pressure.

REMEMBER:

- The size of the cuff needs to be optimized. Too large a cuff will give a false low reading, and too small a cuff will give a false high reading.
- The arm and cuff position should be level with the heart. If the arm is below the heart, the BP will measure higher, and if the arm is above the heart, the BP will measure lower.
- Body position affects blood pressure. If the patient is in supine position, the blood pressure will be higher than if the patient is sitting upright.
- Blood pressures at different sites are NOT interchangeable! The distal readings (wrist, ankle) tend to be higher.
- If there are no contraindications, the upper arm is **always preferred** for cuff pressures.
- The cuff should be correctly sized (the recommended limb circumference is usually printed on the cuff). Most cuffs have index and range marker lines for proper sizing, and the index line should fall between the two range lines when placed around the patient's arm.

(continued)

NOTES

Performing the Square Wave Test

Activate the fast flush device and release. Interpret the response as indicated.

Optimal dampening should have a sharp vertical upstroke and a small overshoot, followed by a straight vertical downstroke with one or two oscillations before a quick return to baseline.

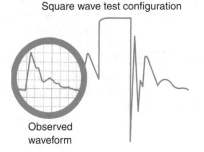

Square wave test configuration

Observed waveform

Underdampening is present if there is a sharp vertical upstroke, a sharp vertical downstroke, extra oscillations (more than three) above and below the baseline, or a prolonged distance (more than two blocks) between bounces. Underdampening is usually caused by small air bubbles in the system or excess tubing.

Square wave test configuration

Observed waveform

Overdampening is due to an obstruction in the line and generates A slightly slurred upstroke and a slurred downstroke with no oscillations above or below the baseline. This will cause the systolic pressure to be artificially depressed and the diastolic pressure to be artificially elevated. Overdampening is usually related to air in the line, blood in the line, or kinks in the tubing.

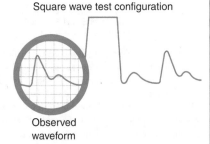

Square wave test configuration

Observed waveform

(*Figures from Hudak, C. M., Gallo, B. M., & Morton, P. B. [1998]. Critical care nursing [7th ed.]. Philadelphia: Lippincott-Raven.*)

(continued)

In general, mean arterial pressure (MAP) is the most stable hemodynamic parameter, providing the most accurate interpretation of a patient's status. It reflects an average pressure throughout the cardiac cycle. MAP is less affected by wave reflection and the response characteristics of the monitoring system than is measured SBP. MAP will generally remain relatively constant when measured at different sites throughout the arterial circuit, whereas measured SBP and DBP may differ.

Normal MAP = 70 to 110 mm Hg

REMEMBER:

MAP is not the **average** between the SBP and the DBP. It is a **mean,** representing CO × SVR. To calculate, **REMEMBER**, 1, 2, 3, … Systolic BP plus diastolic BP times 2, divided by 3.

$$\frac{\text{Systolic BP} + (\text{Diastolic BP} \times 2)}{3}$$

JUGULAR VENOUS DISTENTION

JVD occurs with increased right atrial pressure and is characteristic of right-sided heart failure or pulmonary hypertension. To assess, with head turned to the side, have the patient recline at a 30° to 45° angle to allow visualization of jugular pulsations. Be sure they are venous pulsations, which vary during breathing (as opposed to arterial pulsations, which do not). Measure from an imaginary horizontal baseline from the sternum to the highest point of the venous pulsation. A normal measurement would be approximately 3 cm. Anything greater signals increased venous pressure.

LEAD PLACEMENT *(see EKG Lead Placement, p. 98)*

LEFT VENTRICULAR RESTORATION
(see Dor Procedure, p. 93)

LEVEL 1 VOLUME INFUSER *(see also Hotline Fluid Warmer, p. 116; Ranger Blood/Fluid Warmer, p. 144)*

The SIMS Level 1 System is designed for in-line warming of blood and intravenous fluids administered at flow rates varying from 75 to 60,000 mL/hr. Two pressure chambers, which accommodate all standard blood and solution bags, apply a constant pressure of 280 to 300 mm Hg.

There are four basic disposable tubing sets, each designed for different flow rates and purposes (see figure on p. 130). Setup and priming of all of them is similar; however, the user is urged to review the instructions on the disposable package.

FLUID WARMER SETUP
1. Ensure that water reservoir has adequate water. Add distilled water if required. (Fill above the minimum level mark on System 1000 reservoir.)
2. Plug into power outlet.

DISPOSABLE SETUP
1. Push bottom end of heat exchanger into bottom socket.
2. Slide top socket up.

(continued)

3. Snap heat exchanger into guide. Slide top socket down over heat exchanger.
4. Snap filter with gas vent into holder.
5. Turn on power switch. A green operating light will illuminate, and the water temperature will begin to increase on the display panel.

DISPOSABLE PRIMING

1. Remove all air from fluid bags before spiking.
2. Close clamps above heat exchanger and roller clamp.
3. Remove bag spike cap and spike port of air-free fluid bag.
4. Hang bag from IV pole.
5. (Open clamps below fluid bags on sets D-50 and D-60 HL.) Squeeze drip chamber so that it is one third to one half full.
6. Remove cap on patient line, and open roller clamp. (Open clamps below drip chambers on sets D-100 and D-300.)
7. Close roller clamp when patient line is primed. The filter with gas vent will self prime.
8. Gently tap filter with gas vent against cabinet to release all trapped air. Priming is complete. Make patient connection without entrapping air.
9. To initiate infusion, adjust flow rate using roller clamp.

PRESSURE INFUSION

REMEMBER: Remove all air from containers before use!

1. Set up and prime a D-series tubing.
2. Flip toggle switch on top front of pressure chamber to "off" or "minus" position.
3. Open latch on right side of chamber door, and open door.
4. Hang air-free solution container on door post. Multiple hangers are provided to accommodate fluid bags of different sizes. Fluid container must be hung so as not to occlude container spike port.
5. Close door, and secure side latch.
6. Push toggle switch on top front of pressure chamber to the "on" or "plus" position.
7. Observe pressure gauge to ensure that 280 to 300 mm Hg pressure is achieved.
8. **REMEMBER:** The fluid warmer must be turned on for the pressure system to operate.

   The pressure is not adjustable on this device.

(continued)

NOTES

DISPOSABLES

D-50 & DI-50:
• Normothermic flow rates from 40–400 mL/min
• Sterile fluid path
• 20/case

D-60HL & DI-60HL:
• Normothermic flow rates from 75 mL/hr–530 mL/min
• Sterile fluid path
• 10/case

D-100 & DI-100:
• Normothermic flow rates from 30–950 mL/min
• Sterile fluid path
• 10/case

D-300 & DI-300:
• Normothermic flow rates from 30–1100 mL/min
• Sterile fluid path
• 10/case

■ Rapid volume infuser. (Courtesy SIMS Level 1, Inc., Rockland, MA.)

LOWN-GANONG-LEVINE SYNDROME
(see also Wolff-Parkinson-White Syndrome, p. 165)

The Lown-Ganong-Levine (LGL) syndrome is a variation of the WPW preexcitation syndrome in which accessory fibers are used and the septum is stimulated too early. The pathway associated with this syndrome is thought to join with the atria and bundle of His (rather than with the ventricular myocardium). Thus, the normal impulse from the sinus node can bypass the slow AV conduction. As with WPW, reciprocating tachyarrhythmias can easily occur, and management is directed at them.

Hallmarks of LGL syndrome:
- Normal rate, rhythm, and QRS
- PR interval short (<0.12 sec) with a tendency to PVST, atrial fibrillation, or atrial flutter

MAZE PROCEDURE

The MAZE procedure is used for the surgical treatment of atrial fibrillation, consisting of a series of precise incisions made to the right and left atria. Once the incisions are made, they are sewn together again, causing the conduction of the errant electrical impulses to be eliminated and eradicating the arrhythmia. (The scar tissue generated by the incisions permanently blocks the abnormal conduction pathways.) Historically, this procedure required the use of cardiopulmonary bypass, but more recently, a groundbreaking "minimally invasive" MAZE has been developed, which allows chest access through small, 3-cm incisions. The right lung is collapsed, the right side of the heart is treated, and the lung is reinflated. The same procedure is repeated on the left. The minimally invasive MAZE is not appropriate for every patient with atrial fibrillation but offers an attractive treatment option to acceptable candidates.

MEAN ARTERIAL PRESSURE *(see Intra-arterial Pressure, p. 123)*

MIDCAB *(see Cardiac Surgery, p. 82)*

MITRAL REGURGITATION

In mitral regurgitation (also known as insufficiency), changes of the mitral valve occur that prevent it from closing completely during systole. This allows backflow in the left atrium, which in turn reduces stroke volume and cardiac output. Left atrial pressures increase, causing pulmonary congestion.

Causes:
- Most commonly, history of rheumatic fever
- Infective endocarditis
- Cardiomyopathy
- Ruptured or chordae tendineae
- Leaflet prolapse
- Dilated left ventricle

Assessment:
- Weakness, fatigue (secondary to low cardiac output)
- Pulmonary congestion (related to left ventricular dysfunction)
- In acute cases, pulmonary hypertension (right-sided heart failure with edema, ascites)

(continued)

- Atrial fibrillation
- High-pitched systolic murmur

Diagnosis:
- 2-D echo (shows enlargement of left atrium and ventricle)
- Doppler echo (shows sudden regurgitation of blood into the left atrium during systole)
- Transesophageal echo
- Chest X-ray (shows atrial enlargement and left ventricular hypertrophy)
- ECG (often see "M"-shaped P waves)

Management:
- Medically, much the same as for congestive heart failure. Attempts to reduce afterload to allow more blood to be pumped into the aorta thus reducing the regurgitation into the atrium.
- Surgically, treatment options include valve reconstruction or replacement.

MITRAL STENOSIS

Mitral stenosis is a condition due to severe reduction in the size of the mitral valve opening. As a result, during diastole, blood flow meets resistance and backs up into the pulmonary vasculature, causing the patient to show signs and symptoms of heart failure. If the stenosis is severe enough, the blood may back up all the way to the right ventricle and actually cause right-sided heart failure.

Causes:
- Most commonly, history of rheumatic fever
- Congenital defects (rare)
- Systemic lupus erythematosus
- Infective endocarditis with large vegetations on the mitral valve

Assessment:
- Dependent upon the advancement of the disease and degree of underlying compensation
- Women account for two thirds of the patients; two thirds are younger than 45 years
- Respiratory symptoms (exertional dyspnea, wheezing, coughing)
- Diastolic thrill on palpation over apex
- Loud S_1; low-pitched diastolic murmur

Diagnosis:
- 2-D echo (will show a thickened, calcified, stenotic valve and enlarged left atrium)
- Transesophageal echo (provides a clearer image, more sensitive in detecting left atrial thrombus and useful for detecting vegetation on the valve)
- Doppler echo (most accurate noninvasive results)
- ECG (broad-notched P waves in lead II, and with severe pulmonary hypertension, there will be a right axis deviation and right ventricular hypertrophy)

Management:
- For stenosis due to rheumatic heart disease, prophylaxis (usually penicillin) should be employed prior to certain procedures (i.e., dental).
- Medically, the goal is to control heart rhythm (patients frequently exhibit atrial fibrillation) with beta-blockers and calcium channel blockers as well as providing anticoagulation.

(continued)

- Surgically, treatment options include:
  1. Valvotomy (a balloon passes from the femoral vein to the atrial septum and the mitral valve. The balloon is inflated and enlarges the mitral orifice).
  2. Commissurotomy (open heart surgery is performed, thrombi are removed from the atria, and calcium is removed from the valve leaflets).
  3. Valve replacement (either tissue or mechanical)

MUGA SCAN *(see Muga Scan in Part 10, p. 364)*

MURMURS *(see Heart Sounds: Abnormal, p. 113)*

MYOCARDIAL INFARCTION: EKG PATTERNS
(see also Cardiac Markers in Part 9, p. 342)

Lateral:
- Blockage: Circumflex branch of left anterior descending
- EKG patterns: I, aVL, V_5, V_6 with abnormal Q wave; ST elevation; T-wave inversion
- Watch for: Transient heart blocks (may require temporary pacing) or complication of ventricular aneurysm (7–10 days after infarction).

Inferior:
- Blockage: Right coronary artery
- EKG patterns: II, III, aVF with abnormal Q wave; ST elevation; T-wave inversion
- Watch for: Transient AV blocks, usually Wenckebach block. May require temporary pacing, but rarely is a permanent pacer needed. Watch for right ventricular failure (JVD, hepatojugular reflex, increased CVP, peripheral edema). Check for new systolic murmur (papillary muscle rupture).

Anterior:
- Blockage: Left anterior descending artery
- EKG patterns: I, aVL, V_1 through V_4 with abnormal Q wave; loss of R wave progression; ST elevation; T-wave inversion
- Watch for: Right bundle branch block, Mobitz type II block (indication for permanent pacemaker). Once a block develops, if a significant amount of the anterior wall is damaged, there is a good chance complete heart block will follow. If >50% of the ventricle is damaged, the patient can go into cardiogenic shock with a mortality rate of >85%. Check for a new systolic murmur (ventral septal defect or ventricular aneurysm).

Posterior:
- Rarely seen alone. Usually component of multiple site infarcts.
- Blockage: Right coronary artery, circumflex
- EKG patterns: No leads view the posterior surface directly; therefore, this MI is diagnosed on the basis of reciprocal EKG changes occurring in leads V_1 and V_2 (just the opposite of an anterior wall MI). Tall R wave (rather than a Q wave), ST depression (rather than elevation), and tall symmetrical T wave. Left posterior chest leads V_7, V_8, and V_9 can often diagnose this MI when standard 12-lead is nondiagnostic. (See EKG Lead Placement: Left Posterior Chest Leads.)
- Watch for: Same complications as for inferior, although not as severe.

(continued)

Septal:
- Blockage: Septum
- EKG patterns: V_1 to V_2 possible changes to Q, ST, T. Q waves noted V_3 to V_5.

Anterolateral:
- Blockage: Left anterior descending and circumflex
- EKG patterns: I, aVL, V_1 through V_6 possible changes to Q, ST, T

Anteroseptal:
- Blockage: Left anterior descending
- EKG patterns: V_1 through V_4 possible changes to Q, ST, T. Loss of septal R wave in V_1

Subendocardial (non–Q wave):
- Blockage: Nontransmural
- EKG patterns: No pathologic Q wave, some loss of R wave, depressed ST segment, deep symmetrical T-wave inversion. Diagnosis verified by elevated enzymes.
- Watch for: Extension to Q-wave MI.

Right ventricular:
- Accompanies inferior MI in 30% of cases.
- Blockage: Right coronary artery
- EKG patterns:
    V_1 possible changes to Q, ST, T
    V_4R ST elevation (in patients with inferior wall infarct)
    Possible correlation if ST segment elevation is higher in lead III than in lead II
- Cannot be specifically diagnosed using standard 12-lead. Need V_4R, V_5R, and V_6R. (See EKG Lead Placement Right Chest Leads).
- Watch for: AV block (A fib, A flutter). JVD with clear lungs. BP may drop if preload reduced, so be cautious with morphine, nitroglycerin, and Lasix.

Injury:
ST–T-wave elevation with reciprocal depression

Ischemia:
ST–T-wave depression, T-wave inversion, horizontal ST segments, tall pointed T-waves, inverted U-wave

MYOCARDIAL INFARCTION: RECIPROCAL EKG CHANGES *(see also ST Segment Monitoring, p. 148)*

In the leads opposite to the injured area, reversed or reciprocal changes can be seen. These changes denote the extra workload to the other parts of the heart to compensate for the damaged area. There will be no Q wave, with tall upright Ts and perhaps some increase in height of the R wave. It is impossible to distinguish a reciprocal change of an acute MI from ischemia, because both cause ST depression.

Reciprocal EKG in Changes in Myocardial Infarction	
Primary EKG Change	**Reciprocal Change**
Anterior (V_1, V_2, V_3)	Inferior (II, III, aVF)
Lateral (I, aVL, V_5, V_6)	Inferior (II, III, aVF)
Inferior (II, III, aVF)	Lateral and anterior (I, aVL, V_1 to V_6)
Posterior (V_1, V_2, V_3)	Anterior (V_1, V_2, V_3)

NONINVASIVE CARDIAC OUTPUT MONITORING

Although thermodilution is the most common clinical technique used for cardiac output monitoring, it is expensive, time consuming, and carries the risk of infection and complications. Noninvasive cardiac output monitoring or impedance cardiography (ICG) offers a valuable alternative. It requires two sets of skin electrodes to be placed on the patient; one set on the neck and one set on the thorax, 180° opposite each other. The electrodes emit a constant low-grade (1–4 mA) electrical current. One set of electrodes sends the current, and the other set of electrodes senses the returning current. Changes in thoracic electrical impedance (associated with change in blood flow in the aorta during the cardiac cycle) are recorded as an ICG waveform. Along with the electrocardiogram, algorithms are used to derive hemodynamic parameters.

Another type of noninvasive cardiac output (NICO) monitoring is founded on changes in respiratory CO_2 concentration. It is based on the Fick method, stating that O_2 consumption is proportional to the rate of blood pumped by the heart through the lungs, and it can be measured by monitoring gas exchange and invisibly sampling blood gases. A differential form of this Fick method is used for NICO monitoring. The rebreathing is accomplished through the periodic addition of a rebreathing volume to the ventilator circuit connection. Every 3 minutes, a 50-second rebreathing maneuver causes the patient to inhale only a portion of the exhaled gases. The resulting changes in CO_2 and end tidal CO_2 are used to calculate the cardiac output.

OpCAB *(see Cardiac Surgery, p. 82)*

OXYGEN CONSUMPTION *(see Oxygen Consumption in Part 3, p. 192)*

OXYGEN DELIVERY *(see Oxygen Consumption in Part 3, p. 192)*

PACEMAKERS

There are two types of artificial pacemakers, temporary and permanent.

Permanent pacemakers are implanted under local anesthesia in the operating room or cardiac cath lab. The pulse generator is placed in a subcutaneous pocket in the left pectoral area, and the pacing lead is inserted via the subclavian or cephalic vein and placed within the chambers of the heart. Pacemakers are designed to pace at a set rate if the patient's intrinsic rate falls below a certain number, as seen in bradyarrhythmias. Permanent pacemakers are powered by lithium batteries and have a life span of 7 to 10 years. There are also implantable cardioverter/defibrillator/pacemaker combination devices available, designed to not only pace as necessary, but also terminate an abnormal and fast arrhythmia. Pacemakers may also be used to regulate the atrial rate in atrial fibrillation and coordinate the electrical firing of the atrial and ventricular chambers. A newer form of pacing, cardiac resynchronization therapy (CRT) corrects ventricular electrical dyschrony by simultaneous pacing both the right and left ventricular chambers. Usually used for patients with CHF, synchronizing contractions helps to optimize cardiac output.

Temporary pacemakers are used prophylactically for anticipated dysrhythmias or for transient disturbances and are usually seen in a monitored unit such as a critical care or telemetry unit. The following discussion focuses on the use of these temporary pacing devices.

(continued)

TYPES OF TEMPORARY PACING

- *Transcutaneous* temporary pacemakers provide support in an emergency when there is no time to prepare for an invasive procedure or when invasive procedures are contraindicated. Large surface adhesive electrodes are attached to the anterior and posterior chest wall and are connected to an external pacing unit. The pacing current passes through skin and chest wall structures to reach the heart; therefore, large energies are required to achieve capture.

- *Transvenous* pacing is usually done by percutaneous puncture of the internal jugular, subclavian, antecubital, or femoral vein and threading a pacing wire into the heart (right atrium for atrial pacing, right ventricle for ventricular pacing, and both chambers for dual pacing). The transvenous pacing wire is attached to an external pulse generator.

- *Epicardial* pacing is done via wires that are inserted during surgery, sutured on the epicardial surface of the heart, and brought out through the patient's chest. Atrial wires exit on the right, ventricular wires exit on the left. A connecting cable is used to connect the atrial pacer wire(s) to the atrial pacing poles and ventricular wire(s) to the ventricular pacing poles of an external pulse generator.

REMEMBER:

If there is a problem with sensing or capture, the wires may be reversed so that the positive pole in the atria becomes the negative pole.

Pacing wires should always be encapsulated if not connected to a pulse generator.

TEMPORARY PACEMAKER MODES: FIXED (ASYNCHRONOUS) AND DEMAND (SYNCHRONOUS)

- A fixed rate pacemaker will deliver timed electrical stimuli at a selected rate, regardless of the patient's intrinsic cardiac activity. However, this mode can easily cause V-tach or V-fib if a stimulus occurs during the vulnerable period of the heart (T wave on EKG), and for this reason, this mode is used less frequently than demand pacing.

- A demand pacemaker delivers electrical stimuli only when needed (when the heart fails to depolarize on its own). The pacer will sense intrinsic QRS complexes, and if one is recognized, the pacer will not send out a stimulus. Conversely, if no intrinsic beat is seen, the pacer will initiate a stimulus at a predetermined rate.

PACEMAKER CODING

A universal five-letter code is used to describe the expected pacemaker function, although the older three-letter system is still frequently and more commonly used (utilizing the first three letters of the five-letter code system).

(*continued*)

NOTES

Five-Letter Coding System

Letter 1 = *where pacing takes place*
  V = ventricle
  A = atrium
  D = dual (atrium and ventricle)
  O = none

Letter 2 = *which event the chamber senses*
  V = ventricle
  A = atrium
  D = dual (atrium and ventricle)
  O = none

Letter 3 = *response to the sensed events*
  T = triggers pacing
  I = inhibits firing in response to a sensed intrinsic event
  D = dual (triggers and inhibits)
  O = none

Letter 4 = *program functions; rate modulation*
  P = single programmability
  M = multiple programmability
  C = communication function (telemetry)
  R = rate modulation (pacing rate can vary, rather than being fixed)
  O = absence of programmability or rate modulation

Letter 5 = *antitachyarrhythmia function*
  P = pacing stimulus can be used to convert a rapid rhythm (overdrive pacing)
  S = shock intervention for cardioversion or defibrillation
  D = dual (pacing and shock capabilities)
  O = absence of pacing and shock capabilities

Based on this coding system, the following pacemaker settings are most commonly seen:

- **Atrial fixed rate (AOO) mode:** The atria are paced but not sensed. The pacer fires at a preset rate regardless of the patient's inherent rhythm. Rarely used.
- **Ventricular fixed rate (VOO) mode:** An asynchronous, fixed rate pacing mode whereby the ventricles are paced at a preset rhythm regardless of patient's intrinsic activity and no sensing takes place.
- **Atrial demand (AAI) mode:** Used when the SA node is damaged but AV conduction is unimpaired. In effect, it replaces the sinus impulse. The atria contract and pump blood to the ventricles, causing an "atrial kick," adding 5% to 25% to cardiac output over a ventricular pacemaker. QRS complexes are the same as the intrinsic complexes.
- **Ventricular demand (VVI) mode:** Causes the ventricle to be paced, sensed, and inhibited. The pacer fires if no QRS is sensed during the preset time interval, and intrinsic cardiac activity shuts the pacemaker off. This mode is very popular and is chosen 95% of the time. It is a good mode for use with atrial fibrillation with slow ventricular response and for complete heart block. The QRS complexes appear similar to right-sided PVCs.
- **AV sequential fixed rate (DOO) mode:** Paces both the atria and ventricles, but they are not sensed. The pacing is fixed and occurs at a preset rate regardless of any inherent rhythm.

(continued)

- **AV sequential (DVI) mode:** Causes the atrium to be paced at a programmed rate. Each atrial pace starts an AV interval. If there is no ventricular activity during the interval, the ventricle is paced. Atrial pacing occurs at a programmed rate regardless of intrinsic activity (this mode does not sense P waves) and can therefore cause competitive atrial rhythms. This mode cannot be used when the patient is in atrial fibrillation or atrial flutter. Only ventricular events can be sensed and cause inhibition of the pacemaker. This mode can increase cardiac output by 20% to 50% over the cardiac output produced by ventricular pacing alone and is helpful in decreasing valve regurgitation.

- **Fully automated (DDD) mode:** Paces the atrium and ventricle, senses the atrium and ventricle, and responds to sensed events by inhibiting or triggering. When spontaneous atrial activity occurs at a rate between the programmed and upper and lower rate limits, ventricular pacing is synchronized to atrial activity. When spontaneous atrial activity occurs at a rate below the programmed lower rate limit, the atrium and ventricle are paced AV sequentially. This mode is useful in patients with or without heart block, and with atrial activity that is normal most of the time but may need backup atrial pacing periodically.

- **AV synchronous (VAT) mode:** Causes the atria to be sensed, but pacing takes place in the ventricles if no P wave is seen. If a P wave is sensed, the pacer fires simultaneously with the QRS.

BASIC OPERATION PRINCIPLES FOR TEMPORARY PACEMAKERS

The Medtronic 5375 is the basic model and prototype for most other generations of pacemakers. If you understand the settings and principles of this model, the rationale for use of other models will easily follow.

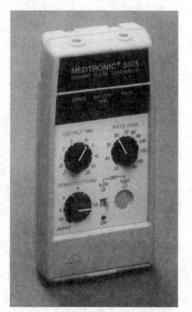

■ Medtronic 5375 Pacemaker, Demand. (Courtesy of Medtronic Inc., Minneapolis, MN.)

(*continued*)

- **Output (mA) or capture** is the setting used for the amount of voltage needed to stimulate the myocardium. **REMEMBER:** Your "mA" gave you a spanking to "stimulate" good behavior. The minimum energy needed for a response is called the pacing threshold. The mA is usually set at three times the threshold, which is normally 1.5 or less (consequently, the mA would be set at approximately 4.5). Factors that increase the threshold are anesthetics, acidosis, hypoxia, fibrosis on the catheter tip, low blood sugar, steroids, catecholamines, and exercise.

To measure the stimulation threshold:*
1. Set rate at 10 beats/min above the patient's inherent rate to obtain 100% pacing. (Pace light flashes regularly at the set rate.)
2. Decrease the mA until 1:1 capture is lost. (Pace and sense lights flash intermittently.)
3. Increase mA until capture is regained. This is the mA threshold. (Pace light flashes and sense light stops flashing.)
4. Reset mA at two to three times the threshold in Step 3 (e.g., if the stimulation threshold is 2.5 mA, set the output at 5.0 mA).
5. Don't forget to restore the pulse generator to the original pacing rate.

- **Sensitivity (mV) or millivolts** determines when the pacemaker fires or inhibits. Imagine a solid brick wall that can lower and raise in height. Also imagine that the heart (patient's intrinsic rhythm) is on one side of the wall, and the pacemaker is on the opposite side of the wall. If the wall is in the lowest position (1 mV) the pacemaker can "see" the heart's intrinsic rhythm very well, and is able to inhibit or pace when required. If, however, the wall is raised to its fullest height (20 mV), the pacemaker is "blocked" by the wall and cannot "see" the heart's intrinsic rhythm very well at all, rendering the pacemaker much less sensitive. **REMEMBER:** The higher the mV setting, the less sensitive the pacing.

To measure the sensitivity threshold:*
1. Set rate at 10 beats/min below the patient's inherent rate. Contraindicated if patient has no intrinsic rate or has symptomatic bradycardia. (Sense light flashes regularly.)
2. Reduce mA to the minimum value. This avoids the risk of competitive pacing.
3. Turn sensitivity control counterclockwise to increase the mV (making the pacer less sensitive) until R-wave sensing is lost and pacer begins firing. (Sense light stops flashing and pace light starts flashing.) **REMEMBER:** Capture is not likely to occur at a minimum output (mA) value.
4. Turn sensitivity control clockwise to decrease the mV (making the pacer more sensitive) until EKG tracing shows that sensing has been restored. (Sense light flashes, pace light stops flashing.) This is the sensitivity threshold.
5. Set the mV at half the threshold in Step 4 (e.g., if the sensitivity threshold is 5.0 mV, set the sensitivity at 2.5 mV).
6. Don't forget to restore the pulse generator to the original pacing rate.

- **Rate** is usually set at 10 beats/min above the patient's intrinsic rate for demand pacing, or at 70 to 100 beats/min for fixed rate pacing.

More sophisticated pacemakers exist, but the same basic principles apply. A popular model is the Medtronic 5330 AV sequential pacemaker. Mentally divide the pacer generator in half vertically. Think of the left side as the atrial settings and the right side as the ventricular settings. In AV sequential pacing, the atrial pacing occurs at a programmed rate regardless of any intrinsic activity, so there is no atrial sensitivity dial.

*In some institutions, RNs are not allowed to perform this function.   (continued)

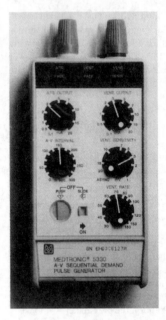

■ Medtronic 5330 Pacemaker, AV Sequential Demand. (Courtesy of Medtronic Inc., Minneapolis, MN.)

Another popular AV sequential pacemaker is the Medtronic 5388, which is digital. The same basic pacing principles apply.

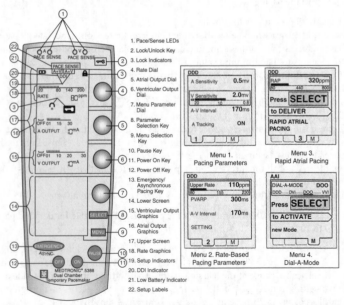

1. Pace/Sense LEDs
2. Lock/Unlock Key
3. Lock Indicators
4. Rate Dial
5. Atrial Output Dial
6. Ventricular Output Dial
7. Menu Parameter Dial
8. Parameter Selection Key
9. Menu Selection Key
10. Pause Key
11. Power On Key
12. Power Off Key
13. Emergency/Asynchronous Pacing Key
14. Lower Screen
15. Ventricular Output Graphics
16. Atrial Output Graphics
17. Upper Screen
18. Rate Graphics
19. Setup Indicators
20. DDI Indicator
21. Low Battery Indicator
22. Setup Labels

Menu 1. Pacing Parameters

Menu 2. Rate-Based Pacing Parameters

Menu 3. Rapid Atrial Pacing

Menu 4. Dial-A-Mode

■ Controls and indicators of the Model 5388.

(continued)

- **To turn on:** Press ON key. Screen lights up, and dual-chamber demand pacing and sensing begin at a preset rate of 80, with atrial and ventricular mA (output) of 10.
- **To turn off:** Press OFF key twice within 5 seconds.
- **Lock/unlock:** This key will unlock the three upper dials (rate, atrial mA, ventricular mA). The padlock icon appears when the dials are locked.
- **Rate and output adjustments:** After unlocking, turn dials clockwise to increase parameters and counterclockwise to decrease parameters.
- **Viewing patient's intrinsic rhythm:** Press and hold PAUSE key to suspend pacing and sensing for up to 10 seconds. To pause again up to 10 seconds, release PAUSE key, then press and hold again.
- **Emergency pacing:** Press EMERGENCY to initiate high-output dual-chamber asynchronous pacing (rate at current setting, or 80 if pacer was off, atrial mA 20, ventricular mA 25).
- **Menus:** Press MENU key to select one of four menus:
  1. **Pacing Parameters**
     Adjusts atrial sensitivity, ventricular sensitivity, AV interval, atrial tracking
  2. **Rate-based Pacing Parameters**
     The following parameters are automatically set whenever rate is adjusted, but if they need manual adjustment, it is done in this screen: Upper rate, AV interval, and PVARP (PVARP is postventricular atrial refractory period, a setting that prevents atrial sensing of crosstalk, which may trigger tachycardia).
  3. **Rapid Atrial Pacing**
     Used for overdrive pacing. *Caution:* This mode is for atrial use only. Be sure leads are connected to the atrium, not the ventricle, before initiating.
  4. **Dial-A-Mode**
     Allows changing pacing mode to DDD, DVI, DOO, or VVI.
- **Battery change:** Replace the old battery when the battery indicator appears during device operation. (A good rule of thumb is to routinely replace every 2–3 days.) While Medtronic recommends disconnecting the pacer from the patient and turning it off before replacing the battery, that is not always possible. If the change is done while the pacemaker is on, pacing will be maintained for 15 seconds (and the device will operate properly, even with battery polarity reversed).
  1. Press the button on the bottom end of the pacer to open the battery drawer.
  2. Remove the old battery and discard.
  3. Insert a fresh battery as shown on the diagram inside the battery drawer.
  4. If the pacer has been shut off, press the ON key to start a power-on self-test. The pace/sense and battery indicator lights flash briefly. If the pacer passes the self-test, dual-chamber demand pacing and sensing begin.

TEMPORARY PACEMAKER TROUBLESHOOTING

- **No output (pacer fails to fire)** could be due to battery exhaustion, a loose set screw, lead wire fracture, the pacer sensing artifact instead of inherent activity (decrease sensitivity to remedy), or the patient inherent rate faster than the rate on the pacer (in which case, it is working properly).
- **Failure to capture (stimuli delivered by pacer fails to depolarize atrium or ventricle)** most likely is due to a low mA (remedy by increasing). Other possibilities: dislodged lead (move patient to left side, gravity may migrate lead to ventricular wall) or a perforated lead, which the physician must replace.

(continued)

- **Oversensing (pacer senses signals that should be ignored)** usually is due to the pacer being too sensitive (increase mA to make pacer less sensitive).
- **Failure to sense (normal pacemaker receives inadequate cardiac signals)** primarily is caused by inadequate amplitude or the shape of the EKG signal. Also could be due to a dislodged lead, lead wire fracture, or the pacer not being sensitive enough (reduce mA to remedy).

PATENT DUCTUS ARTERIOSUS

Normal shunting of blood from pulmonary artery to aorta occurs in fetus and newborn, usually closing 24 to 72 hours after birth. If closing does not occur, the patent ductus causes a pressure load on the pulmonary circuit, resulting in right and left ventricular hypertrophy and constriction of the pulmonary arterioles. If patent ductus is allowed to remain for many years, the pressures in the pulmonary circuit may rise to the point of becoming equal to the pressure of the systemic circuit, causing a "balanced shunt." The right-sided pressures may also exceed the left-sided pressures, in which case there is a reversal of blood and the patient becomes cyanotic. The treatment of choice is surgical intervention.

PERICARDIAL FRICTION RUB *(see Heart Sounds: Abnormal, p. 113)*

PERICARDITIS

Pericarditis is an inflammation of the pericardial sac caused by:
- Viral, bacterial, or fungal infection
- Myocardial infarction
- Cancer, spreading from a nearby tumor in the lung, breast, or blood
- Radiation treatment
- Injury or surgery

Pathophysiology: Disease process → fibrin deposits → effusion (fluid in pericardial sac) → restriction → decreased diastolic filling → increased venous pressure → decreased cardiac output → decreased blood pressure

Diagnosis:
- ST elevation in all leads (then T wave inverts after ST returns to baseline)
- Often a deep PR in AVR only
- Pain on inspiration, relieved by leaning forward
- Positive heart rub
- Positive jugular venous distension

   Right and left heart pressures equalize, resulting in decreased cardiac output. Watch for tamponade. Lab work shows increased sedimentation rate and leukocytosis. An echocardiogram is very diagnostic.

Treatment: Based on underlying cause and severity of condition. Most cases are mild and will self-resolve. NSAIDs may be used to relieve pain and decrease fluid accumulation in the pericardial sac. In recurrent cases, corticosteroids are effective. If the cause is infection, antibiotics are prescribed.

Complications: Include cardiac tamponade and chronic constrictive pericarditis. Pericardiocentesis, a procedure where a thin needle is inserted through the chest wall

(continued)

into the pericardial sac, may be done to evaluate the fluid cytology and remove excess fluid. Chronic constrictive pericarditis may require surgery to remove the pericardium (pericardiectomy).

REMEMBER:

Lovenox is contraindicated. Patient could bleed into the pericardium, causing tamponade.

PHLEBOSTATIC AXIS *(see also Intra-arterial Pressure, p. 123)*

The phlebostatics axis provides an external reference point that approximates the anatomic level of the left and right atria and the pulmonary artery. To correctly determine the leveling point:

1. Draw an imaginary vertical line from the fourth intercostal space at the sternal boarder (nipple line) through the patient's chest.
2. Then draw an imaginary horizontal line that runs half way between the anterior and posterior lateral chest wall.
3. The bisection of these two lines is the phlebostatic axis.

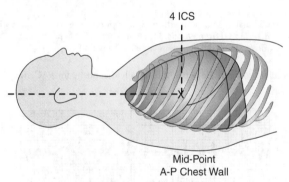

4 ICS

Mid-Point
A-P Chest Wall

■ Phlebostatic axis determination.

Accurate readings require zeroing the stopcock (not the transducer itself) to be level to this axis. Incorrect leveling can cause false readings:

If leveled 1 cm too high, the reading will be 1.86 mm Hg too low.
If leveled 2 cm too low, the reading will be 1.86 cm too high.

Readings should be taken with the patient in the same position each time for comparison. Less than 30° is preferable.

PRELOAD *(see Swan-Ganz: Hemodynamic Algorithm, p. 154)*

PREMATURE VENTRICULAR CONTRACTIONS

PVCs are occasionally present in normal individuals, causing no harmful effects. They are present in 80% of postmyocardial infarction patients; some are benign, and others lead to serious, even fatal, arrhythmias.

(continued)

PVCs can be caused by a change in the excitability of the ventricular tissue, as induced by, for example, anesthetics, hypoxia, or digitalis; or by stimulation of the sympathetic nervous system, as induced by, for example, adrenergic drugs, emotional stress, or amphetamines.

A full compensatory pause is usually diagnostic for PVC. The time between the beat preceding and the beat following the PVC is equal to two normal beats.

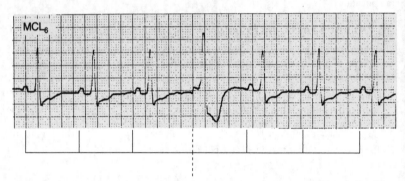

■ Premature ventricular contraction with no interruption to sinus cycle. Lines indicate unchanged cadence. (Adapted from Woods, S. L., Froelicher, E. S., Halpenny, C. J., & Motzer, S. U. [1995]. *Cardiac nursing* [3rd ed.]. Philadelphia: J.B. Lippincott.)

An incomplete compensatory pause is usually diagnostic for PAC. The sinus cycle is reset.

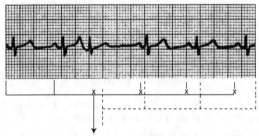

■ Premature atrial contraction resets sinus cycle and causes change in cadence. New regular rhythm starts at arrow. If old sinus cycle had been maintained, beats would fall on dotted lines as indicated. (Adapted from Hudak, C. M., Gallo, B. M., & Morton, P. G. [1998]. *Critical care nursing* [7th ed.]. Philadelphia: Lippincott-Raven.)

In lead MCL1, there is a 90% probability that an ectopic beat will be a PVC rather than an aberrancy if the left "rabbit ear" is taller than the right "rabbit ear."

REMEMBER:

The reverse is not true. If the left "ear" is shorter than the right "ear, " it is not necessarily an aberrancy.

PTCA *(see Angioplasty, p. 73)*

PULMONARY ARTERY PRESSURES
(see Swan-Ganz: Hemodynamic Normals, p. 155)

PULMONARY CAPILLARY WEDGE PRESSURE
(see Swan-Ganz: Hemodynamic Normals, p. 156)

PULMONARY VASCULAR RESISTANCE
(see Swan-Ganz: Hemodynamic Normals, p. 157)

PULSE STRENGTH CLASSIFICATIONS

3+ = full, bounding
2+ = normal
1+ = decreased, thready
0 = absent

PULSUS ALTERNANS *(see also Pulsus Magnus, p. 143;
Pulsus Paradoxus, p. 143; Pulsus Parvus, p. 144)*

Alternating pulses are full and weak; that is, a strong pulse followed by a weak pulse of equal length. It can be seen on the arterial pressure waveform tracing, where the amplitude of the systolic beat differs with every other beat, or on a right ventricular pressure tracing recorded from a Swan-Ganz catheter. Pulsus alternans frequently is a sign of a failing ventricle, although occurrence always warrants further evaluation.

PULSUS MAGNUS *(see also Pulsus Alternans p. 143; Pulsus Paradoxus, p. 143;
Pulsus Parvus, p. 144)*

Bounding pulses of pulsus magnus are usually related to thyrotoxicosis.

PULSUS PARADOXUS *(see also Pulsus Alternans, p. 143;
Pulsus Magnus, p. 143; Pulsus Parvus, p. 144)*

Pulsus paradoxus is the absence of a pulse for >10 mm Hg in arterial systolic pressure during inspiration. If pulsus paradoxus is present, the patient may be developing cor pulmonale, cardiac tamponade, shock, obstructed airway disease, constrictive pericarditis, or pulmonary embolism.

This clinical sign occurs because blood pools in the pulmonary circulation during inspiration, lowering left ventricular preload and thereby lowering cardiac output.

To determine pulsus paradoxus:
1. Place blood pressure cuff on patient, and inflate 15 mm Hg above the highest systolic pressure.
2. Slowly deflate the cuff, and auscultate. The first Korotkoff sound occurs in expiration.
3. After noting the reading when the first sound occurs, continue to release the cuff pressure until sounds are audible throughout the respiratory cycle.
4. The difference between the first and second pressures is the pulsus paradoxus.

PULSUS PARVUS *(see also Pulsus Alternans, p. 143; Pulsus Magnus, p. 143; Pulsus Paradoxus, p. 143)*

Pulsus parvus, a small, weak pulse, is related to aortic stenosis.

PVCS *(see Premature Ventricular Contractions, p. 141)*

QT INTERVAL *(see also Torsade De Pointes, p. 161)*

Normal QT interval is 0.32 to 0.40 seconds, or less than one half the preceding R to R interval.

To correct for rate, divide the QT by the square root of the R to R interval.

RANGER BLOOD/FLUID WARMER
(see also Hotline Fluid Warmer, p. 116; Level 1 Volume Infuser, p. 126)

Blood and fluid warming is used in conjunction with forced-air warming to help protect patients from surgical hypothermia. The Ranger system is a dry heat system that does not use water. Instead, it has a microprocessor-controlled heating unit and utilizes a sensor system to continuously monitor the temperature of the heating surface.

SETUP
1. Slide the warming cassette into the front of machine. Do NOT prime it first.
2. Close clamp on inlet line (blue capped).
3. Hang solution, prime to end of blood tubing (or IV tubing if fluids only), and connect to the inlet line.
4. Open all clamps, turn the bubble trap upside down, and allow it to fill completely.
5. Turn the bubble trap right side up, and place it into holder.
6. Continue to prime the patient line (red capped).
7. Turn the machine on. Alphanumeric display will turn on after a few seconds. It takes less than 2 minutes to warm the machine up to the 41°C set point temperature. You can then begin the infusion. Standard warming cassettes can accommodate fluids up to 9,000 mL/hr.

After use:
1. Close clamp on inlet line (dark blue).
2. Open the clamp distal to the fluid cassette (under the bubble trap), and allow the fluid to flow to the patient for 2 to 3 seconds.
3. Close all clamps, disconnect from the patient, and remove from Ranger warmer.

Troubleshooting:
If you are having difficulty removing the set from the warmer:

1. Close the blue inlet clamp.
2. Squeeze the bubble trap, and close the clamp below the trap.
3. When the bubble trap is released, it will drain out enough fluid to allow the cassette to be removed from the warming unit.

(continued)

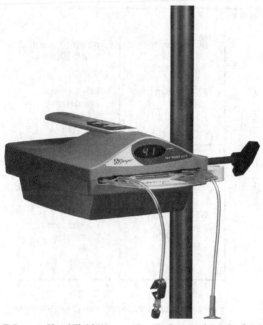

■ Ranger Blood/Fluid Warmer. Ranger is a trademark of Arizant Healthcare Inc., registered or pending in the U.S. Patent and Trademark office and in other countries. (Photograph is reproduced herein with permission. ©2009 Arizant Healthcare Inc. All rights reserved.)

RAPID VOLUME INFUSER *(see Level 1 Volume Infuser, p. 126)*

SEPTIC SHOCK *(see Shock, Septic, p. 147)*

NOTES

SHOCK BOX

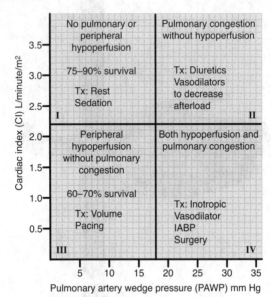

| | No pulmonary or peripheral hypoperfusion 75–90% survival Tx: Rest Sedation **I** | Pulmonary congestion without hypoperfusion Tx: Diuretics Vasodilators to decrease afterload **II** |

■ Shock box. (Adapted from Woods, S. L., Froelicher, E. S., & Motzer, S. U. [1999]. *Cardiac nursing* [4th ed.]. Philadelphia: Lippincott Williams & Wilkins.)

SHOCK, CARDIOGENIC *(see also Shock Parameters, p. 147)*

Cardiogenic shock is related to loss of myocardial contractility.

REMEMBER cardiogenic shock as an "engine malfunction." It occurs mostly in MI or in conditions with deficient heart filling. Look for:

- Increased preload (increase in CVP, PCWP, and positive JVD)
- Increased afterload (increase in SVR)
- Decreased contractility
- Decreased BP; SBP below 80 mm Hg
- Decreased cardiac output

Treatment: Fix heart muscle strength; increase contractility with oxygenation and positive inotropic agents (dobutamine, dopamine, digoxin). Decrease preload and afterload with nitroprusside (vasodilator).

SHOCK, HYPOVOLEMIC *(see also Shock Parameters, p. 147)*

Hypovolemic shock is related to loss of circulating blood volume.

REMEMBER hypovolemic shock as an "empty tank." Look for:

- Decreased preload (decreased CVP, PCWP)
- Increased afterload (increased SVR)
- Increased contractility

(continued)

- Pulsus paradoxus
- Decreased cardiac output

Treatment: Replace fluid loss (vasopressors contraindicated).

SHOCK, NEUROGENIC *(see Shock, Neurogenic, in Part 1, p. 52)*

SHOCK PARAMETERS

Shock Parameters				
	Preload		**Afterload**	
Shock Type	**CVP**	**PCWP**	**SVR**	**Cardiac Output**
Hypovolemic (most common)	↓	↓	↑	↓
Cardiogenic	↑	↑	↑	↓
Distributive—"umbrella" term for the following types:				
Anaphylactic	↓	↓	↓	↓
Neurogenic	↓	↓	↓	↓
Septic (warm or hyperdynamic)	↓	↓	↓	Typically ↑ but can be ↓
Septic (cold or) hypodynamic	↑	↑	↓ (without resuscitation may go ↑)	↓

SHOCK, SEPTIC *(see also Shock Parameters, p. 147)*

REMEMBER **septic shock as a "tank too large."**

Septic shock is clinically defined as the end point in a cascade of five physiologic alterations (described below):

1. Clinical insult
2. Systemic inflammatory response (SIRS)
3. Sepsis
4. Severe sepsis
5. Septic shock

1. First, a **clinical insult occurs,** causing massive infection and massive vasodilation. The insult is related to bacteria, which is usually Gram-negative, and is often *Escherichia coli*. The causes of the insult can be many, for example, head and neck infections, chest pulmonary infections, abdominal and gastrointestinal infections, pelvic and genitourinary infections, bone and soft tissue infections, invasive monitoring, postpartum infections, burns, immunosuppressant therapy, or hyperalimentation.
2. The insult may be followed by a **systemic inflammatory response (SIRS),** which is defined by two or more changes in the following four factors:
   - Temperature higher than 38°C or lower than 36°C
   - Heart rate >90 beats/min
   - Respiratory rate >20 breaths/min
   - White blood cell count higher than 12,000/mm^3 or lower than 4,000/mm^3 with more than 10% immature forms (bands)

(continued)

3. **Sepsis** is the third level of the cascade, defined as the systemic host response to SIRS *plus* a documented infection.
4. The cascade may then progress to **severe sepsis**, which is defined as sepsis *plus* end-organ dysfunction or hypoperfusion.
5. Ultimately, the cascade end point results in **septic shock**, defined as sepsis with hypotension (despite fluid resuscitation) *and* inadequate tissue perfusion.

   Treatment is focused on prompt, aggressive fluid resuscitation with a CVP goal of 8 to 12 cm H_2O as a guideline. Fluid boluses of isotonic crystalloids and colloids (albumin and hetastarch) are given (as tolerated by the patient) to achieve this goal. If ventilator support is required, a higher CVP (>12) is maintained. Other goals are:
- MAP >65 mm Hg
- $S\bar{v}O_2$ >70%
- Urine output 0.5 mL/kg/hr (calculated 0.5 × ___ kg = mL/hr)
- Blood glucose levels of 80 to 120 mg/dL within first 6 hours

   Adequate perfusion is the key to prevention of end-organ damage. Fluid resuscitation is delivered in conjunction with ventilatory support:
- 500 cc 0.9 NS rapid boluses PRN to achieve CVP desired goal;
- If CVP >15, decrease maintenance IV to KVO
- If CVP >20, decrease maintenance IV to KVO, and give diuretic IV

   Prompt pan culturing, followed by antibiotic administration, and treatment of complications is also of major importance. Pressor agents may be considered if the patient remains hypotensive despite reaching the CVP goal. Low $S\bar{v}O_2$ readings may be treated with a positive inotrope infusion such as dopamine.

SIRS *(see Shock, Septic, p. 147)*

ST SEGMENT MONITORING *(see also Myocardial Infarction, p. 131)*

The ST segment is identified as occurring at 0.6 seconds after the J point in the EKG. A change in this segment usually occurs early in MI, then returns to isoelectric in minutes to hours. During acute coronary spasm, ST segment elevation often precedes pain by minutes. Sustained ST elevation (3 months or longer) after an MI usually indicates ventricular aneurysm.

Monitoring tips:
- Leads III and V_3 are most commonly used. However, if the patient has a known "ST fingerprint" that was obtained during STEMI or PCI, the lead(s) that best display this "fingerprint" should be used.
- Lead V_5 is valuable in noncardiac ICU patients for identifying demand-related ischemia.
- Once proper electrode placement has been determined, the skin should be marked with indelible ink, since any variation of lead placement can create false ST segment changes.
- The ST alarm parameter should be set at 1 mm above and below the baseline ST segment in patients who are at high risk of ischemia, and at 2 mm in more stable patients.
- ST elevation or depression that lasts for at least a minute can be clinically significant and warrants further assessment.

(continued)

Conditions that alter ST segment:
- Depressed: Digitalis, hypothermia, suction, pericarditis
- Elevated: Head injury, hyperthyroid condition

STARLING'S LAW

Starling's law states that the greater the stretch of cardiac muscle, the more forceful the heart's contraction and beat. However, when the muscle is overstretched, the force of contraction may decrease below normal level, causing circulatory failure.

REMEMBER:

A rubber band breaks when stretched too far, rendering it useless.

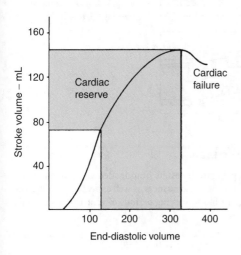

■ The Starling curve. As the end-diastolic fiber length increases, so does the cardiac output. At a self-limited end point, further stretching results in a lessened cardiac output.

STENTS, CORONARY (see also Angiography, p. 71; Angioplasty, p. 73; Atherectomy, p. 78)

Coronary stents are hollow tubes used to "brace open" a narrowed segment of coronary arteries. After predilation with a PTCA balloon catheter, most stents are premounted on a balloon catheter and are inserted through the guide catheter along a guide wire to the lesion site. Once placed across the stenotic lesion, the balloon is inflated, and the stent is expanded and remains in the coronary artery. During the first 3 to 4 weeks after implant, blood clots may form and stick to the metal surfaces of the stent. Thus, anticoagulant and antiplatelet regimens are essential. Over time (usually 6 months), restenosis (blockage within the stent) occurs in about 25% of the patients. This complication led to the development of the newer drug-eluting stents (DES), which are coated with drugs (sometimes imbedded in a thin polymer for time release) to limit the overgrowth of scar tissue at the revascularization site. Currently, three drug-eluting stents have received FDA approval for use in the United States: (1) Cordis CYPHER™ sirolimus-eluting stent; (2) Boston scientific TAXUS™ paclitaxel-eluting system; and (3) Medtronic ENDEAVOR™ zotarolimus eluting stent.

(continued)

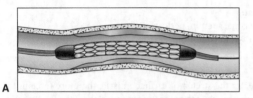

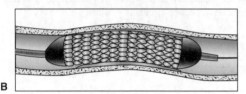

■ Implanting a stent: A, The stent is positioned at the site where the artery was widened. B, The balloon is inflated, and the stent expands. C, The balloon is deflated and removed. The stent will remain in place, keeping the artery open.

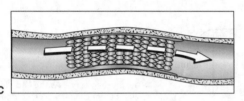

STOKES-ADAMS SYNDROME

In Stokes-Adams syndrome, a syncopal episode results from inadequate cerebral blood flow, which may be accompanied by loss of consciousness as well as seizure activity. The event is precipitated by a high-grade AV block, varying periods of ventricular standstill, or asystole.

STRESS TESTING *(see Stress Testing in Part 10, p. 365)*

STROKE VOLUME

Stroke volume is the amount of blood ejected by the heart into the systemic circulation with each contraction. **Normal:** 60 to 130 mL/beat. To calculate: Divide cardiac output (converted to mL) by heart rate.

$$\frac{CO \times 1000}{HR}$$

STROKE VOLUME INDEX

The stroke volume index is stroke volume adjusted for individual body surface area. **Normal:** 35 to 60 mL/beats/m². To calculate: Divide cardiac index (converted to mL) by heart rate or divide stroke volume by body surface area (obtained from nomogram)

$$\frac{CI \times 1000}{HR} \quad \text{or} \quad \frac{SV}{BSA}$$

SUPERIOR VENA CAVA SYNDROME

SVCS occurs when the superior vena cava is compressed by outside structures, or if a thrombus or clot develops within it, and blood flow is impeded. Venous drainage above the obstruction in the upper thorax is impaired and ultimately there is a "back up" of blood returning to the heart.

Causes: The most common cause is cancer. Primary or metastatic tumors located within the lung or within the mediastinum can cause vein compression. Blood clot (thrombus) formation within the vein itself may be caused by pacemaker wires or intravenous catheters. Rarely, syphilis, tuberculosis, or sarcoidosis may cause this syndrome.

Signs and symptoms:
- Chest, neck, and head vein engorgement (may visualize prominent veins on the skin's surface, particularly in the chest area, increasing in prominence in the flat supine position)
- Chest pain
- Facial, arm, hand edema
- Cyanosis
- Cough, hoarseness, dysphagia, shortness of breath
- Confusion, headache

Treatment is directed toward relieving the underlying cause of the obstruction. To relieve immediate symptoms, a diuretic may decrease circulating volume and make the patient more comfortable. Positioning (45°–90°) may improve respiratory symptoms. Emergency chemotherapy or radiation may be implemented to shrink tumor size. Steroids may also decrease tumor size by decreasing edema. If the cause of the obstruction is a blood clot, anticoagulation in indicated.

$S\bar{v}O_2$ MONITORING

Mixed venous saturation ($S\bar{v}O_2$) reflects the body's ability to provide adequate O_2 in response to tissue oxygen demands. It is affected by cardiac output, hemoglobin, arterial oxygen saturation, and tissue oxygen consumption. It is performed with a fiberoptic pulmonary artery catheter that carries infrared light from the monitor to the distal tip of the catheter. The light from this catheter then scatters off the red blood cells it "sees, " and the measurement of this is converted to a number by the monitor.

- Above 80% = sepsis, left-to-right shunt, excess inotropism, hypothermia, cell poisoning, or wedged catheter
- **Normal = 60% to 80%**
- Below 60% for >3 minutes = O_2 reserve being used, cardiac decompensation
- Below 50% for >3 minutes = O_2 reserve depleted; anaerobic metabolism (lactic acidosis begins)
- Below 30% for >3 minutes = O_2 reserve depleted; insufficient tissue O_2; coma

CAUSES OF DECREASED $S\bar{v}O_2$

1. Less oxygen delivered
   - Fall in cardiac output (heart failure, increased afterload, increased PEEP, dysrhythmias)
   - Decreased arterial saturation (suctioning, disconnect from O_2 source, respiratory failure, abnormal hemoglobin)

(continued)

2. Increased oxygen demand
   - Increased consumption (fever, pain, shivering, seizures, increased work of breathing, exercise)

CAUSES OF ELEVATED S$\bar{v}$O$_2$
1. More oxygen delivered
   - Rise in cardiac output (septic shock, inotropic drugs, IABP support, afterload reducing agents, thyrotoxicosis)
   - Elevated arterial saturation (increased FiO$_2$, hyperoxia)
   - Rise in hemoglobin (polycythemia)
2. Decreased oxygen demand
   - Decreased consumption (anesthesia, hypothermia, paralysis, cyanide toxicity)

MANAGEMENT OF DECREASED S$\bar{v}$O$_2$/LOW CARDIAC OUTPUT
1. Look for correctable causes that are noncardiac (acidosis, electrolytes, respiratory).
2. Optimize preload (PCWP 15–18 mm Hg).
3. Optimize heart rate with pacing if necessary (90–100 beats/min).
4. Control arrhythmias.
5. Assess cardiac output, and give inotropic agents if cardiac index is <2.0 L/min/m^2.
6. Calculate SVR, and give vasodilating agents if SVR is >1,500 dynes/sec/cm^5.
7. Blood transfusions if hematocrit level is <28 to 30 g/dL.

TO CALIBRATE THE S$\bar{v}$O$_2$ MONITOR
First draw waste, then sample from distal port. Compare the monitored S$\bar{v}$O$_2$ value with the mixed venous O$_2$ saturation value (normal 60%–80%). Do NOT use the mixed venous PO$_2$ value (normal 25–40 mm Hg).

SWAN-GANZ: CATHETER INFORMATION

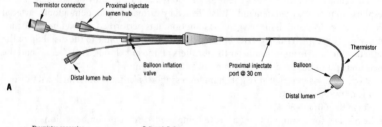

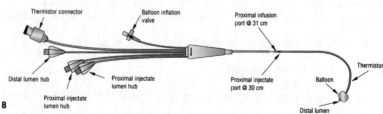

■ Catheter model examples. A, Traditional pulmonary artery (PA) catheter. B, Venous infusion port PA catheter. (*continued*)

(*continued*)

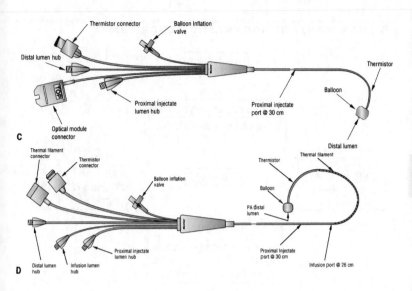

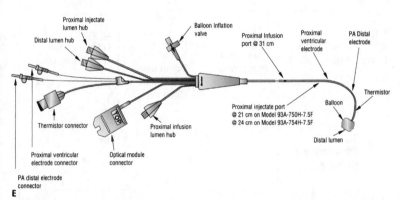

■ (*Continued*) C, Oximetry PA catheter. D, Continuous cardiac output PA catheter. E, Right ventricular ejection fraction oximetry PA catheter. (Courtesy of Baxter Healthcare Corporation, Edwards Critical-Care Division.)

Access choices: Preferred: Right IJ or left SC (left turn, left turn)
    Second choice: Left IJ or right SC (requires right turn before left turn)
Markings: Fat rings = 50 cm; thin rings = 10 cm
Placement: Proximal lumen at approximately 30 cm insert depth; correct placement in right atrium. Venous infusion port (VIP) at 31 cm; superior vena cava at approximately 40 cm. Insertion depth depends on patient size, usually approximately 45 cm with internal jugular access.

SWAN-GANZ: HEMODYNAMIC ALGORITHM

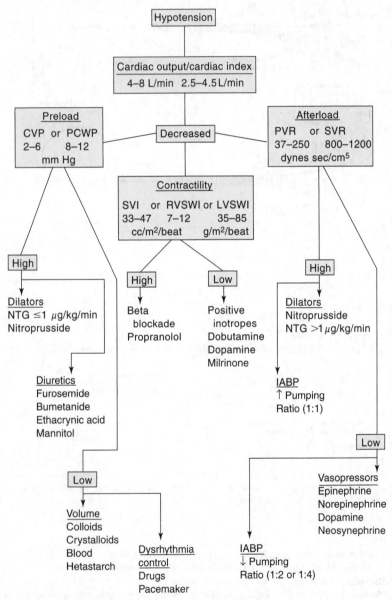

■ Hemodynamic algorithm. (Adapted from Urban, N. [1986]. Integrating hemodynamic parameters with clinical decision making. *Critical Care Nurse, 6* [2]:46–61. Reprinted with permission.)

SWAN-GANZ: HEMODYNAMIC NORMALS
(see also Phlebostatic Axis, p. 141)

RIGHT ATRIAL (CVP) PRESSURES: Normal 4 to 10 cm H₂O; 2 to 6 mmHg

Right side of heart filling pressures = preload (stretch). Contractility affects CVP.

> Poor contractility → Right atrium unable to empty completely → Rise in right ventricular end-diastolic pressure → Rise in CVP

CVP Increases (right ventricle can't pump volume forward) because of:
- Overinfusion of IVs (circulatory overload)
- Venous congestion (tamponade, PEEP, right ventricle failure, late left-side failure)
- Left to right shunt, severe mitral stenosis
- Poor contractility of right ventricle (infarct, pericarditis)
- High pulmonary vascular resistance (PVR) (pulmonary edema, COPD)

CVP decreases (inadequate venous return) because of:
- Hemorrhage
- Third spacing
- Extreme vasodilation (shock)

REMEMBER:

High levels of PEEP will result in a falsely high CVP. To "adjust" the CVP, simply deduct one third of the PEEP value from the CVP value.

For example: PEEP = 12 and CVP = 10 mm Hg

  1/3 of 12 (PEEP) = 4 10 (CVP) − 4 = 6
  6 mm Hg would be "adjusted" CVP value

RIGHT VENTRICLE PRESSURES: Normal $\frac{25-30}{0-5}$ mmHg

On insertion, start recording Swan-Ganz pressures here. Keep catheter moving with balloon inflated; an irritated ventricle causes PVCs.

Systolic pressure increases because of:
- Pulmonary hypertension
- Pulmonary stenosis

Diastolic pressure increases because of:
- Right ventricular failure
- Pericarditis
- Tamponade

PULMONARY ARTERY PRESSURES: $\frac{17-32}{8-10}$ mmHg; Mean <20 mmHg

Right ventricular and pulmonary artery systolic pressure should be the same, but the diastolic pressure is different.

PAP increases because of:
- Left ventricular failure
- Pulmonary vascular disease (e.g., hypertension, embolism, edema)

(continued)

PAP decreases because of:
- Volume depletion
- Drugs
- Aspiration
- Pulmonary stenosis

PULMONARY CAPILLARY WEDGE PRESSURE: Normal 4 to 12 mmHg*

PCWP represents the pressure in the left ventricle when there is no mechanical obstruction; it correlates with pulmonary artery diastolic pressure in the absence of disease. Measure wedge pressure at end expiration. Measure at the waveform peak if the patient is not undergoing ventilation, and measure at the waveform dip if the patient is undergoing ventilation.

REMEMBER: For patient undergoing ventilation, measure waveform in the valley.

Can be normal at 14 to 18 mm Hg in a compromised patient.

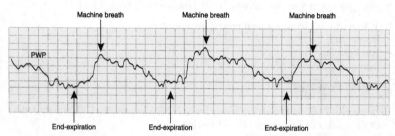

■ Pulmonary capillary wedge pressure (PCWP) tracing showing respiratory variation from positive pressure mechanical ventilation. In this case, PCWP measurement is correctly taken at the mean point of end expiration, not in the valley.

PCWP increases because of:
- Left ventricular failure (audible S_3 with increased left ventricular filling pressure)
- Tamponade
- Pulmonary edema
- Mitral stenosis or insufficiency
- Hypervolemia

PCWP decreases because of:
- Hypovolemia
- Afterload reduction caused by vasodilators

CARDIAC OUTPUT (CO): Normal 4 to 8 L/min

CO is the amount of blood ejected by the heart into the systemic circulation each minute.

$$CO = SV \times HR$$

CO increases because of:
- AV shunt
- Pulmonary edema
- Increased metabolic state (fever, tachycardia, burn)
- Mild hypertension with wide pulse pressure
- Early sepsis

(*continued*)

CO decreases because of:
- PEEP *REMEMBER:* PEEP is deep
- Infarction
- Decreased stroke volume (e.g., caused by dehydration, diuresis, infarction)
- Valve disorders
- Increased PVR
- Poor filling of left ventricle
- Hypovolemia
- Slow heart rate
- Tamponade

CARDIAC INDEX (CI): Normal 2.5 to 4.5 L/min/m^2
<1.5 = grave prognosis
1.5–2.0 = cardiogenic shock
2.0–2.2 = onset of forward failure

Cardiac output should be adjusted for body size (see also Body Surface Area Nomogram) and is known as the cardiac index (CI).

$$CI = CO \div BSA$$

PULMONARY VASCULAR RESISTANCE (PVR): Normal 37 to 250 dyne/sec/cm^5
This provides a measurement of right ventricular afterload. PVR is the force that must be overcome by the right ventricle to produce blood flow through the pulmonary system.

$$PVR = \frac{\text{mean PAP} - \text{PCWP}}{CO} \times 80$$

Pulmonary vessels constrict with a fall in the alveolar PO_2 or a rise in the arterial $PaCO_2$. An obstruction (such as a pulmonary embolus) can also cause the PVR to rise:

Increased PVR → Increased PAP → Right ventricle fails (if CO unchanged) → Increased CVP → Decreased CO

SYSTEMIC VASCULAR RESISTANCE (SVR): Normal 800 to 1,300 dyne/sec/cm^5
SVR is the resistance that must be overcome by the left ventricle to produce blood flow. It is also known as peripheral vascular resistance (not to be confused with PVR, which is pulmonary vascular resistance and a separate entity).

$$SVR = \frac{MAP - CVP}{CO} \times 80$$

REMEMBER:

SVR always moves inversely to the cardiac output.
A *low* SVR means a decreased afterload: Patient is peripherally dilated.
Related to
- Vasodilator therapy
- Early septic shock

(continued)

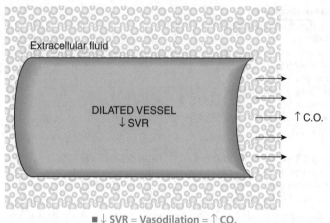

■ ↓ SVR = Vasodilation = ↑ CO.

A *high* SVR means an increase in the afterload: Patient is peripherally constricted.
Related to
- Hypovolemia
- Hypothermia
- Catecholamines
- Hypertension
- Cardiogenic shock
- Massive pulmonary embolism
- Cardiac tamponade
- Any condition causing vasoconstriction

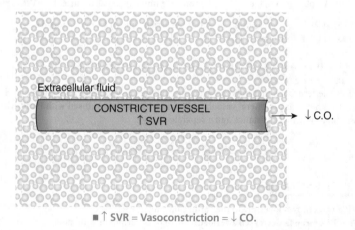

■ ↑ SVR = Vasoconstriction = ↓ CO.

SWAN-GANZ: HEMODYNAMIC WAVEFORMS

A. Catheter advanced to right atrium, balloon is inflated. Pressure is low, usually 2–5 mm Hg.

B. Catheter is floated to right ventricle with the balloon inflated. Waveforms indicate a systolic pressure of 25–30 mm Hg and a diastolic pressure of 0–5 mm Hg.

C. As the catheter moves into the pulmonary artery, the systolic pressure remains the same but the diastolic pressure elevates to 10–15 mm Hg.

D. The balloon is deflated and the catheter is moved until it can be wedged in a smaller vessel. When the balloon is inflated, the pressure recorded is that pressure in front of the catheter. It is an approximate measure of the left ventricular end diastolic pressure.

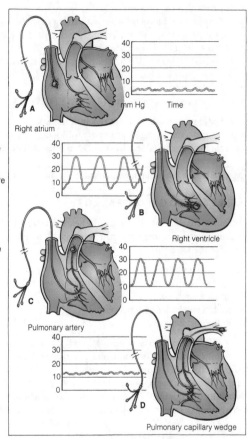

Right atrium

Right ventricle

Pulmonary artery

Pulmonary capillary wedge

■ Insertion of a flow-directed cardiac catheter.

SYNCHRONIZED CARDIOVERSION (see Cardioversion, p. 85)

SYSTEMIC INFLAMMATORY RESPONSE (SIRS)
(see Shock, Septic, p. 147)

SYSTEMIC VASCULAR RESISTANCE (see Swan-Ganz: Hemodynamic Normals, p. 157)

TAMPONADE

Acute compression of the heart, or tamponade, results from the collection of blood or fluid in the pericardial sac. It may occur after blunt or penetrating chest trauma, or by

(continued)

bleeding into the pericardium caused by rupture of the heart or coronary vessel. The "gold standard" for diagnosis is based on echocardiography. Patient has a clinical picture of:

- Narrowing pulse pressure
- Falling systolic blood pressure with rising diastolic pressure
- Pulsus paradoxus >10 to 15 mm Hg (see Pulsus Paradoxus)
- Distant or muffled heart sounds
- Increased preload (CVP >20 mm Hg, PCWP increased)
- Widened mediastinal shadow on chest x-ray film
- Decreased cardiac output
- Cardiac pressures equalizing (RA, PAD, PCWP, LA)

Treatment consists of direct repair of the wound, a thoracotomy or pericardiotomy, or a pericardiocentesis, the insertion of an 18-gauge needle through the xiphocostal angle to aspirate the pericardial sac. Removal of as little as 10 to 20 mL may relieve the symptoms.

TEE *(see Transesophageal Echocardiography in Part 10, p. 366)*

TETRALOGY OF FALLOT

Accounts for 10% of all congenital heart disease, although the defect is rare in adults because successful surgical repair is usually done in early childhood. The classic components of the tetrad are

1. Ventral-septal defect
2. Aorta that overrides the ventral-septal defect and communicates with both the right and left ventricles
3. Right ventricular hypertrophy
4. Pulmonic stenosis

Physical appearance is characterized by small, undeveloped body, clubbing of the extremities, and mild to moderate cyanosis. A loud systolic murmur is heard over the left sternal border. Correction of the defect includes closure of the ventral-septal defect and widening of the right ventricular outflow tract to relieve pulmonic stenosis. Mortality in adults not operated on usually results from cardiac failure, sudden death (related to arrhythmias), cerebrovascular accident, brain abscess, or endocarditis.

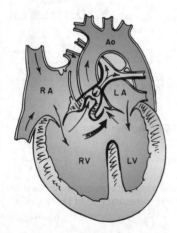

■ Tetralogy of Fallot. (From Finklemeier, B. A. [2000]. *Cardiothoracic surgical nursing* [2nd ed.]. Philadelphia: Lippincott Williams & Wilkins.)

THROMBOLYTIC THERAPY *(see also Alteplase in Part 8, p. 298; Reteplase in Part 8, p. 333; Tenecteplase in Part 8, p. 334)*

Thrombolytic agents work to dissolve the clot that is causing the acute infarction by initiating the conversion of plasminogen to plasmin. Plasmin eats at the fibrin threads holding the clot together, thus leading to its dissolution. The therapy may be used to "buy time" if the treating facility does not have a cardiac cath lab. Reducing the time to treatment, particularly the "door-to-drug" time, has been identified as a critical target to improving outcomes. Initiation of therapy should be within 30 minutes of the patient's presentation.

Absolute contraindications:
- Prior intracranial hemorrhage
- Known structural cerebrovascular lesion
- Known malignant intracranial neoplasm
- Ischemic stroke within 3 months
- Suspected aortic dissection
- Active bleeding (excluding menses) or bleeding tendency
- Significant closed head trauma or facial trauma within 3 months

Relative contraindications:
- History of chronic, severe, poorly controlled hypertension
- Severe uncontrolled hypertension on presentation (SBP >180; DBP >110)
- Traumatic or prolonged CPR (>10 minutes) or major surgery less than 3 weeks
- Noncompressible vascular punctures
- For streptokinase or anistreplase—prior exposure (more than 5 days ago) or prior allergic reaction to these agents
- Pregnancy
- Active peptic ulcer
- Current use of anticoagulant (Coumadin) that has produced an elevated INR of >1.7 or PT of >15 seconds.

There are also risks in using thrombolytics and the benefits must be carefully weighed.
- Main complication is bleeding. Risk is higher for patients who have had recent surgery, trauma, hypertension, liver disease, or recent CVA.
- Most severe bleeding complication within first 24 hours is intracranial hemorrhage.
- Greater benefit with anterior MI than inferior MI.
- Greatest benefit if initiated within 3 hours of onset of symptoms, but can be given within 6 hours of onset.

TISSUE PLASMINOGEN ACTIVATOR *(see Alteplase in Part 8, p. 298)*

TORSADE DE POINTES

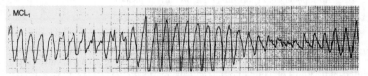

MCL₁

■ Torsades de pointes.

(continued)

Torsade de pointes is a dangerous form of ventricular tachycardia in which the polarity of the ventricular complexes swings between positive and negative. Literally, it is a "twisting of points." The QT is prolonged, and the longer refractory period allows more ventricular ectopic contractions of various kinds. (Normal QT = 0.32–0.40 seconds, or less than one half the preceding R to R interval.) Quinidine, procainamide, disopyramide, or amiodarone is usually the culprit, although anything that lengthens the QT interval could be the cause, for example, hypokalemia, hypomagnesemia, hypocalcemia, profound bradycardia, intracerebral pathologic changes, unilateral alteration of sympathetic tone, or psychotropic drugs. The patient may be conscious, and the tachycardia may be paroxysmal, stopping, and then starting again.

Treatment:

- ACLS protocol for VT
- Overdrive pacing may be necessary, at a rate of up to 140 beats/min.
- Treat hypokalemia (if precipitating factor)
- Magnesium sulfate 1 to 4 g initially, then 1 to 2 g IV diluted in 100 cc D5W over 1 to 2 minutes; may repeat every 4 hours with close monitoring of deep tendon reflexes
  NOTE: Calcium gluconate, 10 to 20 mL IV of 10% solution, can be given as an antidote for clinically significant hypermagnesemia
- If unstable, cardioversion
- Consider lidocaine/phenytoin, isoproterenol, short-acting beta-blockers
- Withdraw all QT-prolonging drugs
- Cardiology consult; possible implantable defibrillator for prophylaxis

TPA (see Alteplase in Part 8, p. 298)

TRANSESOPHAGEAL ECHOCARDIOGRAM
(see Transesophageal Echocardiography in Part 10, p. 366)

TRANSMYOCARDIAL LASER REVASCULARIZATION

Transmyocardial laser revascularization (TMR) is a surgical procedure, usually restricted for use in patients with severe unstable angina who have exhausted all other forms of intervention. TMR is performed through a small left chest incision or through a midline incision, frequently with coronary artery bypass but occasionally alone. The surgeon utilizes a special high-energy computerized carbon dioxide laser to create blood perfusion channels in the heart muscle. The goal is to supplement the function of the coronary arteries and, in effect, allow the heart to "feed itself." TMR usually takes 1 to 2 hours, and recovery is rapid, requiring a 3- to 4-day hospital stay. Long-term follow-up data are not yet available.

TRANSTHORACIC ECHOCARDIOGRAM
(see Transesophageal Echocardiography in Part 10, p. 366)

TRICUSPID REGURGITATION

Tricuspid regurgitation is primarily "functional" rather than structural, occurring secondary to dilation of the right ventricle and the annulus of the tricuspid valve. There is a significant backflow of blood into the right atrium due to the fact that the tricuspid valve literally "billows" during systole, and the leaflets do not close tightly.

(continued)

Causes:

- Rheumatic fever (leaflets and chordae tendineae are scarred, restricting the mobility of the leaflets)
- Congenital abnormalities
- Infective endocarditis
- Right atrial tumor
- Tricuspid valve prolapse

Assessment:

- Fatigue, weight loss, cachexia
- Enlarged liver (hepatomegaly)
- Signs of right-sided heart failure: Jugular venous distention, large V waves on CVP tracing
- Holosystolic murmur along left sternal border

Diagnosis:

- ECG, chest x-ray, echocardiography

Management:

- Mild regurgitation usually requires no treatment, especially if pulmonary hypertension is absent.
- Severe disease may require annuloplasty.

TRICUSPID STENOSIS

The pathophysiology of tricuspid stenosis is similar to mitral stenosis, where there is shortening of the chordae tendineae and fusion of the leaflets at the edges with a fixed opening. Blood cannot get through the valve during diastole, and as a result, pressure builds up in the right atrium, which in time becomes dilated. Ultimately, hypertrophy of the heart wall results.

Causes:

- Usually a result of rheumatic fever. Patients routinely have a long history of the defect, which occurs in conjunction with mitral valve disease.

Assessment:

- Fatigue (related to low cardiac output)
- Hepatomegaly
- Signs of right-sided heart failure: Paroxysmal nocturnal dyspnea, jugular venous distention, prominent A wave on CVP tracing
- Diastolic decrescendo murmur along the left sternal border that increases with inspiration

Diagnosis:

- ECG, chest x-ray
- 2-D echo and TEE to provide data about the valve
- Doppler echo to quantify the stenosis

Management:

- Medically: Intensive dietary sodium restriction, diuretics
- Surgically: Balloon valvuloplasty or valve replacement or repair

VALVULOPLASTY

Valvuloplasty is a procedure done in the cardiac cath lab that is used to widen a stiff, narrowed heart valve. A balloon-tipped catheter is inserted through the groin or a vessel in the arm. Guided by a video monitor and x-ray, the catheter is advanced into the heart and is positioned in the valve opening. The balloon is then repeatedly inflated and deflated in an attempt to split the valve leaflets apart. The procedure is most effective in adolescents and young adults, and while it is indicated for stenosis of the aortic, mitral, and pulmonary valves, the best results are obtained when treating the pulmonary valves. Mitral valve treatment results are generally good, while less success is noted in treating the aortic valve.

VENTRICULAR ASSIST DEVICES

A ventricular assist device (VAD) can take over function for a heart's failing ventricle. It can be

- a left ventricular device (LVAD), providing systemic circulatory support;
- a right ventricular device (RVAD), providing pulmonary circulatory support;
- or a biventricular device (BiVAD) providing both right and left support.

The system consists of a blood pump, cannulas, and a pneumonic or electrical drive console. Blood flows from the patient's heart to the VAD, which then mechanically pumps it back to the body. VADs can be used for short- or long-term support. Most commonly, they are used as a bridge to transplantation, or a support for cardiogenic shock.

VENTRICULAR RESTORATION *(see also Dor Procedure, p. 93)*

Surgical ventricular restoration is a procedure used to treat congestive heart failure caused by myocardial infarction. Following attack, scar tissue or an aneurysm may develop, resulting in an enlarged, rounded heart. The goal of surgical ventricular restoration is to restore the heart to a more normal size and shape, thereby improving function. In this procedure, infarcted muscle is removed with simultaneous reconstruction of the left ventricle by utilizing a balloon mannequin. The mannequin is used as a guide to restore proper size and shape to the left ventricle and also to restore papillary muscle geometry. If necessary, a Dacron patch is placed as part of the "reshaping," and prior to closure, the mannequin is removed. The procedure is usually performed in conjunction with CABG, to ensure optimal blood supply. Rupture of the papillary muscle is a major postoperative consideration.

VENTRICULOGRAM *(see Angiography, p. 71)*

WELLEN'S SYNDROME

A critical stenosis of the proximal anterior descending coronary artery, requiring emergent coronary artery catheterization, because the likelihood of progression to MI is very high. Typically, the patient has chest pain and a normal EKG, only to show the following characteristic EKG changes when asymptomatic:

1. ST/T wave changes in the precordial leads (usually V_2 and V_3 and occasionally V_1–V_4).
2. The EKG may further evolve and the ST/T may turn down to negative at an angle of 60° to 90° in V_2 to V_4 (called the "left anterior descending T-wave syndrome").

(continued)

If the T waves are inverted in V_1 to V_6 at the time of presentation, diagnosis of Wellen's syndrome is difficult, because a differential diagnosis of other T-wave inversion syndromes, such as acute myocarditis, acute pulmonary embolism, or a non–Q-wave MI, is possible.

During subsequent pain periods, the patient may also show a definite ST elevation or depression across the midchest leads, indicative of an anterior MI.

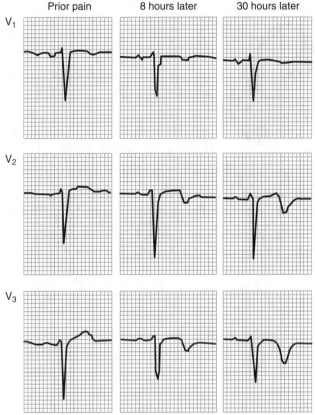

■ Progression of the ST segment/T wave change in the right midprecordial leads in a patient with Wellen's syndrome. (Adapted from Jeff Mann, EM Guidemaps.)

WOLFF-PARKINSON-WHITE SYNDROME (WPW)
(see also Ablation, p. 67; Lown-Ganong-Levine Syndrome, p. 129)

The WPW syndrome is a ventricular "preexcitation" syndrome in which an impulse "sneaks" down a shorter path (via the Kent's bundle or the Mahaim fibers), bypassing the AV node, while at the same time, another impulse from the normal bundle of His pathway is conducted. As a result, the ventricle is stimulated from two directions. This sets

(continued)

up recurrent bouts of supraventricular tachyarrhythmias. Two types of WPW have been identified: Type A on the left side of the heart and type B on the right side of the heart. The hallmarks of the syndrome are twofold: (1) a shortened PR interval (usually <0.12 seconds) because the impulse takes a "shortcut" from the SA to the AV node and (2) an initial slurring on the upstroke of the QRS (delta wave), reflecting the ventricular activation outside the normal conduction system.

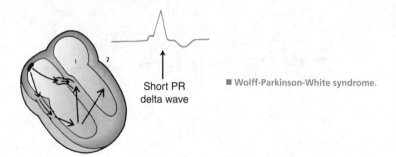

Short PR
delta wave

■ Wolff-Parkinson-White syndrome.

This syndrome is seen most often in young adults and rarely in the elderly. The patient can go in and out of this rhythm, exhibiting entire runs of supraventricular tachyarrhythmias or just experiencing an occasional beat or two. The syndrome may require no treatment if the occurrences are rare. However, recurrent bouts of tachyarrhythmias must be treated as appropriate with vagal maneuvers and, if they are unsuccessful, with vagotonic drugs. Surgical intervention to sever the Kent's bundle or Mahaim fibers bypass tract is often used for those patients who experience frequent, disabling tachyarrhythmias.

PART 3

Pulmonary System

A-a GRADIENT

The A-a gradient indicates whether gas transfer is normal and gives an idea of how well oxygen is moving from the alveoli to the arterial blood. It helps to distinguish hypoventilation from other causes such as $\dot{V}/\dot{Q}$ mismatch, shunting, and/or diffusion abnormalities. The goal is to have a decreased A-a gradient. Although "normal" values change with age, FiO_2 concentration, and barometric pressure, a general rule of thumb is that the gradient should be <10 to 15 mm Hg on room air. A conservative estimate of normal, however, can be made by using the following formula:

$$(Age \div 4) + 4$$

The more exact formula, using the alveolar gas equation, is the following:

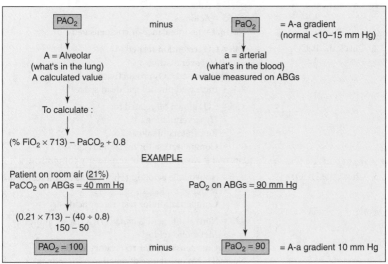

| PAO_2 | minus | PaO_2 | = A-a gradient (normal <10–15 mm Hg) |

A = Alveolar (what's in the lung) A calculated value

a = arterial (what's in the blood) A value measured on ABGs

To calculate :

$$(\% FiO_2 \times 713) - PaCO_2 \div 0.8$$

EXAMPLE

Patient on room air (21%)
$PaCO_2$ on ABGs = 40 mm Hg

PaO_2 on ABGs = 90 mm Hg

$$(0.21 \times 713) - (40 \div 0.8)$$
$$150 - 50$$

$PAO_2 = 100$ minus $PaO_2 = 90$ = A-a gradient 10 mm Hg

■ A-a gradient calculation.

An easier and less complicated method to predict shunting is the PaO_2/FiO_2 (P/F) ratio. It is calculated thus:

$$PaO_2 \div FiO_2$$

Using the criteria from the previous example:

$$90 \div 0.21$$

$$PaO_2/FiO_2 \text{ ratio} = 428 \text{ torr}$$

Normal is 286 torr; lower indicates a shunt.

ABG INTERPRETATION *(see also Base Excess/Deficit p. 174; ABG's in Part 9, p. 340)*

ABG Interpretation			
	pH 7.35–7.45	**PaCO₂ 35–45**	**HCO₃ 22–26**
Respiratory acidosis	↓	↑	—
Respiratory alkalosis	↑	↓	—
Metabolic acidosis	↓	—	↓
Metabolic alkalosis	↑	—	↑
Uncompensated	Abnormal	Either abnormal	
No indication that the opposite system has tried to correct for the other			
Partially compensated	Abnormal	Abnormal	Abnormal
One system has attempted to correct for the other but has not had success			
Fully compensated	Normal	Abnormal	Abnormal
Normal pH indicates that one system has been able to compensate for the other			

Steps to ABG Interpretation

1. Check the pH	>7.45 = Alkalosis <7.35 = Acidosis Normal = no imbalance or compensated
2. Check the PaCO₂	>45 = CO₂ retention related to • *Hypo*ventilation, • Increased CO₂ productivity • Increased physiologic dead space <35 = CO₂ blown off related to: • *Hyper*ventilation • Respiratory alkalosis • Compensation for metabolic acidosis Normal = No imbalance of respiratory component
3. Check the HCO₃	>26 = Nonvolatile acid *lost* (HCO₃ *gained*). Indicates • Metabolic alkalosis or, • Compensation for respiratory acidosis <22 = Nonvolatile acid is *added* (HCO₃ *lost*). Indicates • Metabolic acidosis • Compensation for respiratory alkalosis Normal = No imbalance of metabolic component
4. Determine the imbalance	
5. Determine if compensation exists	

REMEMBER:

pH, PaCO₂ **opposite** direction = respiratory problem
pH, HCO₃⁻ **same** direction = metabolic problem ("M" for "married")
HCO₃⁻, PaCO₂ **same** direction = compensation for abnormal pH
HCO₃⁻, PaCO₂ **opposite** direction = two mixed imbalances present

(continued)

RESPIRATORY ACIDOSIS ($\downarrow$pH, $\uparrow$PaCO$_2$)

Respiratory acidosis is related to stroke, drug overdose, aspiration, pneumonia, acute respiratory distress syndrome (ARDS), cardiac arrest, chronic obstructive pulmonary disease (COPD), hypoventilation, and neuromuscular disorders.

Treatment: Aggressive chest PT, suction. Increase respiratory rate, increase tidal volume.

RESPIRATORY ALKALOSIS ($\uparrow$pH, $\downarrow$PaCO$_2$)

Respiratory alkalosis is related to anxiety, fear, head trauma, brain tumor, hepatic insufficiency, fever, mechanical overventilation, pulmonary embolism, and thyrotoxicosis.

Treatment: Sedation, support, breathe in paper bag for attack of hyperventilation. Decrease respiratory rate, decrease tidal volume.

METABOLIC ACIDOSIS ($\downarrow$pH, $\downarrow$HCO$_3^-$)

Metabolic acidosis is related to renal failure, diarrhea, TPN, acetazolamide (Diamox) (diuretic that prevents carbonic acid formation), ketoacidosis, and lactic acidosis (caused by bicarbonate loss or excess acids in extracellular fluid).

Treatment: Treat underlying cause, monitor intake/output and dysrhythmias, protect against infection.

METABOLIC ALKALOSIS ($\uparrow$pH, $\uparrow$HCO$_3^-$)

Metabolic alkalosis is related to volume depletion (loss of H$^+$, Cl$^-$, K$^+$ from vomiting or diarrhea, gastric suction, or diuretic therapy).

REMEMBER:

al-K$^+$-**low**-sis means potassium value is low when patient is alkalotic.

Treatment: Treat underlying cause, monitor intake/output, potassium replacement therapy.

ABGs, MIXED VENOUS *(see Mixed Venous ABGs, p. 191)*

ACUTE RESPIRATORY FAILURE

Acute respiratory failure is the inability of the respiratory system for adequate gas exchange, namely, sufficient oxygenation, carbon dioxide elimination, or both. Thus, it can be classified as either hypoxemic or hypercapnic.

In practice, it is defined by exhibiting any two of the following four:
- Tachypnea (>35 breaths/min)
- PaO$_2$ <50 mm Hg on room air or <70 mm Hg on 50% O$_2$ mask
- PaCO$_2$ >50 mm Hg
- pH <7.3 (showing significant respiratory acidosis)

Additional criteria include:
- Altered mental status
- Vital capacity <15 mL/kg
- Inspiratory force <25 cm H$_2$O
- PaO$_2$/FiO$_2$ ratio <250

ALBUTEROL *(see Respiratory Inhalation Medications, p. 202)*

ALUPENT *(see Respiratory Inhalation Medications, p. 203)*

AMINOPHYLLINE *(see Part 8, p. 301)*

ANATOMY, PULMONARY

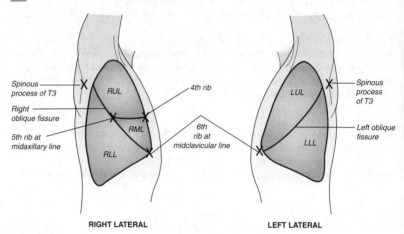

RIGHT LATERAL **LEFT LATERAL**

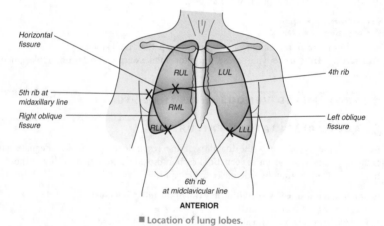

ANTERIOR

■ Location of lung lobes.

ANION GAP *(see Part 5, p. 250)*

ARDS *(see also Prone Positioning, p. 198)*

Acute respiratory distress syndrome (ARDS) (formerly known as adult respiratory distress syndrome until 1994, when it was recognized that the malady is not confined to adults) is a form of severe respiratory failure associated with pulmonary infiltrates originating from several insults involving damage to the alveolocapillary membrane with subsequent fluid accumulation within the air spaces of the lungs. In effect, ARDS is pulmonary edema without volume overload and without depressed left ventricular function.

(continued)

Cause is either a direct or an indirect injury to the lungs:

- Sepsis and systemic inflammatory response (SIRS)—most common reason
- Multiple fractures or long bone fractures (trauma)—related to fat embolism
- Severe head injury—discharge of sympathetic nervous system, resulting in acute pulmonary hypertension and injury to the capillary bed
- Pulmonary contusion—due to direct trauma to the lung
- Multiple transfusions—potential increases with the number of units transfused
- Near drowning, aspiration, and pneumonia—direct insult to lung tissue
- Smoke inhalation—damage from particulate matter inhaled into the lower lung. (These patients should be monitored closely, even if symptoms of ARDS are initially absent.)
- Drug overdoses—tricyclic antidepressants are the most common. (This risk is independent of aspiration.)

Hallmarks of ARDS:

- Bilateral infiltrates on chest x-ray film
- PAWP <18 mm Hg with no evidence of left atrial hypertension
- Impaired oxygenation (regardless of PEEP) with a PaO_2/FiO_2 ratio of <200 torr

The signs and symptoms are usually subtle:

- Chest x-ray film appearance may be normal early in the disease but will digress to show bilateral pulmonary infiltrates (a "ground-glass" appearance) and ultimately a complete whiteout of both lungs.
- ABGs initially show hypoxia with respiratory alkalosis early in the disease and respiratory acidosis as the disease progresses.
- High peak inspiratory pressures
- Increase in the A-a gradient
- Decreased compliance
- Decreased FRC
- P/F ratio <200 torr

The treatment is mainly supportive because there are no specific measures to correct increased vascular permeability or correct the inflammatory process. Mechanical ventilation is generally employed to keep O_2 saturation above 90%. PEEP may be added in small increments to reverse compression atelectasis. Routine or prophylactic use of antibiotics or corticosteroids is not beneficial; in fact, administration of multiple antibiotics may lead to the development of multiple drug-resistant infections. Despite years of research, mortality remains as high as 40% to 60%.

(continued)

NOTES

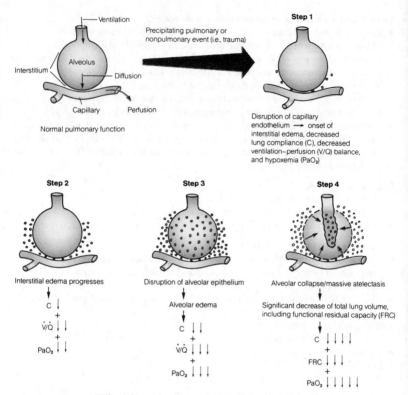

■ Physiology of acute respiratory distress syndrome.

ARTERIAL BLOOD GASES *(see ABG Interpretation, p. 168)*

ARTERIAL O₂ CONTENT

Arterial oxygen content (CaO_2) is primarily determined by the amount of hemoglobin in arterial blood that is saturated with oxygen:

$$CaO_2 = (Hgb \times 1.39 \times SaO_2) + (0.003 \times PaO_2)$$

REMEMBER:

A quicker way to estimate this value: $Hgb \times 1.39 \times SaO_2$

Normal value: 15 to 24 volume percentage

ASSIST/CONTROL VENTILATION *(see Ventilator Modes, p. 212)*

ASTHMA

Asthma is from the Greek for "to pant." Hallmarks are tenacious sputum and reversible airway obstruction. Patient is dehydrated (related to tachypnea) and has decreased

(continued)

vesicular breath sounds with hyperexpansion of chest and decreased chest wall excursion. There is severe airway obstruction and respiratory acidosis. (In less severe attacks, there may be a decrease in the PCO_2 related to hyperventilation and respiratory alkalosis.)

Status asthmaticus is an acute exacerbation of asthma refractory to initial treatment with bronchodilators and is a medical emergency. It can lead to respiratory failure, unconsciousness, and cardiopulmonary arrest. Advanced symptoms include extreme dyspnea, coughing, and wheezing. There are little or no breath sounds, inability to speak, cyanosis, and diaphoresis.

Treatment of choice: Bronchodilators (inhaled or nebulizers), oral or IV steroids, and hydration. Oxygenation with mechanical ventilation may need to be considered. Aminophylline is rarely used, but it may be considered if other therapy fails or if the patient had been using it previously.

ATELECTASIS

Atelectasis refers to the absence of gas in a lung segment or an entire lobe, resulting in lung collapse. Since the right middle lobe is the most narrow and is surrounded by lymphoid tissue, it is the most common area to be atelectatic. While almost always a secondary phenomenon, atelectasis has a direct morbidity linked to it because of hypoxemia. There are four primary causes:

1. Airways have intrinsic obstruction.
2. Airways have extrinsic obstruction (compressed).
3. Lung tissue is compressed.
4. Alveoli incompletely expand and eventually collapse.

Absorption atelectasis is a hazard of high FiO_2 and will most likely occur when there is an obstruction (e.g., a mucous plug) causing blockage of the airways leading to the alveoli. Nitrogen makes up about 80% of the air we breathe but is not absorbed at all by the lung under normal atmospheric conditions. Therefore, nitrogen remains in the lung even after the oxygen has been absorbed, to help keep the alveoli from collapsing. However, if a high concentration of FiO_2 is delivered, the nitrogen is "washed out" (and replaced by the delivered gas.) When this gas is absorbed completely, the alveoli collapse, and atelectasis results.

ATROPINE *(see Respiratory Inhalation Medications, p. 202)*

AUTOPEEP

Normally, end-expiration is a "no-flow" state, and the pressure in the alveoli equals the pressure at the mouth. In conditions of autoPEEP (intrinsic PEEP), however, the pleural and alveolar pressures remain positive at end-expiration, compared with mouth pressures, related to air "trapped" in the alveoli. Subsequently, when the next breath comes, airway pressure increases, and the breaths are "stacked." (This is frequently seen when the respiratory rate and/or minute volume are high, but it can also develop because of a narrow ET tube, water clogging in the exhalation part of the circuit, or a stiff exhalation valve.) AutoPEEP adds to the work of breathing because the patient must generate a negative pleural pressure to initiate inspiration.

How do you know if autoPEEP is present? You can tell this easily in a mechanically ventilated patient by looking at the expiratory airflow. Using the ventilator graphics, if

(continued)

expiratory flow continues until the onset of the next inspiratory cycle, a pressure gradient must exist during the flow, and, by definition, autoPEEP exists.

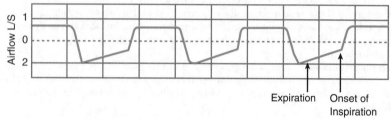

Expiration   Onset of
Inspiration

■ In this example of autoPEEP, expiratory flow continues until the onset of the next inspiratory cycle. Qualitatively this indicates the presence of autoPEEP because the persistent expiratory flow requires a positive pressure gradient from the alveolus to the mouth. (Copyright protected material used with permission of the author and the University of Iowa's Virtual Hospital, www.vh.org.)

Management of the condition is done by adding extrinsic PEEP, thus removing the additional work of breathing required to overcome the positive pressure gradient from the alveolus to the mouth. Expiratory time also needs to be increased. This can be accomplished by decreasing the respiratory rate, setting the I:E ratio in favor of expiration, or increasing peak flow, which will decrease inspiratory time.

BASE EXCESS/DEFICIT

The base excess/deficit is a calculated number that represents the amount of base that must be added to restore the blood to a normal pH of 7.4 (Normal range = −2 to +2 mEq/L).
- Base **excess** is a **positive** number and signifies **metabolic alkalosis.**
- Base **deficit** is a **negative** number and signifies **metabolic acidosis.**

REMEMBER:

Base deficit (acidosis) ← pH 7.4 → Base excess (alkalosis)

The parameter is confusing, in that the terms *excess* and *deficit* are sometimes used interchangeably. To be correct, *excess* should be reported as a positive number, and *deficit* should be reported as a negative number.

BiPAP VENTILATOR SUPPORT

Bilevel positive airway pressure (BiPAP) is a noninvasive, positive pressure ventilation system, usually delivered via face mask (thus eliminating the need for intubation or tracheostomy) and is used to augment breathing for patients who feel that continuous positive airway pressure (CPAP) is unbearable because it is too difficult to exhale against the back pressure. The patient breathes spontaneously, and the circuit is maintained at one pressure during exhalation and a higher pressure during inhalation. It is helpful for patients who have difficulty breathing (often at night) related to COPD, congestive heart failure (CHF), cystic fibrosis, sleep apnea syndrome, and neuromuscular diseases resulting in respiratory insufficiency. It does not provide total ventilation requirements and should never be used as a life-support device.

BLEB (see also Bulla, p. 176)

A bleb is a small bulla, usually found in the subpleural zone of the lung abutting the pleura.

BOYLE'S LAW

When the pressure of a gas is doubled and the temperature remains constant, the volume of the gas is reduced by one half. At a constant temperature (T), the volume of a gas (V) is inversely proportional to the pressure (P) of the volume. That pressure remains constant if the temperature is unchanged.

$$\text{Formula: } P_1V_1 = P_2V_2$$

Example: Think of an inflatable pool raft. When you get on it to relax, initially it will compress under your weight. But at a certain point, the compression ceases and the pressure inside the raft is maintained to keep you afloat.

BREATH SOUNDS, NORMAL

- **Bronchial** breath sounds are normal over the upper third of the sternum and trachea. If they are heard anywhere else, they are abnormal. The sound is produced by the air movement through the larynx, setting up vibrations, not by the air leaving the alveoli. The sound is loud and high pitched.
- **Bronchovesicular** breath sounds are heard over the two lower portions of the sternum, just to either side. They are heard posteriorly between the scapulae. If they are heard anywhere else, the sound is due to partial atelectasis or pulmonary consolidation. The sound is soft with a lower pitch.
- **Vesicular** breath sounds (inspiration) are produced by air entering the alveoli directly, separating the alveoli. They can be heard anywhere anteriorly. Posteriorly, they can be heard anywhere except between the scapulae. The sound is soft and breezy, with the lowest pitch.

BREATH SOUNDS, ABNORMAL

- **Rales** (crackles) can usually be heard only on inspiration and are found wherever the underlying pathologic condition is. The sound is similar to rubbing strands of hair together, next to the ear. They correlate with early left-sided failure, and the degree to which they are audible corresponds to the degree of the failure. They may also be caused by interstitial lung disease and pneumonias. If the rales disappear with three or four breaths or with a cough, they are not due to fluid but to the actual separating of the alveolar walls. They are then known as dry rales, atelectatic rales, or hypostatic rales. Rales are common after the patient has been at bed rest for 24 hours.
- **Rhonchi** are heard predominantly on expiration and are related to secretions in larger airways. The sound is of a continuous snoring quality, similar to rubbing two inflated balloons together.
- **Wheezes** can be heard on inspiration or expiration. When breathing is partially constricted (as in asthma), the sound can be heard primarily on expiration. It has a musical quality, or is likened to creaking or groaning.
- A **rub** is caused by parietal and visceral pleura rubbing caused by inflammation. The sound stops if the patient holds the breath. A rub is usually heard on inspiration and expiration and is a superficial squeaking or grating sound, similar to rubbing two pieces of leather together.

BREATHING PATTERNS *(see Respiratory Patterns, p. 203)*

BRETHINE *(see Respiratory Inhalation Medications, p. 202)*

BRONCHITIS

The patient with bronchitis has recurrent, excessive bronchial mucous secretion, resulting in a productive cough. The increased secretions often render the patient a perfect host for bacteria. The description "blue bloater" is often given because of the presence of hypoxemia resulting in cyanosis and the tendency toward edema. Treatment is aimed at improving alveolar ventilation and relieving the hypoxemia through vigorous pulmonary toilet, postural drainage, intermittent positive-pressure breathing (IPPB) therapy, bronchodilators, and mucolytic agents.

BRONKOSOL *(see Respiratory Inhalation Medications, p. 202)*

BULLA

A bulla is a thin-walled, localized pocket of air in lung tissue. Bullae vary in size from being barely visible on x-ray film to several centimeters in diameter. They may occur in otherwise normal lungs or may be a result of primary emphysema. Secondary infections often develop.

CAPNOGRAPHY

Measured by monitoring samples of expired gas from a circuit attached to an endotracheal tube, CO_2 measured at end-exhalation ($PETCO_2$) can be used to approximate the level of alveolar CO_2, because the percentage of arterial carbon dioxide dissolved in the blood ($PaCO_2$) closely approximates the percentage of alveolar CO_2. As a rule of thumb, $PETCO_2$ values are usually just slightly lower than $PaCO_2$ levels. In fact, the two values tend to move in opposite directions about 22% of the time. A normal capnogram will show a slow rise in CO_2, with a plateau at end-expiration and a steep drop at the beginning of inspiration.

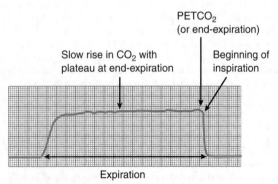

PETCO₂
(or end-expiration)

Slow rise in CO₂ with
plateau at end-expiration

Beginning of
inspiration

Expiration

■ Characteristics of a normal capnogram. (Courtesy of Agilent Technologies and Tom Ahrens, St. Louis, MO.)

(continued)

Measuring the PETCO₂ enables many types of pulmonary assessments to be made:

- **Monitoring patients during weaning from the ventilator.** Because $PETCO_2$ provides continuous estimates of alveolar ventilation, monitoring the values is useful in determining readiness for extubation.

- **Predicting survival during cardiopulmonary resuscitation.** $PETCO_2$ is a noninvasive indicator of cardiac output, with both values moving in the same direction. A $PETCO_2$ <10 mm Hg after 20 minutes of resuscitation is generally considered a reliable indicator that resuscitation will be unsuccessful.

- **Detecting incorrect placement of endotracheal tubes.**
  - When proper tracheal placement occurs, the capnogram will show a waveform. If inadvertent esophageal placement occurs, the waveform will be flat because no CO_2 is eliminated from the esophagus.
  - An alternative device to confirm correct ETT placement is a CO_2 detector. These devices respond quickly to exhaled CO_2 with a simple color change (device specific) from purple/blue to yellow. **REMEMBER:** Yellow is mellow!

- **Disconnection of the patient from the ventilator.** Because capnography directly monitors the patient and not the equipment, disconnection from the ventilator will show an *immediate* flat line on the capnogram.

- **Identifying patient's attempts to breathe while receiving paralytic agents.** There should be no movement of the diaphragm during paralysis; therefore, incomplete paralysis can be detected by a dip in the capnogram waveform, indicating an attempt at a spontaneous breath.

- **Detecting a potential diagnosis of pulmonary embolism.** When there is pulmonary dead space, the relationship between the $PaCO_2$ and the $PETCO_2$ is lost. Thus, in a condition such as a pulmonary embolism, the exhaled air from a poorly perfused part of the lung contains only a small amount of CO_2 and results in a reduced $PETCO_2$.

Two Patients with Shortness of Breath and a Potential Diagnosis of Pulmonary Emboli (PE)		
	Patient 1	**Patient 2**
$PaCO_2$	36 mm Hg	39 mm Hg
$PETCO_2$	32 mm Hg	21 mm Hg
Interpretation	No significant PE Normal $PaCO_2$–$PETCO_2$ gradient	PE should be considered Widened $PaCO_2$–$PETCO_2$ gradient

CO_2 detection during nasal cannula oxygen delivery is possible via flow through *mainstream* or sidestream capnometry, in nonintubated patients. Normal $EtCO_2$ values are 35 to 45 mm Hg, with some experts stating that as low as 30 mm Hg can be normal. Accurate measurements are often difficult in patients who are mouth breathers or who have obstructed nares, and a special sampling cannula should be utilized in this situation.

CARBON MONOXIDE POISONING *(see also Hyperbaric Oxygen, p. 186; Oxyhemoglobin Dissociation Curve, p. 194)*

Carbon monoxide, with affinity for hemoglobin 210 times greater than oxygen, combines with hemoglobin (Hgb) to form carboxyhemoglobin (COHb). Carbon monoxide impairs oxygen unloading at the tissue level, and the oxyhemoglobin dissociation

(continued)

curve shifts to the left. This results in decreased O_2 available to tissues, creating cerebral hypoxia. The patient has a characteristic cherry-red skin color and flu-like symptoms, such as headache, nausea, vomiting, fatigue, and weakness. Treatment is with 100% oxygen until all signs and symptoms resolve. Hyperbaric oxygen (HBO) therapy can be used to decrease the half-life, but because of the poor availability of HBO chambers, its use is limited.

Carboxyhemoglobin Levels

Carboxyhemoglobin Level	Symptoms
0–5%	Normal
<15%	Often in smokers, truck drivers
15–40%	Headache, some degree of confusion
40–60%	Loss of consciousness, Cheyne-Stokes respirations
50–70%	Mortality >50%

CHARLES'S LAW

Known as the law of volumes, Charles's law states that at a constant pressure, the volume of a given mass of an ideal gas will expand as the temperature rises, and likewise, the volume of the gas will contract as the temperature decreases.

$$Formula: V_1T_2 = V_2T_1$$

Example: Think of a warm can of soda. When opened, there is usually enough pressure built up within the container to cause the contents to spew all over. (Some containers will spontaneously explode if exposed to heat or direct sunlight.) Conversely, if the container were cold, very little pressure would be released.

CHEST TUBES *(see also Effusion, p. 182; Heimlich Valve, p. 184; Pneumothorax, p. 197)*

Chest tubes are used in patients who require removal of air, blood, or fluid from the pleural or mediastinal space. Tube sizes are in French (F). The smaller ones (16F–20F) are used for removing air, whereas the larger ones (22F–40F) are used for removing blood and thick drainage. The proximal end of the chest tube has eyelets to drain the air or fluid, and the distal end connects to the drainage unit. There are five basic components of the system:

1. **Collection chamber**
   Capacity 2,000 to 2,500 cc depending on model used. More than 200 mL/hr drainage usually signals a bleeding complication. Drainage fluid will overflow from one compartment to the next. When reading, note that there may be a decrease in original volume of the first compartment after fluids spill over into the next, attributed to surface tension "buildup." The actual volume of the previous compartment should be checked for accuracy if the total output is critical.
2. **Suction chamber**
   Suction is applied to the chest tube unit as ordered, usually −20 cm of water. The suction source needs to be set at typically 80 mm Hg to achieve −20 cm of water suction. If multiple chest tubes are pulling from one suction canister, increased amounts

(continued)

of wall suction may be required to achieve the ordered suction amount on all chest tube units.

- **Dry suction system set-up**
  This set up does NOT require water to be added to establish suction. Suction is achieved by dialing a suction control knob to the desired amount and applying wall suction as described above. Various chest tube suction indicators, such as floats, bellows, or displays are available on differing models, but they will all "activate" when suction is applied, confirming that the system is operational.

- **Wet suction system set-up**
  Older systems DO require the addition of water to the suction chamber to establish the prescribed suction level. Increments on the suction chamber indicate the water fill level for different amounts of suction. Apply wall suction and when gentle bubbling is noted in the suction chamber, the correct amount of suction has been applied. Excessive suction/bubbling will not achieve greater amounts of suction and will evaporate the water more quickly, requiring replacement of water more often to maintain the ordered suction level. On some systems, like the dry suction, various indicators such as floats will confirm activation of suction.

3. **Water seal chamber or one-way valve**
   Chest tubes of varying models will require either water to be added to establish a water seal, or have a one-way valve that allows air to leave the pleural cavity, but preventing it from returning and thereby maintaining a negative pressure system. If the model requires water to be added, it must be filled to a minimum of the 2-cm mark.

4. **Air leak meter**
   Some drainage units provide an air leak meter (not to be confused with a water seal) that permits air leak detection. The air leak chamber must be filled with water, usually 30 mL, to the level indicated on the unit. The meter is labeled from low (1) to high (7) on most models. The higher the numbered column through which the bubbling occurs, the greater the degree of air leak. The column beside the air leak meter usually fluctuates with breathing, which represents normal tidaling. Negative pressure can build up in this column, which may be reflected by a rising fluid level. Continuous bubbling may indicate a leak in the system (check connections), whereas intermittent bubbling that fluctuates with respirations is mostly likely caused by the lung.

5. **High negativity relief valve**
   This valve is provided to vent excessive negativity. If pressed, filtered air will enter the unit. Use caution! If suction is not operative (gravity drainage), depressing this valve can reduce the negative pressure within the collection chamber to zero (atmosphere) and result in a possible pneumothorax. The need for use of this valve is rare. Stripping or milking thoracic chest tubes can cause excessive negativity, and using this valve will restore prescribed levels. Some units feature an indicator window with a picture of a palm tree or the word "yes" when proper negativity exists. This icon should appear continuously while the patient is to suction but may appear intermittently during gravity drainage.

TROUBLESHOOTING

1. **Specimen collection**
   Using a standard luer lock syringe, specimens should be taken from the needleless self-sealing sampling port found *in the connector* on the chest tube. The connector and the syringe can be inverted to facilitate sample collection. (*Important:* DO NOT take the

(*continued*)

specimen from the tubing itself, as tubing is NOT self-sealing, and a needle puncture could cause an air leak.)

2. **Accidental removal of chest tube, from insert site**
   Cover the site with a dry, sterile dressing. If you hear air leaking from the site, tape the dressing on only three sides to allow the escape of air and to prevent a tension pneumothorax. Call the physician, and prepare for a new chest tube insertion.

3. **Inadvertent disconnection from drainage unit**
   Submerge the distal end of the chest tube in about 1 inch of sterile 0.9% NaCl to create a liquid seal until a new drainage unit can be prepped and attached. DO NOT CLAMP.

4. **Drainage unit is full and needs to be changed**
   After prepping a new drainage unit, remove the current one from suction. Clamp the chest tube with a rubber-tipped hemostat, or the clamp provided on the tubing, and disconnect from the old unit. (*Caution:* Be sure that suction is OFF before you clamp the tube! Clamping while suction is still on could cause a pneumothorax.) Quickly connect to the new unit, unclamp the tube, and resume suction.

5. **Unit has tipped; drainage spilled into other compartments of collection chamber**
   There are two alternatives. One is to change the drainage unit to a new one, another is to mark each chamber appropriately and add all the amounts together to determine total drainage.

CHEST X-RAY FILM *(see Part 10, p. 360)*

CHRONIC OBSTRUCTIVE PULMONARY DISEASE

Chronic obstructive pulmonary disease (COPD) is a group of respiratory diseases that obstruct the pathway of normal alveolar ventilation, by either spasm of the airways, mucous secretions, or morphopathologic changes of airways and/or alveoli. The three most common are (1) chronic bronchitis, (2) pulmonary emphysema, and (3) bronchial asthma.

Signs typically include elevated pulmonary artery pressures, peaked P on electrocardiograph (EKG) tracing (pulmonary hypertension causes right atrial enlargement and position change), incomplete right bundle branch block, increased functional residual capacity (and barrel chest), multifocal atrial tachycardia (due to hypoxia and right ventricular strain), and compensatory polycythemia (increase in red blood cells [RBCs] to increase the hematocrit).

Treatment is to first treat the hypoxia with vigorous pulmonary toilet and postural toilet, then give IPPB therapy (to aerate alveoli and remove CO_2), bronchodilator therapy, mucolytic agents, antibiotics (usually ampicillin), or steroids. The Venturi mask delivers most controlled O_2 for patient.

CLOSED PNEUMOTHORAX *(see Pneumothorax, p. 197)*

CO₂ MONITORING *(see Capnography, p. 176)*

COMBITUBE

The combitube is a unique device used to facilitate emergency or difficult intubation of a patient. It does not require visualization of the larynx and is a double lumen tube, with

(continued)

one blind end. Once placed, inflation of the cuff allows the device to function as an endotracheal tube, and closes off the esophagus allowing for ventilation and preventing reflux of gastric contents.

COMPLIANCE

Static compliance is a measurement of the elastic properties of the lung, usually measured while patient is using the ventilator. Reduction in compliance also tends to reduce patient's tidal volume and increase breathing frequency to overcome the work of moving large volumes of air. To calculate:

Tidal volume ÷ (peak plateau pressure − PEEP)
Normal: (textbook) 100 mL/cm H_2O
       (usually) 50 mL/cm H_2O

Dynamic compliance is a measurement to evaluate the work of breathing or the amount of force needed to overcome airway resistance. To calculate:

Tidal volume ÷ (peak inspiratory pressure − PEEP)
Normal: 45 to 50 mL/cm H_2O

Studies have shown that as ratios of dead space to tidal volume are increased, compliance falls, which indicates that the patient's status is deteriorating.

CONTROLLED MANDATORY VENTILATION
(see Ventilator Modes, p. 212)

COPD *(see Chronic Obstructive Pulmonary Disease, p. 180)*

CPAP *(see Ventilator Modes, p. 212; BiPAP Ventilator Support, p. 174)*

CUFF MEASUREMENT *(see Endotracheal Tube Placement, p. 183)*

DALTON'S LAW

Known as the law of partial pressures, Dalton's law states that the total pressure of a mixture of gasses is equal to the sum of the partial pressures of each individual component of the gas mixture.

Example: Think of a bag filled with an equal amount of marbles and popcorn. You squeeze the bag tightly, over and over again. Eventually, the popcorn will compress more than the marbles, and the proportion of marbles to popcorn kernels will change. Dalton's law says this will NOT happen with gases. Mixed gases will *always* stay in the same proportion under pressure, and *none* will compress any more than others.

$$\text{Formula: Pressure}_{total} = \text{Pressure}_1 + \text{Pressure}_2 + \cdots + \text{Pressure}_3$$

DEAD SPACE

Dead space is a measurement to determine total wasted ventilation, or that which is ineffective in gas exchange. It is normally one third of tidal volume, but this may increase markedly in the late phase of ARDS or in pulmonary embolism.

DEEP VEIN THROMBOSIS *(see Pulmonary Embolism, p. 200)*

DYNAMIC COMPLIANCE *(see Compliance, p. 181)*

EBUS (Endobronchial Ultrasound) *(see Part 10, p. 363)*

EFFUSION *(see also Pneumothorax, p. 197; Thoracentesis in Part 4, p. 241)*

Also known as hydrothorax, effusion is clinically the same as pneumothorax, but an effusion has fluid infiltrates instead of air. An empyema has pus-like fluid. On x-ray film, a pleural effusion shows blunting of the costophrenic angle, silhouetting of the diaphragm, and meniscus sign (a crescent-shaped inclusion of air surrounded by consolidated lung tissue).

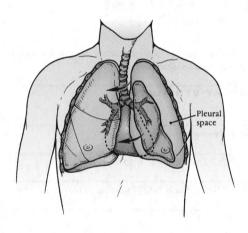

Pleural space

■ Pleural effusion. Fluid has collected in the pleural space and has displaced lung tissue. Also note shift of fluid into the mediastinum and torsion of the bronchus.

EMBOLISM *(see Pulmonary Embolism, p. 200)*

EMPHYSEMA *(see also Chronic Obstructive Pulmonary Disease, p. 180)*

From the Greek for "inflation," emphysema is an obstructive respiratory disorder characterized by air trapped in overdistended alveoli and by collapse of bronchioles on expiration, causing prolonged expiratory outflow. The lungs are hyperresonant on chest percussion. Even if disease is severe, patient maintains a normal gas exchange and often has an elevated hematocrit; thus, the term "pink puffer" is often applied.

EMPYEMA *(see Effusion, p. 182)*

END TIDAL CO$_2$ MONITORING *(see Capnography, p. 176)*

ENDOBRONCHIAL ULTRASOUND *(see Part 10, p. 363)*

ENDOTRACHEAL TUBE PLACEMENT

Nasotracheal tube size: Usual 7.5 internal diameter (ID)
Endotracheal tube size: Adult female: Usual 7.0 to 8.0 ID (internal diameter)
Adult male: Usual 7.5 to 8.5 ID (internal diameter)
Endotracheal tube placement: 2 to 3 cm above the carina

Rule of thumb: Depth = 3 × the ID (internal diameter)

REMEMBER:

21 (cm) is lots of fun
22 (cm) will sometimes do
23 (cm) will seldom be

Cuff pressures: Usual 20 to 25 mm Hg; optimum is enough air to barely seal trachea

<20 mm Hg = risk of aspiration, VAP
>25 mm Hg = risk of tracheal damage

EXTUBATION CRITERIA *(see Weaning Parameters, p. 215)*

FICK PRINCIPLE *(see also Swan-Ganz: Hemodynamic Normals in Part 2, p. 156)*

Gas diffusion in the lung is described by Fick as "the total uptake or release of a substance by an organ is the product of the blood flow to the organ and of the arteriovenous concentrations of the substance."* This principle implies, then, that the cardiac output per minute from the right ventricle (and consequently the left ventricle) can be determined by measuring the amount of blood pumped by the right ventricle into the lung capillaries in 1 minute. Hence the formula:

$$\frac{O_2 \text{ absorption mL/min} (\dot{V}O_2)}{\begin{array}{cc} O_2 \text{ content of} & - & O_2 \text{ content of} \\ \text{arterial blood} & & \text{mixed venous blood} \\ (CaO_2) & & (C\bar{v}O_2) \end{array}} = \text{Cardiac output (CO)}$$

Fick, 1870.

FLAIL CHEST

Flail chest is an injury in which two or more ribs are fractured in several places, causing instability of the chest wall and subsequent respiratory impairment. Because the injured portion of the chest wall no longer has a bony connection with the rest of the rib cage, when the chest wall expands during inspiration, the detached part of the chest (flail segment) is drawn in, and the mediastinum shifts away from the affected side. On expiration, the positive pressure pushes the flail segment outward, pulling the mediastinum toward the affected side and causing difficulty in exhaling. Usually, the injured ribs heal without intervention.

REMEMBER:

Inspiration: Chest wall moves **in.** Mediastinum moves **away** from affected side.
Expiration: Chest wall moves **out.** Mediastinum moves **toward** affected side.

(continued)

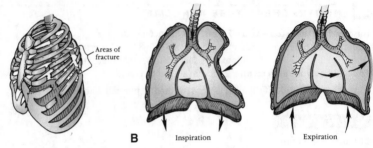

A   **B**   Inspiration   Expiration

■ A, Chest wall injury that can produce flail chest abnormality. B, Physiology of flail chest abnormality, resulting in paradoxical breathing.

Treatment: Chest tube insertion may be required particularly in patients receiving positive pressure ventilation, as they are at increased risk of developing a pneumothorax. Effective analgesia is mandatory to help prevent respiratory decompensation caused by atelectasis and retained secretions.

FORCED VITAL CAPACITY *(see Weaning Parameters, p. 215)*

FREMITUS

Fremitus is a vibration that can be palpated when a patient speaks. Sound is best produced through solid material, therefore:

Increased fremitus = lung consolidation, atelectasis
Decreased fremitus = pneumothorax, emphysema, effusions

REMEMBER:

If you knock on a solid table, the sound is greater than if you knock on air.

FUNCTIONAL RESIDUAL CAPACITY *(see Lung Volumes, p. 189)*

GREENFIELD VENA CAVA FILTER *(see Inferior Vena Cava Filter, p. 188)*

HEIMLICH VALVE *(see also Chest Tubes, p. 178)*

If a patient has a small, uncomplicated pneumothorax with little or no drainage that does not require suction, the chest tube frequently is connected to a Heimlich valve instead of a traditional drainage unit. The Heimlich is a small, mobile, one-way flutter valve, composed of a piece of latex rubber tubing inside a round plastic housing with connectors on both ends. The blue end should connect to the chest tube, with the arrow pointing *away* from the patient's chest. (Incorrect placement could cause the tube to trap air, resulting in a life-threatening pneumothorax.) The clear end of the valve either hangs free or is connected to a vented bag, allowing air to escape. As the patient exhales, the positive pressure generated by the air leaving the chest enters the tubing, causing the valve to open so that air can be released. During inspiration, the tube collapses on itself, preventing air from reentering.

(continued)

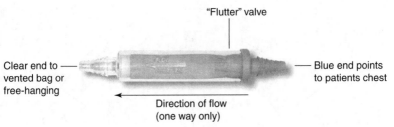

"Flutter" valve

Clear end to vented bag or free-hanging

Blue end points to patients chest

Direction of flow (one way only)

■ Heimlich valve. (Courtesy and © Becton, Dickinson and Company.)

HELIOX THERAPY

Helium and oxygen mixtures (heliox) have a lower gas density than air or air mixed with supplemental oxygen. Thus, heliox therapy is thought to be of benefit to obstructive lung diseases because the low density will result in a decrease in resistive forces and improve the delivery of oxygen to distal airways. Usually administered via a nonrebreathing oxygen mask, and sometimes with supplemental oxygen via a nasal cannula, the helium/oxygen mixture can range from a high of 80:20 to a low of 50:50 before being weaned off.

HEMOTHORAX *(see Pneumothorax, p. 197)*

HENDERSON-HASSELBALCH EQUATION

The Henderson-Hasselbalch equation is a method of calculating the pH of a buffer system. In medicine, it is used to calculate any one of the three parameters of acid-base balance: pH, $PaCO_2$, or bicarbonate.

$$pH = 6.1 + \log \frac{(HCO_3^- \ mEq/L)}{(0.03 \times PaCO_2)}$$

As long as the ratio of carbonic acid (H_2CO_3) to bicarbonate (HCO_3^-) is approximately 1:20, the pH of blood is normal. It is this ratio that determines the blood pH, rather than the absolute values of each.

(continued)

NOTES

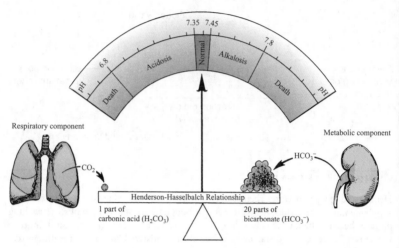

■ Henderson-Hasselbalch relationship, demonstrating mechanisms for the defense against changes in body fluid pH.

HENRY'S LAW

Simply stated, this law of physical chemistry proposes that at a constant temperature, the weight of a gas dissolved by a liquid is directly proportional to the pressure of the gas on the liquid. Example: Think of a bottle of champagne. Prior to opening, CO_2 contained inside the bottle is at a pressure slightly higher than atmospheric. However, when the cork is "popped," the gas escapes and the pressure above the liquid in the bottle decreases. Eventually, if the champagne is allowed to remain open, the concentration of CO_2 in the bottle will equilibrate to the CO_2 in the air (and the champagne will go flat!).

HYDROTHORAX *(see Effusion, p. 182)*

HYPERBARIC OXYGEN

Hyperbaric oxygen therapy (HBOT) is a treatment used to saturate the tissues with oxygen and hopefully reverse any areas of hypoxia. It is administered by placing the patient in a sealed chamber and having them breathe 100% oxygen while under increased atmospheric pressure. It is effective against tissue infection such as chronic leg ulcers or gas gangrene. Unfortunately, after prolonged use, it induces endarteritis obliterans of small arterioles, defeating the benefits of the therapy. It is used occasionally in life-threatening cases of carbon monoxide poisoning by increasing the dissolved oxygen to maintain life while the carbon monoxide is displaced from hemoglobin.

HYPERCAPNIA

Hypercapnia is increased carbon dioxide in the blood resulting from hypoventilation caused by respiratory muscle weakness, neurologic disease states, or drugs. With an increase in CO_2 production, the CO_2 diffuses rapidly into the blood. The pH falls, respirations increase, and respiratory acidosis results. Treatment is based on increasing alveolar ventilation.

HYPOCAPNIA

Hypocapnia is caused by hyperventilation resulting from pain, anxiety, liver disease, or central nervous system (CNS) events. The increased alveolar ventilation results in decreased CO_2 and increased pH. Treatment is to slow the respiratory rate and decrease the tidal volume, if the latter is high.

HYPOXEMIA *(see also Hypoxia, p. 187)*

Hypoxemia is a deficiency of O_2 tension in arterial blood, threatening tissue oxygenation. However, normal tissue oxygenation, even though hypoxemia is present, is possible through the compensatory mechanisms of (1) right shift of the oxyhemoglobin dissociation curve, (2) increase in hemoglobin, or (3) increase in cardiac output.

HYPOXIA *(see also Hypoxemia, p. 187; Carbon Monoxide Poisoning, p. 177)*

Hypoxia is a deficiency of O_2 at the cellular level caused by low cardiac output, arterial hypoxemia, or severe anemia. It results in anaerobic metabolism and lactic acidosis (regional or systemic). Treatment is to restore the O_2 deficiency with supplemental oxygen.

INCENTIVE SPIROMETRY

An effective exercise for prophylaxis against respiratory complications in high-risk patients. There is increased retention of how to perform the exercise if taught preoperatively.

Incentive Spirometry Do's and Don'ts

Do's
- Prior to starting IS exercises:
  - Provide oral care.
  - Manage pain.
  - Sit the patient as upright as possible.
  - Educate that the reason for IS is to fully inflate the lungs, thereby preventing pulmonary complications.
- Complete IS every hour; 5–10 consecutive times.
- Begin therapy as soon as possible.
  NOTE: Atelectasis can begin within one hour after surgery.
- Teach to:
  - breathe in with a controlled effort.
  - maintain the reading within the optimal range on the flow rate guide or indicator.
  - hold breath for 3–5 seconds at maximum inspiration.
  - splint incision to decrease pain during cough effort
- Assess breath sounds before and after therapy.
- Clean mouthpiece with water after use.

Don'ts
- Allow patient to use IS without proper instruction.
- Place the device out of reach.
- Allow more than two hours to lapse without reassessing IS efforts and attainment of inspiratory goal.
- Allow patient to take short, sharp inspiratory breaths . . . this is ineffective!

(continued)

Incentive Spirometry Nomogram

Height	58" (147 cm)	62" (158 cm)	66" (168 cm)	72" (183 cm)	76" (193 cm)
Age	Expected inspiratory capacity (mL) male/female				
20	2,350/2,250	2,700/2,550	3,050/2,900	3,550/3,350	3,900/na
40	2,200/1,950	2,550/2,250	2,900/2,600	3,400/3,050	3,750/na
60	2,050/1,650	2,400/1,950	2,750/2,300	3,250/2,750	3,600/na
80	1,900/1,350	2,200/1,650	2,550/2,000	3,100/2,450	3,450/na

INFERIOR VENA CAVA FILTER

An IVC filter is a small metal device implanted in the vena cava designed to protect against pulmonary embolism by trapping blood clots before they can be transported to the lung. Blood can still flow around the filter, and any clots that are "captured" eventually dissolve through the natural process of lysis. While 80% of the filters placed are because of deep vein thrombosis, other conditions such as failure/contraindication to anticoagulation, or a high risk of pulmonary embolism are accepted criteria. Typically done in the Interventional Radiology Department, the procedure is relatively noncomplicated and requires less than an hour to complete. The filter is inserted percutaneously, usually through the internal jugular or femoral vein, and complications are rare. Most filters are permanent, but more recently, some filters are available that are "retrievable." They are fitted with a "snaring" device (which varies from model to model) to allow them to be pulled back into a sheath and removed from the body. Previously, filters that were in the IVC for less than 3 weeks were considered retrievable, but with advanced technology, some models can now remain for as long as a year.

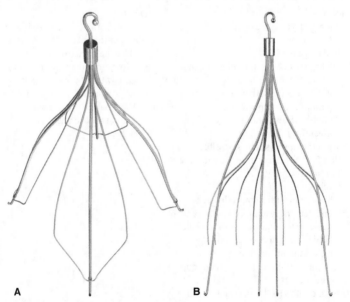

A   B

■ Cook inferior vena cava filters. A, Tulip. B, Celect. (Courtesy of Cook Medical, Bloomington, Indiana.)

(continued)

REMEMBER:

- The filter is made of a metal that has been used for years to make surgical implants such as hip, knee, and heart valves. The body will NOT reject the filter.
- The small amount of metal in the filter is MRI compatible; however, the technician needs to know that it exists.
- The filter will NOT trigger a metal detector.

INHALATION MEDICATIONS
(see Respiratory Inhalation Medications, p. 202)

INTERMITTENT MANDATORY VENTILATION
(see Ventilator Modes, p. 213)

INVERSE RATIO VENTILATION *(see Ventilator Modes, p. 213)*

ISOETHARINE *(see Respiratory Inhalation Medications, p. 202)*

ISUPREL *(see Respiratory Inhalation Medications, p. 202)*

IVC FILTER *(see Inferior Vena Cava Filter, p. 188)*

LACTATE LEVELS *(see Part 9, p. 355)*

LEVALBUTEROL *(see Respiratory Inhalation Medications, p. 202)*

LUNG SOUNDS *(see Breath Sounds, p. 175)*

LUNG VOLUMES *(see also Weaning Parameters, p. 215)*

Lung volumes are divided into four "volumes" and four "capacities." A capacity is a calculated value, based on the sum of two parameters. The most important for adequate gas exchange are (1) inspiratory reserve volume (IRV), (2) tidal volume (VT), and (3) functional residual capacity (FRC).

(continued)

NOTES

Residual Volume (RV)
Air that remains in the lungs at the end of maximum exhalation. Approximately 1,200 mL.

Expiratory Reserve Volume (ERV)
Maximum volume of air that can be exhaled after a normal exhalation to residual volume. Usually one third of VC, or approximately 1,200 mL.

Functional Residual Capacity (FRC)
Sum of RV + ERV
Volume of air in lungs after normal expiration. Serves as a gas reservoir and maintains alveoli in their partially expanded state. Approximately 2,400 mL.

Inspiratory Reserve Volume (IRV)
Maximum volume of air that can be inhaled after a tidal breath has been taken. Allows for a sigh to reinflate partially collapsed alveoli. Approximately 3,600 mL.

Total Lung Capacity (TLC)
Sum of all lung volumes
Volume of air in lungs after a maximal inspiration. Approximately 6,000 mL.

Inspiratory Capacity(IC)
Sum of IRV + VT
Maximum volume of gas inspired from resting expiratory level. Usually two thirds of VC, or approximately 3,600 mL.

Tidal Volume (VT)
The volume of gas moved in or out of the lungs in a normal resting breath. Inspiration delivers new atmospheric gas to the lungs, and expiration removes carbon dioxide. A general estimate of normal VT is 10 mL/kg of body weight, or approximately 500 mL.

Vital Capacity (VC)
Sum of ERV + IC
Maximum volume of air exhaled after maximum inspiration. Can be approximated at 65 mL/kg of body weight, or approximately 4,800 mL. (A decrease of VC in the neuromuscularly diseased patient indicates that the patient is unable to cough or move secretions. Not true, however, if decrease is due to restrictive lung disease.)

■ Lung volumes.

(*continued*)

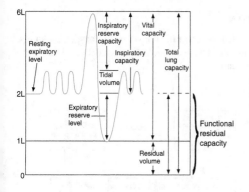

■ Pulmonary function test measurements showing normal lung volumes and capacity.

MECHANICAL VENTILATION *(see Ventilator Modes, p. 212)*

METAPROTERENOL SULFATE
(see Respiratory Inhalation Medications, p. 203)

MINUTE VENTILATION *(see Weaning Parameters, p. 215)*

MIXED VENOUS ABGs *(see also S$\bar{v}O_2$ Monitoring in Part 2, p. 151)*

Mixed venous ABGs refers to blood gases in a blood sample that indicate a complete mixing of the blood, that is, blood returned from the extremities to the right ventricle. This may sometimes be sampled from a central venous line, though even in the superior vena cava or right atrium, the mixing is incomplete. To be accurate, the sample must be obtained from the distal lumen of a pulmonary artery catheter.

Mixed Venous ABG Values	
pH	7.31–7.41
PCO$_2$ mm Hg	41–51
PO$_2$ mm Hg	35–42
O$_2$ saturation%	68–77
HCO$_3^-$ mEq/L	22–26

NITROGEN WASHOUT *(see Atelectasis, p. 173)*

OBSTRUCTIVE DISEASES *(see Chronic Obstructive Pulmonary Disease, p. 180)*

OPEN PNEUMOTHORAX *(see Pneumothorax, p. 197)*

OXYGEN CONSUMPTION

Oxygen consumption calculation is used to determine the volume of oxygen consumed by the body tissues per minute, as indicated by the amount of oxygen delivered minus the amount of oxygen returned after circulation.

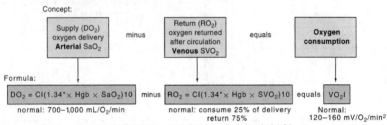

Concept:

| Supply (DO_2) oxygen delivery **Arterial** SaO_2 | minus | Return (RO_2) oxygen returned after circulation **Venous** SVO_2 | equals | **Oxygen consumption** |

Formula:

$$DO_2 = CI(1.34^* \times Hgb \times SaO_2)10 \quad minus \quad RO_2 = CI(1.34^* \times Hgb \times SVO_2)10 \quad equals \quad VO_2I$$

normal: 700–1,000 mL/O_2/min   normal: consume 25% of delivery   Normal:
                                                        return 75%   120–160 mV/O_2/min^2

*Some sources cite 1.39 as oxygen carrying capacity instead of 1.34.

Transport pattern examples:

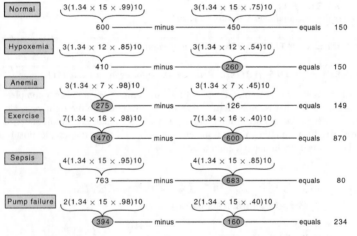

Normal	$3(1.34 \times 15 \times .99)10$		$3(1.34 \times 15 \times .75)10$		
	600	minus	450	equals	150
Hypoxemia	$3(1.34 \times 12 \times .85)10$		$3(1.34 \times 12 \times .54)10$		
	410	minus	(260)	equals	150
Anemia	$3(1.34 \times 7 \times .98)10$		$3(1.34 \times 7 \times .45)10$		
	(275)	minus	126	equals	149
Exercise	$7(1.34 \times 16 \times .98)10$		$7(1.34 \times 16 \times .40)10$		
	(1470)	minus	(600)	equals	870
Sepsis	$4(1.34 \times 15 \times .95)10$		$4(1.34 \times 15 \times .85)10$		
	763	minus	(683)	equals	80
Pump failure	$2(1.34 \times 15 \times .98)10$		$2(1.34 \times 15 \times .40)10$		
	(394)	minus	(160)	equals	234

■ Oxygen consumption. Circled numbers indicate parameter out of balance.

OXYGEN DELIVERY SYSTEMS AND CONVERSIONS

Oxygen Delivery Systems and Conversions

Low Flow FiO_2/Lpm (Gross Estimates)

Nasal Catheter or Cannula

1 Lpm	24%
2 Lpm	28%
3 Lpm	32%
4 Lpm	36%
5 Lpm	40%
6 Lpm	44%

Mask (Simple)

5–6 Lpm	40%
6–7 Lpm	50%
7–8 Lpm	60%

Partial Rebreather

Similar to simple face mask but has side ports covered with discs to prevent room air from entering the mask. Also has a soft reservoir bag that conserves the first 1/3 of exhaled air but allows the remaining 2/3 to escape.

6 Lpm	35%
8 Lpm	50%
10 Lpm	60%

Nonrebreather

Similar to partial rebreather, with side ports covered with discs to prevent room air from entering the mask. However, the nonbreather differs in that the nonrebreather reservoir bag has a one-way valve to prevent the exhaled air from entering the bag and facilitating a larger concentration of O_2 to collect for the patient to inhale.

6 Lpm	60%
8 Lpm	80%

Venturi Mask

A mask similar to the simple face mask, but the tubing that connects to the O_2 source is larger and has interchangeable colored adapters to change the O_2 concentration, allowing for a more controlled delivery of FiO_2.

4 Lpm	24%
6 Lpm	28%
8 Lpm	35%
10 Lpm	40%

Lpm, liters per minute.

OXYGEN TOXICITY

Oxygen toxicity is best thought of as the truly poisonous effect of the drug oxygen on the whole body. It develops after a person has breathed 100% oxygen for longer than 12 hours. It can occur with an FiO_2 below 100%, but a longer time. An FiO_2 below 60% is probably safe for weeks. To avoid toxicity, however, the PaO_2 should be maintained at the lowest concentration possible, and the use of PEEP should be considered. Transfuse red blood cells to patients with anemia.

Symptoms of oxygen toxicity include dyspnea, decreased compliance, an increase in the A-a gradient, and paresthesia in the extremities. Retrosternal pain occurs in some patients after they have received 100% oxygen for as little as 6 hours. Complications from oxygen toxicity are on the decline with the sophisticated ventilation systems of today, although occasionally edema and ARDS may result.

OXYHEMOGLOBIN DISSOCIATION CURVE

The oxyhemoglobin dissociation curve, a graph of great physiologic importance, demonstrates the relationship between PO_2 and O_2 saturation. The shape of the curve represents the protective mechanisms in health and disease. When there are large changes in the arterial PO_2 (upper portion of graph), there are only small changes in the oxygen saturation. The lower, steeper portion of the curve shows that as hemoglobin becomes desaturated from 70% downward, large amounts of O_2 are released for use by tissues with proportionally less change in PO_2. Thus, the significance of the curve shows that

- A shift to the *left* means the RBCs hold on to oxygen (difficult to unload), less O_2 is delivered to the tissues, and therefore the *O_2 saturation increases.*

Causes: Alkalosis, hypothermia, decreased $PaCO_2$, drop in 2,3-DPG, hyperventilation, high altitude breathing, carbon monoxide poisoning, methemoglobinemia (abnormal hemoglobin).

REMEMBER:

Left = aLkaLosis (coLd and Low) or "left latches on" (holds on to O_2 and does not release it to tissues).

- A shift to the right means the RBCs readily release oxygen (better unloading at tissue level), and therefore the O_2 saturation readings decrease *(tissues* are OK, even though PO_2 and SaO_2 are low).

Causes: Acidosis, fever, increased $PaCO_2$, or a rise in 2,3-DPG

REMEMBER:

A shift to the **right** is **right** for the patient or "right releases." (The O_2 saturation may be down, but less oxygen is bound to the RBCs and more oxygen is available to the tissues.)

(*continued*)

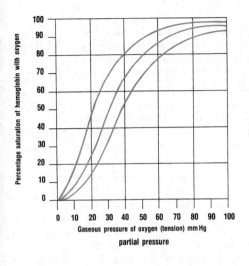

■ Right and left shifts of oxyhe-moglobin dissociation curve.

OXYMIZER OXYGEN CONSERVING DEVICE

With the Oxymizer oxygen conserving device, oxygen is usually administered via a nasal cannula, with flow continuing throughout the respiratory cycle. However, the greatest benefit of oxygen therapy occurs during early inspiration, with much of the remaining oxygen lost to the surrounding environment. The Oxymizer is a device worn in the same manner as a cannula but includes a collapsible reservoir, which captures incoming oxygen during expiration. The oxygen captured in this reservoir is then inhaled by the patient during the first instant of the next inspiration, providing an extra-rich supply of oxygen and conserving the supply as well. Flow rates may be one fourth to one fifth the amount used with a nonoxygen conserving cannula.

P/F RATIO *(see A-a Gradient, p. 167)*

PEEP *(see Ventilator Modes, p. 213)*

PICKWICKIAN SYNDROME

Initially, "Pickwickian" was used to describe obese, hypersomnolent patients. In 1956, however, the obesity hypoventilation syndrome (OHS), or Pickwickian syndrome, was identified as having principal clinical features. It has since remained the focus of much physiologic interest.

Patients are identified by:
- Marked increase in abdominal contents, raising the diaphragm
- Increased chest wall weight
- Fatty deposits within the diaphragm and intercostal muscles, resulting in decreased strength of respiratory effort
- Chronic hypercapnia (decreased FVC, RLV, ERV, FRC, usually without obstruction to flow)

(continued)

- Often associated with sleep apnea
- Marked polycythemia (leading to risk of venous thrombosis and PE)
- Chronic hypoxemia (resulting in severe pulmonary hypertension, cor pulmonale, valvular insufficiency, acute hepatic engorgement, massive peripheral edema)
- Elevated pulmonary artery wedge pressure (suggesting left ventricular dysfunction)

Although many obese patients have chronic hypercapnia and low ventilation, true "Pickwickians" are unable to have their CO_2 corrected with treatment. They represent a syndrome of chronic alveolar hypoventilation of unknown cause, without intrinsic lung disease. Whether the defect is acquired, results from a congenital abnormality of ventilatory control, or represents an extreme in the spectrum of the normal population has not yet been determined.

PLEURODESIS

When a patient has *severe, recurrent* pleural effusions (frequently related to a diagnosis of cancer) chemical pleurodesis is performed to deliberately cause the membranes of the lung to "stick together" and thus prevent reaccumulation of fluid. Initially a chest tube is placed and all fluid is drained over the course of 2 to 5 days. A sclerosing agent is then injected into the pleural space via the chest tube, and the tube is closed. Ultimately, the pleura will become irritated, inflamed, and as an end result, "stick together." The chest tube is then reopened and the sclerosing agent is removed. However, the chest tube will remain in place for a period of several days, to ensure that all the fluid has drained. Once the drainage has ceased, the chest tube is removed, and the wound edges are sutured. The procedure is a painful one, and patients are generally premedicated with a sedative and analgesic. Sometimes a local anesthetic is instilled into the pleural space, or an epidural catheter may be placed. Successful performance of this procedure, however, will relieve patient symptoms of pleural effusion and improve the quality of life.

Pleurodesis Common Sclerosing Agents

Agent	Success Rate (%)
Talc	90–96
Nitrogen Mustard	52
Doxycycline	90
Bleomycin	84
Quinacrine	70–90

PNEUMONIA *(see also Effusion, p. 182)*

Pneumonia is an acute inflammation of the lung(s) caused by a respiratory infection. Best positioning for oxygenation is with good lung **down.**

Pathophysiology: Inflammation (infection) of alveoli leads to consolidation of lung. Exudates fill the alveoli. VQ mismatch and shunt may result and pleural effusions may develop.

Treatment: Antibiotic therapy (preferably starting <6 hours after presentation), antivirals for influenza or varicella, antifungals, and supportive therapy to include oxygenation, hydration, antipyretics, and analgesics.

(continued)

Nosocomial pneumonia is associated with a morbidity and mortality rate in excess of 30%. Studies have shown that patients with pneumonia caused by *Pseudomonas aeruginosa* and *Staphylococcus aureus* are at greatest risk for treatment failure. Accordingly, early identification becomes increasingly important, and prevention is primary.

PNEUMOTHORAX

A pneumothorax is a collection of air in the pleural space that disrupts negative pressure. There are several forms.

An **open pneumothorax** ("sucking chest wound") occurs when the outer chest wall is damaged and allows air to enter the lung. If the size of the hole in the chest wall is significantly smaller than the trachea, the patient can usually tolerate it for a short time. The air moving in and out contributes nothing to gas exchange, however, and inhibits lung expansion and increases the work of breathing. Treatment includes placement of chest tubes and an occlusive chest wall dressing.

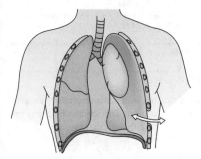

■ Open pneumothorax. (Hood, R. M. [1989]. Pre-hospital management, initial evaluation, and resuscitation. In R. M. Hood, A. D. Boyd, & A. T. Culliford [Eds.], *Thoracic trauma* [p. 14]. Philadelphia: WB Saunders. Reprinted with permission.)

A **closed pneumothorax** (spontaneous) occurs when the outer chest wall is intact, but damaged visceral pleura allow air to enter with no place to exit. It is usually caused by the rupture of a small bleb (an enlarged air sac) on the surface of the lung, overdistension of alveoli, rupture of diseased lung, or trauma during central line placement. If the initial leak is small and no more air enters, the pneumothorax resolves spontaneously in a few days. If, however, the leak continues, more air enters, the pressure builds, and a tension pneumothorax results.

A **tension pneumothorax** occurs when air cannot be evacuated from the pleura, and the mediastinum is forced to the opposite side, sometimes causing collapse of the opposite lung as well. There is decreased cardiac output and decreased venous return. A tension pneumothorax is often related to PEEP, usually >15 cm H_2O (if the tidal volume used is too large).

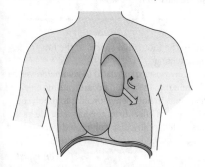

■ Tension pneumothorax. (Hood, R. M. [1989]. Pre-hospital management, initial evaluation, and resuscitation. In R. M. Hood, A. D. Boyd, & A. T. Culliford [Eds.], *Thoracic trauma* [p. 14]. Philadelphia: WB Saunders. Reprinted with permission.)

(*continued*)

A **hemothorax** is the same as a pneumothorax, but with a collection of blood instead of air.

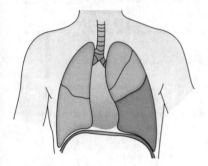

■ Massive hemothorax. (Hood, R. M. [1989]. Pre-hospital management, initial evaluation, and resuscitation. In R. M. Hood, A. D. Boyd, & A. T. Culliford [Eds.], *Thoracic trauma* [p. 14]. Philadelphia: WB Saunders. Reprinted with permission.)

PRESSURE CONTROL *(see Ventilator Modes, p. 214)*

PRESSURE SUPPORT *(see Ventilator Modes, p. 214)*

PRONE POSITIONING *(see also ARDS, p. 170)*

This technique is used to improve oxygenation in patients with acute respiratory distress syndrome (ARDS) who are receiving mechanical ventilation. The specific mechanisms responsible for oxygenation improvements are uncertain, although there are several possibilities:

- Improved ventilation-perfusion matching
- Changes in lung mass and shape
- Alterations in chest wall compliance
- Mobilization of secretions
- Improvement in functional reserve capacity

The optimal length of time a patient is required to remain in the prone position and the frequency of repositioning to supine have not yet been determined, although studies show that a prone position of 6 or more hours daily for 10 days improves oxygenation but does not improve survival. Overall, prone positioning improves oxygenation for 60% to 70% of ARDS patients.

PROVENTIL *(see Respiratory Inhalation Medications, p. 202)*

PULMONARY EDEMA

Pulmonary edema is the accumulation of fluid in the interstitial spaces of the lung or in the air spaces themselves, causing impaired gas exchange.

High-pressure pulmonary edema (cardiogenic, hydrostatic) is related to volume/pressure overload of pulmonary system. Transudation of fluid into the alveoli occurs, causing an elevation of colloid osmotic pressure. This, in turn, results in fluid being forced into the alveoli. One cause of the increased capillary pressure is the dam effect from the left ventricle back through the pulmonary circulation that occurs in left ventricular failure and pericardial disease. The cornerstone of treatment is 100% O_2, furosemide (Lasix), and morphine.

(continued)

Low-pressure pulmonary edema (neurogenic [NPE], noncardiogenic) is related to the increased permeability of the pulmonary capillary membrane caused by ARDS, increased intracranial pressure, hemorrhage, trauma, or stroke. It usually develops within a few hours of a well-defined neurologic insult. Although the pathophysiology is not completely understood, because the most common neurologic events are associated with increased intracranial pressure, intracranial hypertension is considered a key etiologic factor. The treatment strategy focuses on the underlying cause rather than on morphine or Lasix. Some institutions use agents such as α-adrenergic antagonists, β-adrenergic blockers, dobutamine, and chlorpromazine, but assessment of their effectiveness is difficult because NPE usually resolves spontaneously within 48 to 72 hours in most affected persons.

Both types of edema are characterized by dyspnea, cough, orthopnea, anxiety, cyanosis, sweating, pink frothy sputum, and, very often, chest pressure.

Pathophysiology of pulmonary edema (oversimplified):

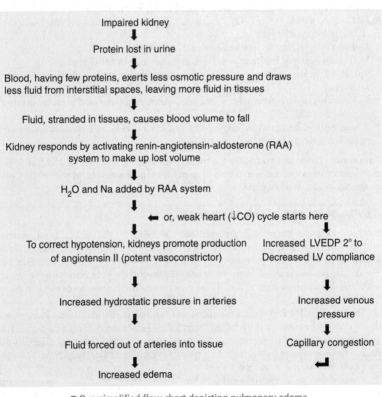

Impaired kidney
↓
Protein lost in urine
↓
Blood, having few proteins, exerts less osmotic pressure and draws less fluid from interstitial spaces, leaving more fluid in tissues
↓
Fluid, stranded in tissues, causes blood volume to fall
↓
Kidney responds by activating renin-angiotensin-aldosterone (RAA) system to make up lost volume
↓
H_2O and Na added by RAA system
↓
← or, weak heart (↓CO) cycle starts here

To correct hypotension, kidneys promote production of angiotensin II (potent vasoconstrictor)   Increased LVEDP 2° to Decreased LV compliance
↓
Increased hydrostatic pressure in arteries   Increased venous pressure
↓
Fluid forced out of arteries into tissue   Capillary congestion
↓
Increased edema

■ Oversimplified flow chart depicting pulmonary edema.

PULMONARY EMBOLISM *(see also V̇/Q̇ Ratio, p. 210; Inferior Vena Cava Filter, p. 188; Alteplase in Part 8, p. 298; Deep Vein Thrombosis in Part 7, p. 284)*

A pulmonary embolism (PE) is a sudden mechanical obstruction of the pulmonary arterial bed related to ventilation/perfusion imbalance and shunting. A 50% occlusion will produce a massive PE, which often develops into a pulmonary infarction and can further evolve into PEA. About 90% of pulmonary emboli are due to DVTs (deep vein thrombosis) arising from the iliac or femoral veins, or from the vena cava. (Once a clot that has formed in one these large, deep veins breaks free and travels to the lung, it is termed an embolus.)

Diagnosis:
- **ABGs**—Decreased PaO_2 (although a normal value does *not* exclude the diagnosis) and a decreased PCO_2 with respiratory alkalosis. The patient will experience tachypnea and dyspnea.
- **Chest x-ray**—Pleural effusion, and a blunted costophrenic margin
- **EKG**—Inverted or depressed ST segment, right axis deviation, atrial fibrillation, or right bundle branch block
- **D-dimer**—90% negative predictive value if <500 mg/L
- **V̇/Q̇ scan**—Low or indeterminate result does not exclude the diagnosis
- **Spiral CT scan**—High accuracy for detection in the main or lobar pulmonary arteries
- **Echocardiography**—New onset severe tricuspid regurgitation and pressure overload in right ventricle
- **Assessment**—Chest pain to varying degrees, hemoptysis (with massive pulmonary embolism), pleural friction rub, pleural pain

Treatment: Based on anticoagulation therapy and keeping the PTT 1.5 to 2 times normal. Inferior vena cava filters and embolectomy are sometimes used, as well as the tissue plasminogen activator, alteplase.

PULMONARY HYPERTENSION

Emerging as one of the most underdiagnosed conditions on the medical front, pulmonary hypertension (PH) is characterized by increased pressure in the pulmonary arteries of at least double normal pressures: >25 mm Hg at rest and >30 mm during exercise. The disease process results in narrowing and stiffening of the pulmonary arterial lumen walls and causes an obstruction of blood flow, which (over time) leads to right-sided heart failure.

The New York Heart Association Functional Classification System assigns four categories to classify the extent of the resultant heart failure (see Heart Failure in Part 2, p. 110), and this information is frequently used to estimate prognosis and determine eligibility for clinical trials. Symptoms of PH include dyspnea, fatigue, chest pain, tachycardia, syncope, peripheral edema, and possibly cyanosis.

While definitive diagnosis is difficult, the "gold standard" for identification is right-sided cardiac catheterization. Treatment is aimed at slowing disease progression and decreasing the workload of the heart by allowing blood to flow more easily through the pulmonary arteries. The IV drug Flolan (epoprostenon) and the IV/SQ drug Remodulin (treprostinil) are commonly used, although there are many other drugs available. More recently, the FDA has approved Tyvaso (treprostinil) Inhalation Solution for treatment, administered via a specialized inhalation system.

PULMONARY VASCULAR RESISTANCE
(see also Swan-Ganz: Hemodynamic Normals in Part 2, p. 157)

The force needed by the right ventricle to produce blood flow through the pulmonary system is the pulmonary vascular resistance (PVR). Normal is 37 to 250 dyne/sec/cm. The pulmonary vessels constrict with a fall in alveolar PO_2 or a rise in arterial PCO_2. Also, an obstruction (such as a pulmonary embolus) causes the PVR to rise.

RACEMIC EPINEPHRINE *(see Respiratory Inhalation Medications, p. 203)*

RAPID SEQUENCE INTUBATION

RSI is a technique used to quickly sedate, paralyze, and intubate a patient without waiting to see the effect of the preprocedure drugs administered. It is generally reserved for trauma patients or for patients at risk of aspiration of stomach contents into the lungs. The protocol is frequently institution specific, and the reader is advised to review individual policy. The following, however, provides a generalized overview.

BEFORE PARALYSIS
- It is NOT conventional to premedicate RSI patients. The reason is that if you are unable to intubate the patient, when anesthetic agents wear off (usually within 5 minutes), the airway will NOT be at risk. The exception, however, is in blunt head injury patients. Lidocaine 1 mg/kg may be given in an effort to decrease the intracranial pressure that will occur with intubation.
- Begin Sellick maneuver (cricothyroid pressure to prevent vomiting and aspiration)

INITIAL SEDATION
- The patient goes to "sleep" with the aid of an IV induction agent, usually propofol, midazolam, thiopental, ketamine, etomidate, or diazepam.

INDUCTION
- To rapidly intubate, it is important to have a high degree of relaxation quickly. Succinylcholine (1–1.5 mg/kg IV) is the drug of choice, causing every muscle in the body to contract then subsequently relax. Widespread muscle contraction (rather like cramping) is common, and often patients will complain of muscle pain the next day. Succinylcholine also causes a sudden release of potassium into the bloodstream, and for this reason, it is contraindicated for use in patients with hyperkalemia. Other contraindications for its use include burns (24 hours to 2 years post), stroke or spinal cord injury (1 week to 6 months postinjury); multiple sclerosis, amyotrophic lateral sclerosis, and crushed muscles (7–90 days postinjury).
- Alternately, rocuronium (0.6–1.2 mg/kg IV) or vecuronium (0.10 mg/kg IV) may be used. Neither cause cardiac toxicity, and both are nondepolarizing.

INTUBATION
- Have an elastic bougie at the bedside to "railroad" the endotracheal tube if there is difficulty with tube placement.
- The patient is preoxygenated (to wash nitrogen out of the lungs and to create a reservoir for O_2).
- The tube is placed and secured and the cuff is inflated. Placement is assessed, and sedation continues as required.

RENIN-ANGIOTENSIN SYSTEM
(see Renin-Angiotensin System in Part 5, p. 261)

RESPIRATORY FAILURE *(see Acute Respiratory Failure, p. 169)*

RESPIRATORY INHALATION MEDICATIONS

ALBUTEROL (PROVENTIL, VENTOLIN)

Albuterol is a bronchodilator with minor β_{-1} and strong β_{-2} adrenergic receptor effects. Usual dose by aerosol: 0.5 mL of 0.5% solution in 3 mL normal saline. Usual dose by inhaler: Two puffs three times a day or four times a day. Onset is in about 15 minutes, peak occurs in 30 to 60 minutes, and duration ranges from 3 to 8 hours. It is useful in patients with asthma or COPD. It can cause tachycardia, palpitations, or insomnia. There is no advantage to administering albuterol for bronchoconstriction.

ALUPENT *(see Metaproterenol Sulfate, p. 203)*

ATROPINE

Atropine has an anticholinergic action to block acetylcholine and is useful for drying secretions. Onset is in 15 minutes, peak occurs in one half to 1 hour, and duration is 3 to 4 hours. Usual dose by aerosol: 0.05 to 0.1 mg/kg of a 1% solution. It can cause pupil dilation, increased CNS stimulation, and tachycardia.

BRETHINE (TERBUTALINE)

Brethine is a long-acting bronchodilator. It stimulates some β_{-1} adrenergic receptors, but mostly β_{-2}. Onset is in 5 to 30 minutes, peak occurs in 30 to 60 minutes, and duration is 3 to 6 hours. Usual dose by aerosol: 0.25 to 0.5 mL in 2.5 mL normal saline every 4 to 8 hours. Usual dose by inhaler: Two puffs every 4 to 6 hours. It can cause vasodilation, with decrease in blood pressure and increase in heart rate.

BRONKOSOL *(see Isoetharine, p. 202)*

ISOETHARINE (BRONKOSOL)

Isoetharine has some β_{-1} and moderate β_{-2} properties. Onset is in 1 to 5 minutes, peak occurs in 5 to 60 minutes, and duration is 1 to 3 hours. Usual dose by aerosol: 0.5 mL in 2.5 mL normal saline four times daily. Usual dose by inhaler: One to two puffs four times daily. This is a good choice for patients with cardiac arrhythmias.

ISUPREL (ISOPROTERENOL)

Isuprel is a potent bronchodilator with strong β_{-1} and β_{-2} properties. It relaxes the smooth muscles of the bronchial tree and is a good drug choice for acute bronchospasm. Onset is in 2 to 5 minutes, peak occurs in 5 to 60 minutes, and duration is 1 to 3 hours. Usual dose by aerosol: 0.25 to 0.5 mL of a 5% solution in 2.5 mL normal saline four times daily. Usual dose by inhaler: One to two puffs four times daily. Frequent side effects occur, including palpitations, tachycardia, and flushing of skin.

LEVALBUTEROL (XOPENEX)

In low doses, levalbuterol acts relatively selectively at β_{-2} adrenergic receptors to cause bronchodilation and vasodilation. (At high doses, β_{-2} selectivity is lost, and the drug also

(continued)

acts at β_{-1} receptors to cause typical sympathomimetic cardiac effects.) The usual dose is by nebulization, 0.63 mg (available in 0.63 mg/3 mL or 1.25 mg/3 mL) every 6 to 8 hours. Onset is within 5 minutes, peak occurs in 1 hour, and duration is for 6 to 8 hours. Levalbuterol does not increase the heart rate as much as albuterol; thus, it is beneficial for patients with ischemic heart disease who also have reactive airway disease.

METAPROTERENOL SULFATE (ALUPENT)
Metaproterenol sulfate is a long-lasting bronchodilator that stimulates both β_{-1} and β_{-2} adrenergic receptors. Onset is in 1 to 5 minutes, peak occurs in one half to 1 hour, and duration is for 2 to 6 hours. Usual dose by aerosol: 0.3 mL of a 5% solution in 2.5 mL normal saline four times daily. Usual dose by inhaler: Two to three puffs every 4 hours. It can cause tachycardia.

MUCOMYST (ACETYLCYSTEINE)
Mucomyst is a mucolytic agent indicated for tenacious secretions. Liquefaction is apparent within 1 minute after administration, and maximum effect occurs in 5 to 10 minutes. Can cause bronchoconstriction. Usual dose by aerosol: 3 to 5 mL of 20% Mucomyst in a 5 mL solution given three times daily or four times daily. Usual dose by instillation: 1 to 2 mL of 20% Mucomyst or 2 to 4 mL of 10% Mucomyst.

PROVENTIL *(see Albuterol, p. 202)*

RACEMIC EPINEPHRINE
Racemic epinephrine is a strong β_{-1} bronchodilator, useful for laryngospasm and immediate postextubation in children. Onset is in 3 to 5 minutes, peak occurs in 5 to 20 minutes, and duration is for 1 to 3 hours. Usual dose by aerosol: 0.125 to 0.5 mL in 2.5 mL normal saline. Usual dose by inhaler: One to two puffs four times daily.

VENTOLIN *(see Albuterol, p. 202)*

RESPIRATORY PATTERNS

APNEUSTIC BREATHING
Apneustic breathing is characterized by a prolonged inspiratory hold. There may be expiratory pauses. Typically, it has a very slow rate. It is related to midbrain or low pons conditions.

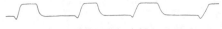

■ Apneustic breathing.

ATAXIC *(see Biot's Respirations, p. 203)*

BIOT'S RESPIRATIONS
Biot's respirations are irregular and random, with no pattern. Several short breaths of equal depth are followed by long, irregular periods of apnea. They are related to lesions at the midbrain or medullary level.

■ Ataxic breathing (Biot's respirations).

(continued)

CENTRAL NEUROGENIC HYPERVENTILATION

Central neurogenic hyperventilation looks like hiccups. There are sustained, regular, rapid respirations with forced inspiration and expiration at a rate of >60 per minute. It is related to lesions in the low midbrain or pons.

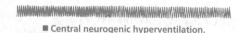

■ Central neurogenic hyperventilation.

CHEYNE-STOKES RESPIRATIONS

Cheyne-Stokes respirations are characterized by initial shallow respirations that increase in depth, reach a peak, then decline. A period of apnea follows, and the cycle is repeated. The apnea gives the PCO_2 time to build up again (after being blown off by the rapid respirations) and triggers the breathing pattern to start again. Cheyne-Stokes respirations occur with upper brainstem involvement.

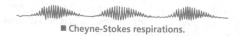

■ Cheyne-Stokes respirations.

CLUSTER BREATHING

Cluster breathing denotes a lesion in the low pons. Periods of irregular respirations alternate with periods of apnea.

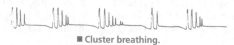

■ Cluster breathing.

KUSSMAUL'S RESPIRATIONS

Kussmaul's respirations are characterized by deep, regular, sighing respirations, with an increase in respiratory rate. They are caused by metabolic acidosis.

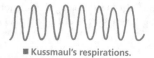

■ Kussmaul's respirations.

RESPIRATORY PHYSIOLOGY TERMS

GENERAL

PaO_2	partial pressure of oxygen in arterial blood
$PaCO_2$	partial pressure of carbon dioxide in arterial blood
PAO_2	partial pressure of oxygen in inspired gas
P_B	barometric pressure
V_T	tidal volume
V_D	volume of dead space
$\dot{V}_E$	volume of expired gas per unit of time (minute ventilation)
$\dot{V}_A$	volume of alveolar gas per unit of time (alveolar ventilation)

(*continued*)

LUNG VOLUMES

VC	vital capacity	VT	tidal volume
IC	inspiratory capacity	TLC	total lung capacity
IRV	inspiratory reserve volume	EEP	end-expiratory pressure
ERV	expiratory reserve volume	EPAP	end-positive airway pressure
FRC	functional residual capacity	PIP	peak inspiratory pressure
RV	residual volume		

PULMONARY MECHANICS

MEFR	maximal expiratory flow rate	IE	inspiratory/expiratory ratio
MMFR	maximal midflow rate	FEF	forced expiratory flow rate
MIFR	maximal inspiratory flow rate	FVC	forced vital capacity
MVV	maximal voluntary ventilation	ECMO	extracorporeal membrane oxygenation
FEV	forced expiratory volume		
CV	closing volume	NIF	negative inspiratory force
CC	closing capacity	IRV	inverse ratio ventilation
FVC	forced vital capacity		

RESPIRATORY SYSTEM ANATOMY *(see Anatomy, Pulmonary, p. 170)*

RESTRICTIVE DISEASES

Restrictive diseases are respiratory diseases that restrict movement of the thorax and/or lungs, resulting in decreased chest expansion and therefore a reduction in volume of air inspired and expired. They may be associated with interstitial fibrosis, thoracic deformities, or neurologic factors such as myasthenia gravis or Guillain-Barré syndrome.

REVERSE I:E RATIO *(see Ventilator Modes, p. 213)*

RHABDOMYOLYSIS *(see Part 5, p. 262)*

SARS

Severe acute respiratory syndrome (SARS), first identified in humans in 2003, is a febrile, infectious, severe lower respiratory disease caused by a newly described coronavirus named SARS-associated Coronavirus (SARS-CoV). The disease is spread primarily by close human contact when droplets are released into the air by an infected person. Typically, SARS begins with flu-like symptoms (high fever, headache, muscle aches, cough, diarrhea) and frequently progresses to pneumonia. Many studies are under way to determine if there are specific laboratory tests that can be used to distinguish SARS from other febrile respiratory illnesses, but to date, diagnosis is based on a combination of clinical and epidemiologic findings. The vast majority of patients with SARS have a clear history of exposure to either a SARS patient or to a setting in which SARS transmission is occurring and develop pneumonia. Mortality is about 9%, although to date, only eight confirmed cases have been reported in the United States, with no confirmed deaths. Since no medical regime has been developed that shows consistent improvement in outcomes, treatment at this time remains strictly supportive.

SPONTANEOUS PNEUMOTHORAX *(see Pneumothorax, p. 197)*

STATIC COMPLIANCE *(see Compliance, p. 181)*

STATUS ASTHMATICUS

An acute exacerbation of asthma refractory to initial treatment with bronchodilators, leading to respiratory failure, unconsciousness, and even cardiopulmonary arrest. It is considered a medical emergency.

Symptoms: Include extreme dyspnea, restlessness, anxiety, and if sufficient airflow, coughing and wheezing. Advanced symptoms include little or no breath sounds, inability to speak, cyanosis, and diaphoresis. The bronchial smooth muscle contraction (bronchospasm), vascular leakage, increased airway inflammation, and mucous secretion all lead to airway obstruction and ultimately respiratory failure.

Treatment: Includes bronchodilators (inhaled or nebulizers), corticosteroids, anticholinergics, Heliox therapy, ketamine, beta-agonists, magnesium sulfate, hydration, and oxygen. Mechanical ventilation may be considered. Aminophylline is rarely used, although it may be considered in conjunction with other therapies.

$S\bar{v}O_2$ MONITORING (see $S\bar{v}O_2$ Monitoring in Part 2, p. 151)

SYNCHRONIZED INTERMITTENT MANDATORY VENTILATION (see Ventilator Modes, p. 214)

TENSION PNEUMOTHORAX (see Pneumothorax, p. 197)

TIDAL VOLUME (see Lung Volumes, p. 189; Weaning Parameters, p. 215)

TRACHEOSTOMY

A tracheostomy is a surgery used to create an opening in the windpipe to facilitate breathing, although the opening itself is commonly termed a tracheostomy. The tube that is inserted into the opening is known as a tracheostomy (trach) tube, and consists of three parts:

1. The outer cannula. This consists of a neck plate, extending from the outer sides of the tube, and slots at the outer edge of the flange to secure the tube in place around the patient's neck. The purpose of the outer cannula is to hold the tracheostomy open.
2. The inner cannula. This piece fits inside the outer cannula and has a twist lock to secure it in place. It is removed for cleaning.
3. The obturator. This is utilized when first inserting the tracheostomy tube. It serves as an initial "guide" and provides a smooth surface for entry. It is usually retained and kept at the bedside after initial use, in case the tracheostomy tube should become dislodged.

   Although there are many different manufacturers of trach tubes, it should be noted that a *specific type of tube* will be the same, no matter who makes it.

DISPOSABLE CUFFED TUBES

The inflatable cuffs on these tubes are low pressure, and often "DCT" (disposable cuff tube) is marked on the neck plate. The initials ID on the flange indicate inner diameter of the cannula and the initials OD indicate the outer diameter. The length is the distance from the neck plate to the distal end of the tube. The cuff should always be inflated when using with ventilators but may be deflated if the patient uses a speaking valve.

(continued)

Tracheostomy Tube Diameters and Conversion			
Outside Diameter (mm)	French	Jackson	Approximate Inside Diameter (mm)
6.0	18.0	2	4.0
7.0	21.0	3	4.5–5.0
8.0	24.0	4	5.5
9.0	27.0	5	6.0–6.5
10.0	30.0	6	7.0

CUFFED TUBE WITH REUSABLE INNER CANNULA

Same as the disposable cuffed tube, but in this case, the inner cannula is NOT disposable, and meant to be reused after thorough cleaning.

CUFFLESS TUBE WITH DISPOSABLE INNER CANNULA

This type of tube is used for patients who are ready to be decannulated. The patient may be able to talk without a speaking valve. The inner cannula is disposable.

CUFFLESS TUBE WITH REUSABLE INNER CANNULA

Same as the disposable cuffless tube, but in this case, the inner cannula is NOT disposable, and meant to be reused after thorough cleaning.

FENESTRATED CUFFED TUBE

These tubes allow the patient to speak, but when capping a fenestrated cuffed tube, be sure to *deflate the cuff and remove the inner cannula*. This allows air to pass by the larynx instead of the stoma, so the patient can speak. There is a high risk for aspiration of secretions with this tube, and it may be difficult to ventilate the patient adequately.

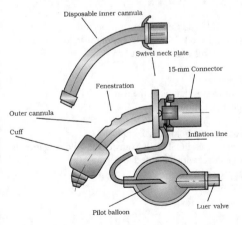

Disposable inner cannula
Swivel neck plate
15-mm Connector
Fenestration
Outer cannula
Cuff
Inflation line
Pilot balloon
Luer valve

■ Shiley fenestrated tracheostomy tube. (Courtesy of Mallinckrodt Medical, Irvine, CA.)

PASSY-MUIR VALVE

This is a one way valve that fits on the tracheostomy tube to allow the patient to vocalize. When breathing in, the valve opens so air enters the lungs through the trach tube. When breathing out, the valve closes, making the air from the lungs flow around the tube,

(continued)

through the vocal cords. This air movement causes the sounds. Some patients find it diffi-cult to adjust to the use of this valve since the work of breathing is increased when the valve is in place. A weaning program with lengthening time periods of usage may be required.

TRALI *(see Part 7, p. 294)*

TRANSBRONCHIAL NEEDLE ASPIRATION (TBNS) *(see Part 10, p. 366)*

TUBERCULOSIS

One of the world's deadliest diseases, tuberculosis is an infection caused by an aerobic bacterium (*Mycobacterium tuberculosis*) that has a unique lipid layer that renders it resistant to antibiotics and host defense mechanisms. It is spread via airborne droplets (in the form of coughing, sneezing, talking, or singing) by any person who has an active infection. The droplets can remain airborne for minutes to hours after expectoration, and can transition from the lungs to other organs of the body. Infection can be detected 2 to 12 weeks after exposure by a positive Mantoux tuberculin skin test (TST).

To administer Mantoux tuberculin skin rest (TST):
- Inject 0.1 mL of tuberculin purified protein derivative (PPD) into the intradermal layer of the inner surface of the forearm.
- The injection should be made with a tuberculin syringe, with the needle bevel facing upward. When placed correctly, the injection should produce a pale elevation of the skin (a wheal) 6 to 10 mm in diameter.
- Read between 48 and 72 hours after administration. (If the time frame expires, the test must be repeated.)
- Measure induration (palpable, raised, hardened area or swelling) in millimeters *across*, not down, the forearm. Do NOT measure erythema (redness).

To interpret TB skin test:
- **15 mm or greater induration** is considered POSITIVE in any person.
- **10 mm or greater induration** is considered POSITIVE in any of the following groups:
  Persons who frequent high-risk "congregate" settings
  IV drug users
  Mycobacteriology lab employees
  Persons with clinical disease processes that place them at risk
  Recent immigrants from high-risk countries
  Children younger than 4 years
  Infants and children exposed to adults in high-risk groups
- **5 mm or greater induration** is considered POSITIVE in any of the following groups:
  Persons who have had recent contact with TB-infected person
  Persons who are immunosuppressed
  Persons with CXR changes consistent with TB
  HIV infected persons
  Persons with organ transplant

Tuberculosis stages:
- LATENT. The patient is infected, but does not have active TB. The organism is alive, but inactive. The patient is *not* infectious to others and is asymptomatic but will show a positive reaction to the TB skin test. It must be noted, however, that a positive TB test

(continued)

only tells that a person has been infected with the TB bacteria. It does *not* tell whether or not the person has progressed to the TB disease. Other tests, such as CXR and sputum tests, are needed to determine whether the person has TB disease.

- ACTIVE. Approximately 5% to 10% of persons exposed to the TB bacteria will develop active TB. This progression may occur soon after infection, or much later in life (especially in the setting of immunosuppression). *The patient is considered infectious and may spread the TB bacteria to others.*

Guidelines for preventing transmission:

- Negative pressure isolation room (negative pressure causes air to rush *into* the room when a door is opened).
- Personnel to wear N-95 respirator mask (see below) at all times. Visitors should be offered respiratory protection and instructed on use as well.
- Ultraviolet germicidal irradiation (UVGI) and room air recirculation units.
- Room door closed at all times.
- Diagnostic and treatment procedures should be performed in the room when possible. If patient requires transport to another area, have the patient wear a surgical mask during transport and bypass waiting areas. Workers transporting the patient are advised to mask during transport as well.

N-95 disposable filter respirator guidelines:

- Fit testing is required.
- Wear the mask for only one patient and only as long as the structural integrity of the mask is maintained.
- Between uses, store the mask in a clean/dry plastic bag.
- One mask for each individual healthcare worker. They are not to be shared.
- Never use an N-95 mask on a patient.
- Check the mask before entering the room. Place both hands completely over the mask, but don't disturb the position and exhale deeply. If air leaks around the nose, tighten the nose piece. If air leaks at the respirator edges, adjust the straps until the air leak is resolved.

NOTES

V̇/Q̇ RATIO

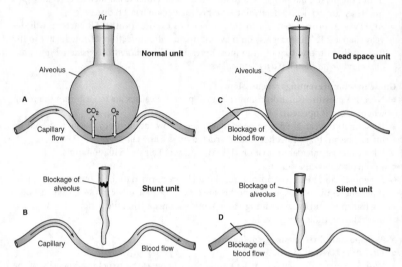

■ Ventilation-perfusion situations: A, Normal ventilation, normal perfusion. B, Shunting with no ventilation, normal perfusion. C, Dead space with normal ventilation, no perfusion. D, silent with no ventilation, no perfusion.

Optimum gas exchange between blood and the alveolus and occurs when ventilation and perfusion correspond equally. Normally, a ratio of 4 L/min ventilation to 5 L/min perfusion occurs in a healthy individual, yielding a $\dot{V}/\dot{Q}$ ratio of 0.8:1. A mismatch exists when there is inadequate ventilation, inadequate perfusion, or both. Anything that interferes with ventilation (e.g., bronchospasm, emphysema, asthma) will decrease the $\dot{V}/\dot{Q}$ ratio, and anything that interferes with perfusion (e.g., pulmonary embolus, changes in pulmonary artery pressures) will increase the $\dot{V}/\dot{Q}$ ratio.

VENTILATOR-ASSOCIATED PNEUMONIA

VAP is the leading cause of nosocomial infection in the ICU and develops shortly after intubation with subsequent mechanical ventilation. It results in significant morbidity and mortality, and the focus is *prevention*—aimed at modifiable risk factors as outlined in the following table.

(continued)

NOTES

Ventilator-Associated Pneumonia (VAP)

Risk Factors for VAP	Nursing Interventions to Prevent/Minimize VAP
Mechanical ventilation/intubation <24 hours = 3-fold ↓ in VAP >24 hours = 6- to 21-fold ↑ in VAP	• Orotracheal rather than nasotracheal intubation • Aggressive weaning: Creation of "fast track" weaning protocols; CPAP/weaning trials as soon as is feasible • Maintain ETT cuff pressures at ≥20 mm Hg • Suction/clear secretions from above the ETT cuff prior to deflating the cuff for ETT positioning or prior to ETT removal
*HOB flat or <30 degrees	• HOB at 30–45 degrees at all times, unless medically contraindicated *Significantly decreases VAP
**Pooling of tracheal/upper airway secretions in the subglottic area	• Intubate using an ETT with a dorsal lumen above the cuff, placed to continuous suction to drain pooled secretions **This intervention alone decreases VAP incidence by 45–50%
Decreased level of consciousness/ sedated/delirium	• **Sedation vacation** at least once Q24 hours • Limit benzodiazepine/sedation use • Administer analgesics prn to control pain • Allow fully awake state as frequently as possible NOTE: Wakefulness decreases incidence and severity of delirium, another risk factor for VAP
Poor oral hygiene	• Aggressive/regular oral care • May consider oral antiseptics such as chlorhexidine 0.12% oral solution 15 mL BID until 24 hours after extubation
Poor infection control practices	• Regular hand washing with soap or alcohol disinfectant • Wear gloves when handling the ventilator equipment or during procedures involving the ETT/airway and/or when handling respiratory fluids
Transport from the ICU for diagnostic or therapeutic procedures	• Minimize out-of-ICU transports • Transport with HOB at 30–45 degrees • Suction mouth and oropharynx prior to laying flat • Lay flat for as brief a time period as possible
Contaminated respiratory equipment/medications etc.	• Decrease frequency of opening circuit • Do not change circuit routinely, based on duration of use only
Paralytic Agents	• Limit use • Train-of-four to accurately assess effect
Gastric irritation/gastric or small intestinal tubes/gastric distention and aspiration	• Gastric pH modifying agents/H_2 antagonists/antacids • Routinely verify placement of feeding tubes • Verify amount of gastric residual at regular intervals—notify physician if not tolerating feeds/high gastric residual • Monitor for signs/symptoms of infections of the upper respiratory tract; i.e., sinusitis. Remove tube if complication noted and replace in alternate orifice, if possible

VENOUS O₂ CONTENT

Venous oxygen content ($C\overline{v}O_2$) is primarily determined by the amount of hemoglobin in venous blood that is saturated with oxygen.

$$C\overline{v}O_2 = (Hgb \times 1.39 \times S\overline{v}O_2) + 1.39 \times S\overline{v}O_2$$

REMEMBER: This faster calculation for a quick approximation:

$$C\overline{v}O_2 = (Hgb \times 1.39 \times S\overline{v}O_2)$$

Normal value: 12 to 15 volume percent

VENTILATION/PERFUSION RATIO (see V̇/Q̇ Ratio, p. 210)

VENTILATOR MODES

ASSIST CONTROL

Ventilator provides a breath with either a preset tidal volume or preset peak pressure every time the patient initiates a breath. In the past, only preset tidal volumes were able to be used for this setting, but with the advent of newer technology, presetting a peak pressure is an option. When using a preset peak pressure, the mode is sometimes termed Intermittent Positive Pressure Ventilation (IPPV). A minimum "back up" rate is usually set to be sure the patient does not become apneic, and a maximum rate (although used infrequently) can be set if the patient is breathing too rapidly.

CONTROLLED MANDATORY (MECHANICAL) VENTILATION

The frequency of breaths is determined by the ventilator alone, with no option available to the patient. It is an uncomfortable mode for patients who are conscious and therefore indicated for use in only unconscious or paralyzed patients, those who have experienced a neurologic event, or those with sedation on board.

CONTINUOUS POSITIVE AIRWAY PRESSURE

Continuous positive airway pressure (CPAP) is pressure that is maintained throughout inspiration and expiration during spontaneous breathing. It is usually 5 to 15 cm H_2O. Patient may generate own rate of breathing and own tidal volume; thus, CPAP may be used alone or with intermittent mandatory ventilation at low rates for weaning.

FLOW-BY VENTILATION

Flow-by ventilation, like pressure support, produces a continuous flow of gas through the circuit, which can meet the patient's demands but not assist the patient's ventilation. However, because the ventilator circuit is not closed (as in pressure support), flow-by ventilation cannot ventilate as high-pressure support levels can. Because it is not pressurized, however, there is no risk of barotrauma. It is often used as a weaning mode in conjunction with assist/control or pressure support. (It converts the system from pressure to flow triggered.) A flow-by of 15/3 means that 15 L of O_2 are "flowing by" but that the flow decreases to 3 L when the patient exhales, thus decreasing resistance.

HIGH-FREQUENCY VENTILATION

High-frequency ventilation (HFV) is most frequently used in the setting of ARDS, is referred to as "lung protective ventilation" and utilizes very high respiratory rates (up

(*continued*)

to 900 breaths per minute) and small tidal volumes in an attempt to reduce ventilator-assisted lung injury. There are three "sub" classes of this mode:

- **High-frequency oscillatory ventilation** (HFOV or HFO) utilizes rates up to 900 breaths per minute and causes pressure to oscillate around the constant distending pressure (equivalent to the PEEP). It pushes gas into the lung during inspiration and pulls it out during expiration. Frequently used on patients who have hypoxia that is not responsive to normal mechanical ventilation.
- **High-frequency jet ventilation** (HFJV) is a support system used with rates of approximately 100 to 200 breaths per minutes, with tidal volumes of one to three times predicted anatomic dead space. An endotracheal tube "adaptor" is used in place of the normal 15 mm ET tube adaptor, allowing a "jet" of gas to flow out of the adaptor and into the airway at a high pressure for a brief duration. Jet ventilators utilize I:E ratio settings (sometimes "reversed") to allow for maximum passive exhalation.
- **High-frequency positive pressure ventilation** (HFPPV) is rarely used, since advancing technology has allowed the development of HFOV and HFJV. This mode utilizes a rate of 90 to 100 breaths per minute on a conventional ventilator but employs tidal volumes that would be higher than HFOV of HFJV.

INTERMITTENT MANDATORY (MECHANICAL) VENTILATION

Intermittent mandatory ventilation (IMV) requires the ventilator to deliver a predetermined number of breaths and a set tidal volume. It allows the patient to breathe spontaneously between machine breaths, but the patient receives only his or her own spontaneous tidal volume. IMV can be used for weaning.

INVERSE RATIO VENTILATION

The normal inspiratory/expiratory ventilation ratio (I:E ratio) in most ventilators is 1:1.5 to 1:3, producing a short inspiratory time and a long expiratory time. This increases venous return and right atrial filling and allows time for air to leave the lungs. Inverse ratio ventilation reverses this ratio to produce an inspiratory time equal to or even longer than expiratory time—as high as 4:1. Although it is useful in ARDS (by expanding stiff alveoli slowly and preventing their collapse with a rapid expiratory time), this mode is unnatural and requires the patient to be either heavily sedated or, more frequently, medically paralyzed.

NEURALLY ADJUSTED VENTILATORY ASSIST

Neurally adjusted ventilatory assist (NAVA) is a new positive pressure mode of mechanical ventilation, which permits the respiratory center in a patient's brain to control the ventilator by means of electrodes mounted on an NG tube and positioned in the esophagus at the level of the diaphragm. The electrical activity of the diaphragm is captured, fed to the ventilator via a computer, and used to assist the patient's breathing, both with a given breath as well as assist between breaths. This means that the patient's respiratory center is in direct control of ventilation, and any variation in demand is responded to immediately. This new method strives to increase patient comfort, reduce the risk of iatrogenic hyperinflation, respiratory alkalosis, and hemodynamic impairment. Training is required to learn to position the electrode, adjust the trigger, and determine the level of ventilatory assist.

POSITIVE END-EXPIRATORY PRESSURE

Positive end-expiratory pressure (PEEP) is positive pressure, usually 5 to 20 cm H_2O, added at the end of expiration. It prevents closure of the alveoli and promotes better

(continued)

oxygen exchange. It is used as an adjunct to assist control ventilation, intermittent mandatory ventilation, synchronized intermittent mandatory ventilation, and pressure support modes. High levels of PEEP may cause barotrauma to weak lungs and may result in tension pneumothorax, or they may decrease cardiac output by increasing intrathoracic pressure, causing compression of the heart and decreased venous return. The patient usually responds to volume to maintain adequate preload.

REMEMBER:

PEEP is DEEP (high levels of PEEP will decrease cardiac output).

PRESSURE CONTROL

In pressure control (PC) setting, pressure and respiratory rate are predetermined. The ventilator delivers a flow of gas until the preset pressure is attained. It can be used with inverse ratio ventilation to allow alveoli a prolonged duration of positive inflation. This, in turn, shortens expiratory time and prevents loss of the patient's tidal volume.

PRESSURE-REGULATED VOLUME CONTROL

Pressure-regulated volume control (PRVC) requires rate, FiO_2, and pressure limit to be preset. The patient may take spontaneous breaths. During breathing, if the ventilator senses that the entire tidal volume cannot be delivered without violating the pressure limit, it will alter the flow to allow the whole tidal volume to be delivered. Breath by breath, the ventilator continuously adapts the inspiratory pressure to changes in the volume/pressure relationship. This mode is appropriate for patients who initially need high flow rates to open up closed lung compartments, those in whom unnecessarily high airway pressures should be avoided, and those with lung conditions such as asthma, chronic obstructive bronchitis, and lung injury.

PRESSURE SUPPORT

Pressure support (PS) is a weaning method whereby the patient initiates inspiration, and the ventilator supports (assists) it to achieve a predetermined peak pressure level. This eases the flow of gas into the lungs and increases tidal volume.

SYNCHRONIZED INTERMITTENT MANDATORY VENTILATION

Synchronized intermittent mandatory ventilation (SIMV) is essentially the same as IMV, but the ventilator is synchronized so that if a patient initiates a breath, the ventilator does not deliver a breath at the same time. It is a method of weaning that is more comfortable for the patient than IMV. It is often combined with pressure support (see above).

VOLUME-ASSURED PRESSURE SUPPORT

Volume-assured pressure support (VAPS) is a combination of pressure control and volume control. It provides the fast flow response to patient demand of pressure control, along with the assured volume delivery of volume control.

VENA CAVA FILTER (*see Inferior Vena Cava Filter, p. 188*)

VENTOLIN (*see Respiratory Inhalation Medications, p. 202*)

VITAL CAPACITY (*see Lung Volumes, p. 189*)

WEANING PARAMETERS *(see also Lung Volumes, p. 189)*

Not All Criteria Need be Satisfied	
Parameter	**Ideal**
Respiratory Rate	<12 and >30 breaths/minute
Tidal volume (VT)	>5 mL/kg
f/VT ratio (Tobin index) Calculated by dividing respiratory rate (spontaneous) by tidal volume (L) Example: RR = 25 VT = 300	<100 24 ÷ 0.3 = 80
Forced vital capacity (FVC) Max exhalation after max inhalation	10–15 mL/kg
Negative inspiratory force (NIF) Normal = –80 cm to –100 cm	At least –25 cm to maintain MV
PaO$_2$	>80%
SaO$_2$	>90%
FiO$_2$	<50%
PEEP	<5 cm H$_2$O
Minute volume (MV) Amount of air in/out in one minute	<10 L/min
Heart rate	Within 20 bpm of baseline and >60 bpm
Blood pressure	Within 20 mm Hg of baseline
PCWP	<20 mm Hg

PART 4

Gastrointestinal and Urinary Systems

ANATOMY: DIGESTIVE SYSTEM

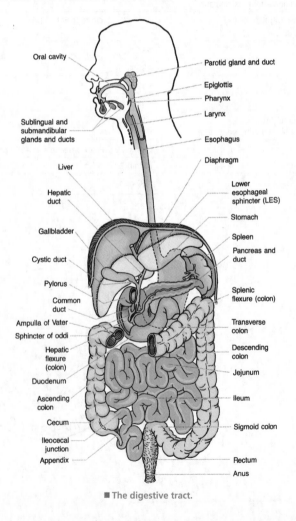

Oral cavity

Parotid gland and duct

Epiglottis

Pharynx

Larynx

Sublingual and submandibular glands and ducts

Esophagus

Diaphragm

Liver

Lower esophageal sphincter (LES)

Hepatic duct

Stomach

Gallbladder

Spleen

Cystic duct

Pancreas and duct

Pylorus

Splenic flexure (colon)

Common duct

Ampulla of Vater

Transverse colon

Sphincter of oddi

Descending colon

Hepatic flexure (colon)

Jejunum

Duodenum

Ascending colon

Ileum

Cecum

Ileocecal junction

Sigmoid colon

Appendix

Rectum

Anus

■ The digestive tract.

ANATOMY: LIVER FUNCTION *(see also Hepatic Encephalopathy, p. 232; Hepatic Failure, p. 232; Bilirubin in Part 9, p. 340)*

The liver is the largest internal organ. It stores fat-soluble vitamins and conjugates bilirubin to make it water soluble for excretion by the kidneys. In hepatic failure, the liver is unable to conjugate bilirubin, leading to an increase in both direct and indirect bilirubin, as well as a buildup of ammonia.

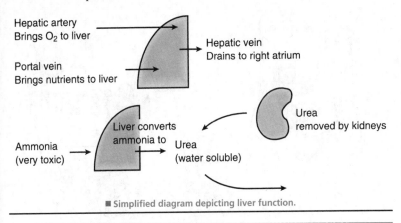

Hepatic artery
Brings O_2 to liver

Hepatic vein
Drains to right atrium

Portal vein
Brings nutrients to liver

Urea
removed by kidneys

Liver converts ammonia to

Ammonia
(very toxic)

Urea
(water soluble)

■ Simplified diagram depicting liver function.

ASCITES

Ascites, an accumulation of fluid in the abdominal cavity, is caused by decreased protein content and an increase in osmolarity. It is a common complication of advanced hepatic disease. Pressure from the ascites frequently results in dyspnea. Sodium restriction is the cornerstone of therapy, along with diuretics. Paracentesis (removal of fluid from the abdominal cavity) is rarely used because it may precipitate hepatic coma, shock, or hypovolemia (see Paracentesis).

BARIATRICS

Bariatrics is a collective term describing one of several surgical procedures performed on the stomach and/or intestines to help a patient with extreme obesity lose weight. It is usually reserved for those with a body mass index (BMI) of >40 (which equates to at least 100 lb over recommended weight) but also is indicated for those with a BMI of >35 who have secondary problems such as heart disease or type 2 diabetes.

To calculate body mass index:

$$(\textbf{weight in pounds} \times 700) \div (\textbf{height in inches, squared})$$
<18 = not enough fat   18–25 = normal   >25 = too much fat

The surgeries fall into two categories for reducing caloric intake:

1. *Restrictive only.* The stomach is made smaller during surgery. The patient feels full faster and learns to decrease the amount eaten.
2. *Malabsorptive and restrictive combined.* Not only is the stomach size reduced, but part of the stomach and/or intestines are bypassed so that fewer calories are absorbed (unfortunately, nutrients are lost as well).

(continued)

- **Biliopancreatic diversion (BPD)** (malabsorptive and restrictive): Portions of the stomach are surgically removed, leaving only a small pouch that is connected directly to the final segment of the small intestine. The duodenum and jejunum are completely bypassed. A common channel, allowing bile and pancreatic digestive juices to mix prior to entering the colon, is left remaining. Weight loss occurs because calories go directly to the colon, where no absorption takes place.

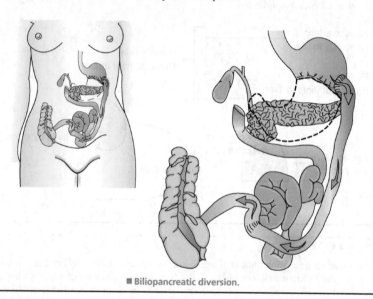

■ Biliopancreatic diversion.

- **Biliopancreatic diversion with duodenal switch (BPD/DS)** (malabsorptive and restrictive): This surgery allows a larger portion of the stomach to be left intact, including the pyloric valve that regulates the release of contents from the stomach into the small intestine. The duodenum is divided near the pylorus, and the small intestine is divided as well. The portion of the small intestine connected to the large intestine is attached to the short duodenal segment next to the stomach. The remaining segment of the duodenum, connected to the pancreas and gallbladder, is attached to this limb, closer to the large intestine. Where contents from these two segments mix is called the common channel, and it dumps into the large intestine. Since this surgery fosters less nutrient absorption, a higher amount of weight loss is accomplished.

(continued)

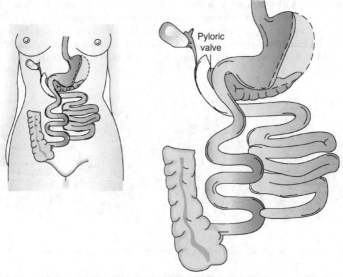

■ Biliopancreatic diversion with duodenal switch.

- **Laparoscopic adjustable gastric banding** (restrictive only): Accomplished laparoscopically, a hollow band is placed around the stomach near its upper end, creating a small pouch and a narrow passage into the larger remaining portion of the stomach. The creation of this small passage delays the emptying of food and causes a feeling of fullness. The band can be tightened or loosened over time to change the size of the passage. Initially, the pouch holds about 1 oz. of food and later expands to hold 2 to 3 oz. This surgery has minimal metabolic effects because it does not interfere with digestion.

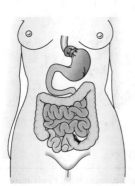

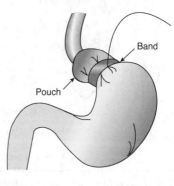

Band can be tightened or loosened over time to change the size of the passage

Band

Pouch

■ Laparoscopic adjustable gastric banding.

(*continued*)

- **Roux-en-Y gastric bypass** (malabsorptive and restrictive): Performed laparoscopically since 1993, this is the most frequently performed bariatric surgery in the United States. In the following figure, the stomach is divided into two parts (**A**), and the small intestine is carefully measured and cut (**B**). The small intestine is then connected to the small pouch (**C**), and the bypassed part of the small intestine is reconnected, forming a "Y" (**D**).

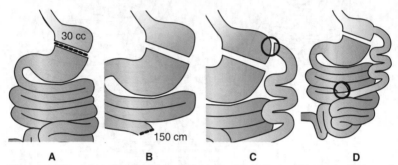

A   B   C   D

■ Roux-en-Y Procedure. (Adapted from Bariatric Treatment Centers™ [www.bariatric.com] and Forest Health Services LLC.)

- **Vertical banded gastroplasty (VBG)** (restrictive only): The upper stomach near the esophagus is stapled vertically to create a small pouch along the inner curve of the stomach. The outlet from the pouch to the rest of the stomach is restricted by a band. This band delays emptying of food from the pouch, creating a feeling of fullness. Because this surgery does not interfere with the normal digestive process, its success is defeated by continuance of a junk food diet.

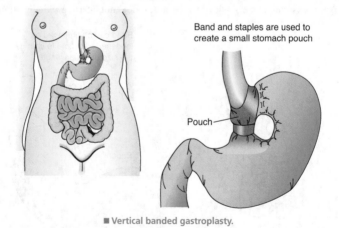

Band and staples are used to create a small stomach pouch

Pouch

■ Vertical banded gastroplasty.

- **Vertical sleeve** (restrictive only): The left side of the stomach (greater curvature) is surgically removed, leaving a new stomach that resembles the size and shape of a banana.

(*continued*)

Surgically, it is a simpler operation than laparoscopic adjustable gastric banding or biliopancreatic diversion with duodenal switch, since both ends of the stomach and the small intestine remain intact. The procedure is sometimes performed in one step, but more frequently, it is a two-part procedure reserved for the extremely obese or those who have so many health problems that they do not qualify for gastric bypass surgery. The first step of the procedure is to create the "sleeve," which helps the patient begin to lose weight. After enough weight has been lost (usually 80–100 lb and sometimes requiring longer than a year), the second step can be undertaken. The "sleeve" is converted into a formal gastric bypass or duodenal switch, promoting additional weight loss and offering the patient a more permanent result.

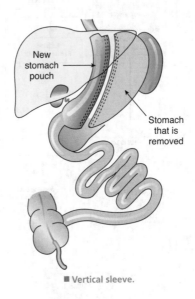

New stomach pouch

Stomach that is removed

■ Vertical sleeve.

(continued)

BARIATRIC DECISION TREE

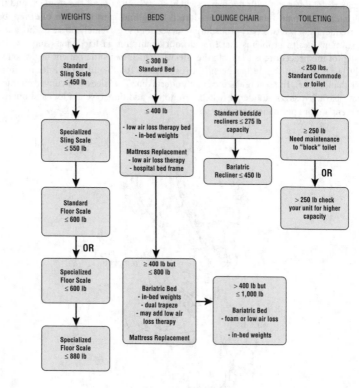

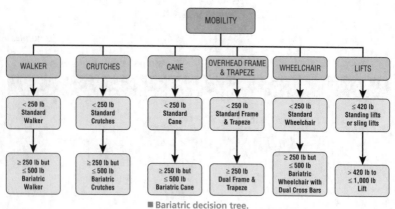

■ Bariatric decision tree.

BASAL METABOLIC RATE

The basal metabolic rate is a calculated value (in k/cal) that reflects the minimal caloric requirement that a resting individual needs in order to sustain life (amount of energy the body would burn if the person were sleeping for 24 hours).

- General calculation: Body weight (in lb) × 10 kcal/lb
- Harris Benedict equation:
   Males: 66 + (13.7 × weight in kg) + (5 × height in cm) − (6.8 × age in years)
   Females: 655 + (9.6 × weight in kg) + (1.7 × height in cm) − (4.7 × age in years)

BILIRUBIN *(see Part 9, p. 340)*

BILLROTH PROCEDURE *(see Ulcers, p. 242)*

BOWEL MANAGEMENT SYSTEMS

Several fecal containment systems are currently available to collect and contain liquid stool and thus preserve the integrity of the skin. They can be either external (a pouch is applied directly to skin of perianal area and attached to a gravity drainage bag) or internal (a pliable catheter is inserted into the anorectal cavity and attached to gravity drainage). Some of the newer internal systems (Zassi, ActiFlo, DigniCare, Flexi-Seal) also have irrigation and/or enema access. Containment of feces becomes increasingly important when dealing with organisms such as *Clostridium difficile* and vancomycin-resistant enterococci.

- 29 days is the general rule for maximum indwelling days.
- May not be effective if distal rectum is surgically altered.
- Weak sphincter tone may cause the catheter to expel or have increased leakage of stool.
- Not to be used if impacted stool present.
- Excessive, prolonged traction on the catheter could result in sphincter dysfunction.

BOWEL OBSTRUCTION *(see also Colostomy, p. 224; Ileostomy, p. 234)*

Bowel obstruction develops when intestinal contents cannot pass through the lumen of the bowel as a result of mechanical causes, neurogenic causes, or vascular abnormalities.

TYPES

- Simple: No interference with blood supply.
- Strangulated: Blood supply to obstructed segment decreases; ischemia occurs; may progress to necrosis and gangrene.
- Incarcerated: Blood supply severely altered. Necrosis and gangrene occur.

(continued)

Large Bowel Versus Small Bowel

Characteristic	Large Bowel	Small Bowel
Stool	None	Intermittent until bowel clears, then none
Distension	Pronounced	Minimal
Vomiting	Not common	Occurs if obstruction proximal to ileum
Pain	Mild, steady	Cramping in upper abdominal area

CECOSTOMY *(see Colostomy, p. 224)*

CIRRHOSIS *(see also Bilirubin in Part 9, p. 340)*

Cirrhosis is a disease in which liver damage is followed by scarring. Fibrous tissue forms and compresses blood, lymph, and bile channels. It is the final stage of many types of liver injury.
- **Portal cirrhosis (Laennec's disease):** Associated with alcoholism; the most common type. It has three components: (1) destruction of hepatic tissue, (2) diffuse increase in fibrous tissue, and (3) disorganized regeneration. The liver is enlarged and firm. An important secondary factor is the development of portal hypertension and esophageal or gastric varices (see Esophageal Varices).
- **Posthepatitic cirrhosis:** Associated with viral or toxic hepatitis. The liver is shrunken and irregular, with large regeneration nodules and fibrous tissue.
- **Biliary cirrhosis:** Associated with intrahepatic cholestasis. There is scarring around the ducts and lobules, and immune mechanisms may be disturbed.

COLOSTOMY *(see also Bowel Obstruction, p. 223, Ileostomy, p. 234)*

A colostomy is the opening of some portion of colon to the abdominal surface. It is named for the section of the colon that is cut into.

SIGMOID AND DESCENDING COLOSTOMY

The stoma is normally in left area of colon. The rectum, anus, and damaged portion of large intestine are removed. Elimination is fecal material. Surgery is permanent; prognosis is good.

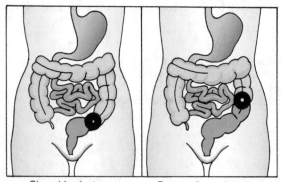

Sigmoid colostomy   Descending colostomy

■ Sigmoid and descending colostomy. Shaded area indicates section of bowel removed.

(continued)

TRANSVERSE COLOSTOMY

The stoma is usually slightly above and to one side of navel. Only the damaged portion of large intestine is removed. It usually is a "resting" process, and closure is performed later. Management can be with irrigation, which gives 50% control (stays clean 6–10 hours). Two types of colostomy are performed along the transverse colon:

Double-Barrel Transverse Colostomy

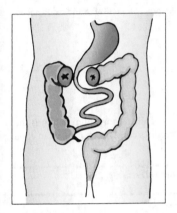

■ Double barrel transverse colostomy. (Courtesy of United Ostomy Association, Irvine, CA.)

There are two stomas: One active, one inactive. Active stoma diverts feces to outside (bypassing injury or inflammation), and inactive stoma drains mucus until healing is complete. It requires constant wearing of an appliance. The ostomy is usually closed within 6 months, and the bowel is rejoined.

Loop Transverse Colostomy

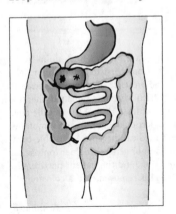

■ Loop colostomy. (Courtesy of United Ostomy Association, Irvine, CA.)

An intact loop of bowel is brought through abdomen and held in place by a plastic bridge or anchor. It is temporary for as little as 10 days or as long as 9 months.

(continued)

ASCENDING COLOSTOMY (CECOSTOMY)

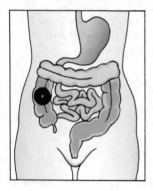

■ Ascending colostomy. Shaded area indicates section of bowel removed.

The stoma is in right lower quadrant. It functions like an ileostomy: Elimination is thin and filled with gastric juices. Flow is constant and requires constant wearing of an appliance. Surgery is temporary.

CROHN'S DISEASE *(see Inflammatory Bowel Disease, p. 235)*

CULLEN'S SIGN *(see also Pancreatitis, p. 236)*

Cullen's sign, ecchymosis around the umbilicus, is associated with severe intraperitoneal hemorrhage.

REMEMBER:

C· ← Umbilicus   "C" shape for Cullen's

CYSTOSTOMY *(see Urinary Diversions, p. 244)*

DIVERTICULITIS

A diverticulum of the colon is an outpouching of mucosa through a weak point in the muscular layer of the bowel wall. It generally results from persistent and abnormally high intracolonic pressure. (Note: **Diverticulosis** is the presence of many *diverticula* in the sigmoid and the ascending colon. When the diverticula become inflamed, then the term "diverticulitis" is used.) The cause is unknown. At least 10% of the middle-aged population is affected. No treatment is necessary for diverticula that cause no symptoms; however, symptomatic diverticula generally require medical therapy. A possible complication is perforation with resultant abscess formation or generalized peritonitis. The inflammatory process may also cause bowel obstruction, and the patient may require surgery. Occasionally, a portion of the involved bowel is removed, and a colostomy is placed.

(continued)

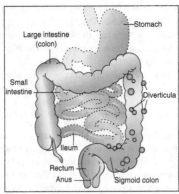

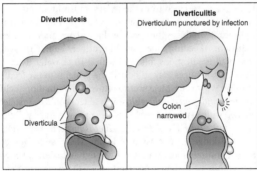

■ (Top) Location of diverticula in the sigmoid colon. (Bottom left) Diverticulosis. (Bottom right) Diverticulitis. (Courtesy of National Digestive Diseases Information Clearinghouse. [1989]. *Clearinghouse fact sheet: Diverticulosis and diverticulitis.* NIH publication no. 90–1163. Washington, DC: US Department of Health and Human Services.)

DUODENAL ULCER *(see Ulcers, p. 242)*

ENCEPHALOPATHY *(see Hepatic Encephalopathy, p. 232)*

ENTERAL NUTRITION *(see also Parenteral Nutrition, p. 238)*

Enteral nutrition is an alternative method to support patients who are unable to meet their nutritional needs orally by placing a feeding tube into the gastrointestinal tract.

NASOGASTRIC (NG) TUBE
Size: 8 to 12 French (F) when tube feeds are anticipated for <6 weeks; 14 F or larger for medications, gastric decompression, or short-term tube feeding (1–2 weeks)
Placement: Predetermined distance (usually 40–45 cm). Measure from the tip of nose to ear lobe, and from ear lobe to the tip of xiphoid process for gastric placement.

(continued)

Evaluating correct placement: *Radiology remains the only reliable method to verify initial placement of blindly inserted feeding tubes.* The older traditional practices of verification should be discontinued because of their lack of efficacy and potential for harm:

- The audible "pop" over the epigastrium with auscultation may lead to a false assumption of correct placement.
- A pH of <5.0 with aspirate inspection *may* indicate gastric placement but is not helpful in detecting esophageal placement (aspirate could be gastric reflux).
- Placing the tube in water to check for "bubbling" lacks consistency, as no bubbling may be observed with pulmonary placement if the tube ports are occluded.

Other options: More recently, the CORTRAK™ тмenteral access system has evolved, consisting of a computer monitor, receiver unit, and an electromagnetic transmitter stylet.

The system allows for a real-time representation of NG tube placement and affords the clinician the luxury of responding immediately to a misplaced tube (i.e., into a lung, or coiled in the stomach). A receiver is placed on the patient's xiphoid process, and the NG tube is advanced. A signal is received from the stylet's transmitter, and the real-time location of the tube is displayed. The system negates the need for multiple chest x-rays during placement, and significantly reduces the need for fluoroscopy and/or endoscopy.

Relieving tube occlusion: Feeding tubes should routinely be flushed with 30 cc of water every 4 hours and all medications followed with a 10 cc water flush (per institution policy). Nonetheless, gastric juices may still cause the proteins in the feeding solutions to reflux, and an occlusion will occur. Measures to remedy this situation include:

- *If there is still flow in the tube but it is sluggish,* warm water should be instilled into the feeding tube and agitated with a syringe. Frequently this measure alone will clear the tube.
- *If there is still flow in the tube and the warm water is ineffective,* a number of products have been used to dislodge the occlusion: Adolph's Meat Tenderizer, cranberry juice, Coke, Pepsi, Sprite, and/or Mountain Dew. Although occasionally effective, the most consistent result comes with the administration of the pancreatic enzyme Viokase. When dissolved in 5 cc of water, injected, and allowed to dwell for 5 minutes, it will usually relieve the occlusion.
- *If the tube is completely occluded* and it is impossible to instill water or enzyme, the last option is to insert a flexible wire, in an attempt to clear the tube.

GASTROSTOMY TUBE

- Percutaneous endoscopic gastrostomy is the mainstay of long-term enteral feeding.
- *R E M E M B E R :* With the G/J tube, use the "G" port for medications; use the "J" port for H$_2$O and tube feeds ONLY.

SMALL BOWEL FEEDING TUBE (DOBBHOFF, ENTRIFLEX)*

- To insert:
  1. Determine the length for gastric placement (usually 50–65 cm). Measure from the tip of nose to ear lobe and from ear lobe to the tip of xiphoid process for gastric placement. Then, add approximately 10 inches (25 cm) for intestinal placement.
  2. Secure stylet inside the feeding tube, and instill 10 to 30 cc warm water to activate the *internal* lubricant.
  3. Dip the weighted tip in warm water to activate the *external* lubricant.
  4. Pass through the nostril and into the patient. Once inserted, do not pull stylet back and forth to manipulate it within the tube. (This avoids damage or puncture of the lung, should the tube be in the tracheobronchial tree.)

(*continued*)

5. Confirm tube placement, then remove the stylet.
6. Spontaneous transpyloric passage of the weighted tip to the intestine occurs within 24 to 48 hours. Placing patient in a semi-Fowler's and positioning to the right side may expedite this process.

Some institutions do not allow RNs to pass enteral tubes requiring a stylet. The reader is advised to refer to institution-specific policy.

Enteral Nutrition Formulas

Indication/Characteristics	Nutritional Formulas
1 kcal/mL	Jevity, Isocal HN, Entrition HN, Osmolite, Promote
1.5 kcal/mL	Ensure Plus, Jevity 1.5, Nutren 1.5, Isosource 1.5, Osmolite 1.5, Boost Plus
2.0 kcal/mL	Resource 2.0, Deliver 2.0, Two Cal HN
1 kcal/mL *(Fiber, Low Osmo)*	Jevity, Jevity 1.2, Promote with Fiber
Low Residue/Low Fiber	Vital High Nitrogen (Vital HN)
Low Residue/Isotonic	Osmolite/Osmolite 1.2
Isotonic, High Protein, High Nitrogen *(High proportion of calories from protein)*	Promote
High Protein, Gluten Free, Low Residue *(Wound healing)*	Impact with Glutamine (1.3 kcal)
High Nitrogen	Two Cal HN, Isocal HN
Low Fat	Vivonex TEN
Low Carb/High Fiber—Diabetes Management	Glucerna 1.0, Glucerna 1.2, Glucerna 1.5, DiabetiSource AC
Renal/Dialysis *(High Protein)*	Nerpo—Carb Steady, Suplena—Carb Steady, Novasource Renal
Renal (Reduced Kidney Function) *(Low Protein)*	Suplena, RenalCal
Pulmonary—COPD/Cystic Fibrosis/ Respiratory Failure	Pulmocare, Nutren Pulmonary
Pulmonary—SIRS/AIDS/ALI/Ventilator Dependent *(Low Residue)*	Oxepa
Pulmonary—ALI *(Low CHO, High Fat, Caloric Dense ALI—1.5 cal/mL)*	Nutren Pulmonary
High Calorie/Low Residue/Gluten and Lactose Free	Hi-Cal
High Fiber/High Protein	Fibersource HN/Promote with Fiber
Fiber	Promote with Fiber, Jevity 1.0, Jevity 1.2, Jevity 1.5, Benefiber Powder

more . . .

(continued)

Enteral Nutrition Formulas (Continued)

Indication/Characteristics	Nutritional Formulas
Modular Components	Glutasolve (90 kcal/pkg with 15 g L-glutamine) Juven (78 kcal/pkg with 14 g protein) MCT oil (115 kcal/Tbsp (15 mL) with 14 g fat) Protein Powder (25 kcal/mL)
Elemental Formulas *(High-nitrogen, low-fat elemental formulas for malabsorptive disease states)*	Crucial, Vivonex Plus, Vivonex RTF, Vivonex TEN, Peptamen, Tolerex
Semielemental Formulas *(Immune Enhancing)*	Perative (1.3 kcal)
Burns/Malabsorptive/Pancreatitis	Optimental
High Protein/Immune Support	Pivot 1.5, Perative
Hepatic Support	Nutrihep, Osmolite, Jevity 1.0, Suplena
Wound Healing	Crucial, Arginaid, Impact, Juven
General Supplement	Ensure Plus, Ensure, Boost, Boost Plus

Abbott-Nutrition and Nestle'-Nutrition are currently the main suppliers of the tube feeding products. Additional research may be obtained online to select the product that best meets the patients' nutritional requirements.

ERCP *(see Part 10, p. 363)*

ESOPHAGEAL VARICES *(see also Cirrhosis, p. 224; Gastrointestinal Bleeding, p. 231; Shunt, p. 240)*

In a scarred cirrhotic liver, the intrahepatic veins may be squeezed shut so that blood backs up into the portal vein and into diverting channels around the esophagus, causing the life-threatening complication of varices. Restoration of blood volume with RBCs is primary. After evaluation of clotting status, FFP and platelets may also be used.

Management to control bleeding:
- **Octreotide (Sandostatin),** a synthetic analogue of somatostatin with a longer half-life. It decreases portal pressure, and it decreases the blood transfusion requirement by 50%. Usually given as a 50-μg IV bolus, followed with a drip at 25 μg/hr.
- **Vasopressin** 0.1 to 0.4 units per minute is sometimes used; however, octreotide is preferable because of fewer side effects.

Once patient's condition is stable, preferred methods of treatment are:
- **Endoscopic sclerotherapy:** A sclerosing agent is infused through a special channel on an endoscope and injected into or around the varices to seal them off.
- **Banding:** A suction tool is attached to the endoscope, the vein is "sucked up," and a small elastic band is placed around it to seal it off.

Emergency measures to tamponade bleeding:
- **Sengstaken-Blakemore** tube (or Minnesota tube)

FECAL DIVERSION *(see Bowel Management Systems, p. 223)*

FEEDING TUBES *(see Enteral Nutrition, p. 227)*

GASTRECTOMY *(see Ulcers, Gastric, p. 242)*

GASTRIC BANDING *(see Bariatrics, p. 217)*

GASTRIC pH

Use Nitrazine paper (phenaphthazine) for pH determination. Apply several drops of nasogastric (NG) aspirate to paper, and shake off excess. Read immediately from comparison chart on side of dispenser.

REMEMBER:

Nitrazine paper becomes inactive if it becomes wet from other fluids. If gastric contents have antacids in them, flush NG with saline and reaspirate.
- Normal pH is 4.5 to 7.5. Usual treatment for pH 5.0 or below is with antacid (Mylanta).

GASTRIC ULCER *(see Ulcers, p. 242)*

GASTROINTESTINAL BLEEDING *(see also Esophageal Varices, p. 230; Shunts, p. 240)*

Upper GI bleeding may be due to:
- Duodenal or gastric ulcer, erosive gastritis
- Esophageal varices, esophagitis, esophageal tear
- Tumors (occasionally)

Lower GI bleeding may be due to:
- Ruptured diverticulum
- Ischemic bowel
- Polyps, tumors (occasionally)
- Ulcerative colitis
- Eroding aortic aneurysm

REMEMBER:

The rapidity of the blood loss is often more important than the amount.
Treatment involves replacing lost fluid and controlling bleeding with lavage, a Sengstaken-Blakemore tube, and/or IV vasopressin (Pitressin). Sclerotherapy or variceal banding is indicated for small varices, and a TIPS (transjugular intrahepatic portosystemic shunt) procedure for large varices.

GASTROJEJUNOSTOMY *(see Ulcers, Gastric, p. 242)*

GASTROSTOMY TUBE *(see Enteral Nutrition, p. 227)*

GREY TURNER'S SIGN

Grey Turner's sign is a bluish color of the flank caused by retroperitoneal bleeding.

HARRIS BENEDICT EQUATION *(see Basal Metabolic Rate, p. 223)*

HEPATIC ENCEPHALOPATHY

Encephalopathy is a disorder related to the abnormalities that occur only with significant liver dysfunction. It is characterized by an increase in the blood ammonia level (the liver is no longer available to remove it by converting it to urea). Any increase in the ammonia level has a toxic effect on the brain, and the patient will have impaired mentation, neuromuscular disturbance, and an altered level of consciousness.

Stages of Hepatic Encephalopathy

Stage	Impairment
I	Slight personality change, impaired mentation
II	Mental confusion, asterixis (hands "flap")
III	Lethargic
IV	Unresponsive (high mortality)

TREATMENT
- Restrict dietary protein.
- Administer oral neomycin (alters gut flora so blood is not broken down and changed to ammonia).
- Administer lactulose (promotes ammonia secretion).
- Peritoneal dialysis or liver transplant may be necessary.
- Monitor potassium levels (kidneys retain ammonium ions along with potassium ions).
- Do not administer lactated Ringer's solution via IV (diseased liver converts this to lactic acid and produces more ammonia).

HEPATIC FAILURE *(see also Bilirubin in Part 9, p. 340)*

Caused by a long list of various insults (viral infections, drug-related toxicity, metabolic conditions, autoimmune diseases, cancer), hepatic failure renders the liver unable to conjugate bilirubin and thus results in a wide range of possible abnormalities:
- Elevated indirect and direct bilirubin
- Elevated PT with INR >1.5
- Elevated ammonia levels
- Elevated AST and ALT levels
- Labile blood glucose levels
- Decreased phosphorus and magnesium levels
- Thrombocytopenia
- DIC

Treatment is supportive, with lactulose to decrease ammonia levels, H2 blockers to manage any GI bleeding, FFP and platelets to manage coagulopathies, and maintenance of hemodynamic, respiratory, and electrolyte stability.

HEPATITIS

Hepatitis is the widespread inflammation of liver cells and edema, which leads to distortion of the liver's lobular shape. The liver becomes enlarged, exhibiting a smooth edge and tenderness on palpation.

HEPATITIS A (INFECTIOUS HEPATITIS)

Hepatitis A can be transmitted by the fecal or oral route. Because the organism is also food- and water-borne, shellfish are often associated with transmission. Clinical course of infection is usually over 1 to 3 months, with a complete recovery. Enteric precautions should be maintained, although after jaundice disappears, the patient is no longer infectious.

HEPATITIS B (SERUM HEPATITIS)

Hepatitis B can be transmitted via contact with blood or blood products, requiring a break in the skin for actual transmission to occur. Hepatitis B is the leading cause of fulminant liver failure. Isolation and enteric precautions are required. After jaundice subsides, isolation can be discontinued, although the patient is considered infectious as long as an antigen can be identified in the serum. (Approximately 4% of patients who have recovered from hepatitis B are still infectious after 6 months.) The patient is then considered a carrier.

LAB PROFILE

- Serum glutamic-oxaloacetic transaminase (SGOT) and serum glutamic-pyruvic transaminase (SGPT) increase. Levels rise during prejaundice phase to peaks of >500 U/L by the time jaundice appears, followed by a rapid fall over several days. SGOT and SGPT levels return to normal 2 to 5 weeks after onset of jaundice.
- Albumin is slightly decreased.
- Serum globulin is increased.
- Bile pigments are altered (see Bilirubin).

Treatment consists of a long period of rest, lactulose to promote ammonia secretion, and decreased dietary protein (protein breaks down in the GI tract to ammonia).

HEPATITIS C (NON-A, NON-B)

Hepatitis C is caused by a virus and is usually transmitted via blood, blood products, and shared needles, although there is some evidence that it may also be transmitted sexually. It has a better prognosis than hepatitis B. The hepatitis C antibody does not confer immunity, and infection may become chronic.

HEPATITIS D (DELTA VIRUS)

Hepatitis D is a defective virus that needs the hepatitis B virus to exist. In humans, it occurs only in the presence of a hepatitis B infection. Hepatitis D, like B, is transmitted by blood and blood products, and it carries the same risks as hepatitis B. It most commonly affects IV drug users.

A patient can become infected with the hepatitis D virus at the same time an infection of hepatitis B is acquired. This is termed "coinfection." Or, a patient can become infected with hepatitis D at any time after an acute hepatitis B infection. This is termed "superinfection."

(continued)

Hepatitis D superinfection should be considered whenever the condition of a patient with hepatitis B suddenly deteriorates. It can be diagnosed by the presence of antibodies against the hepatitis D virus. IgM antibodies indicate acute infection.

Treatment consists of administration of interferon-α, and some studies suggest that a dose higher than that used for hepatitis B patients may be beneficial.

HEPATITIS E

Hepatitis E is transmitted in much the same way as hepatitis A, primarily the fecal-oral route, and from fecally contaminated drinking water. Unlike hepatitis A, however, it does not appear to be transmitted by person-to-person contact, although nosocomial infection has been occasionally reported. Hepatitis E is rare in the United States; the few cases in this country are seen in travelers returning from areas where hepatitis E is endemic.

The typical clinical signs and symptoms of hepatitis E are similar to those of other types of hepatitis. They include abdominal pain, anorexia, dark urine, fever, hepatomegaly, jaundice, malaise, nausea, and vomiting. The period of incubation ranges from 15 to 60 days (mean 40 days), and the period of infectivity following acute infection, although not definitely proven, appears to be up to 14 days after the onset.

No products are available to prevent hepatitis E. Prevention relies primarily on clean water supplies and good hygienic practices.

HYPERALIMENTATION (*see Parenteral Nutrition, p. 238*)

ILEAL CONDUIT (*see Urinary Diversions, p. 244*)

ILEOCECAL POUCH (*see Urinary Diversions, p. 245*)

ILEOSTOMY (*see also Bowel Obstruction, p. 223; Colostomy, p. 224*)

Ileostomy is the opening of the ileum onto the abdominal surface, usually performed for ulcerative colitis and sometimes for Crohn's disease or cancer of the bowel. The entire large intestine and rectum are removed (total colectomy). Discharge liquid flows constantly. The stoma is one half to 1 inch long and is usually formed to protrude so the discharge doesn't flow directly onto the skin.

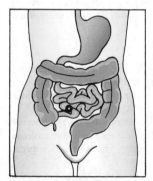

■ Ileostomy. Shaded area indicates section removed.

Ileostomy

ILEUS

Although there can be many causes, this condition most frequently occurs after abdominal surgery and is characterized by an obstruction of the intestine due to it being paralyzed, or at least, inactive enough to prevent the passage of intestinal contents. On auscultation, there are no bowel sounds present and the patient may complain of abdominal distention (bloating), abdominal pain, and constipation. Diagnosis is confirmed by a CT scan of the abdomen and pelvis, or with a GI series. Treatment is aimed at decompressing the abdomen via placement of an NG tube, and attempting to restore peristalsis. If the obstruction is severe, intestinal infection and gangrene are possible and surgery may be required.

INDIANA POUCH (see Urinary Diversions, p. 245)

INFLAMMATORY BOWEL DISEASE

Inflammatory bowel disease is a collective term that refers to two chronic diseases that cause inflammation of the intestines: Crohn's disease and ulcerative colitis. *It is not to be confused with irritable bowel syndrome, or IBS, which affects the motility of the colon, is much less serious, and bears no relationship to either Crohn's or ulcerative colitis.*

- Ulcerative colitis is an inflammatory disease that affects only the colon. The inflammation involves the entire rectum and extends up the colon in a continuous manner. There are no areas of normal intestine between the areas of diseased intestine. It is marked by ulceration of only the innermost lining of the colon, resulting in bleeding and production of pus and mucous. There is frequent diarrhea. If the disease progresses to the point that symptoms are severe and are unable to be helped with drugs, surgical removal of the large intestine may be necessary.
- Crohn's disease causes inflammation to any area of the digestive tract from the mouth to the anus, although it most commonly affects the small intestine. All layers of the intestine are affected, and there can be normal healthy bowel in between patches of diseased bowel. Every attempt is made to avoid surgery, as there is a concern that an aggressive surgical approach will lead to further complications, such as short bowel syndrome (which involves a reduced ability to absorb nutrients).

The symptoms of these two illnesses are similar: diarrhea and abdominal pain. Diagnosis is based on endoscopy, colonoscopy, barium study, and biopsy. Treatment is aimed at relieving the symptoms because both maladies are chronic, characterized by remissions and exacerbations. Anti-inflammatory drugs are used to decrease the inflammation, and immunosuppressive agents work to restrain the immune system from attacking the body's own tissues and causing further inflammation.

IRRITABLE BOWEL SYNDROME (IBS)

IBS is a long-term condition that affects the motility of the colon. It is much less serious than inflammatory bowel disease and bears no relationship to either Crohn's or ulcerative colitis. Symptoms include recurrent abdominal pain, discomfort, cramping, bloating, and alteration in bowel function (diarrhea, constipation, or both). The cause is unknown, but certain foods, stress, hormonal changes, and some antibiotics may trigger symptoms. Treatment focuses on lifestyle modifications.

KEHR'S SIGN

Kehr's sign is pain in the left shoulder caused by diaphragmatic irritation related to splenic rupture. An increase in white blood cells (WBCs) is common.

KOCK POUCH (see Urinary Diversions, p. 246)

LIVER ENCEPHALOPATHY (see Hepatic Encephalopathy, p. 232)

LIVER FAILURE (see Hepatic Failure, p. 232)

MALLORY-WEISS SYNDROME

Mallory-Weiss syndrome is painless GI hemorrhage related to weakness in the esophageal wall, causing rupture during coughing or vomiting (or any increase in abdominal pressure).

MCBURNEY'S POINT

McBurney's point is one third the distance from the anterior superior iliac spine to the umbilicus. McBurney's sign is tenderness at the site and is associated with acute appendicitis.

MESOCAVAL SHUNT (see Shunts, p. 240)

MURPHY'S SIGN

Murphy's sign is severe pain and inspiratory arrest with palpation of the right upper quadrant. It is indicative of cholecystitis.

NEOBLADDER (see Urinary Diversions, p. 246)

NEPHROSTOMY (see Urinary Diversions, p. 244)

NASOGASTRIC TUBE (see Enteral Nutrition, p. 227)

PANCREATITIS

Pancreatitis is an autodigestive disease related to escape of activated enzymes from acinar cells. About 60% of cases are related to alcoholism, 20% to biliary tract disease, and less than 10% to gallstones or posttraumatic injury to the pancreas.

SYMPTOMS
- Severe epigastric pain radiating to the back
- Abdominal distension, nausea, vomiting
- Absent bowel sounds
- Fatty, foul-smelling stools
- Increased serum amylase (2–3 days)
- Increased urine amylase (5–7 days)
- Increased lipase
- No rebound tenderness

(continued)

The patient may also have hypocalcemia (resulting in twitching and seizures), HHNK, bilateral rales, atelectasis of base of left lung, and pleural effusion. ARDS is sometimes an end result because of the enzymes released by the pancreas, causing loss of surfactant.

Hemorrhagic pancreatitis causes blood to pool retroperitoneally, producing a bluish color of the flank (Grey Turner's sign) and around the umbilicus (Cullen's sign).

TREATMENT

- Research shows that morphine is a better choice for pain control rather than Demerol.
- Fluid replacement (for loss due to vomiting)
- Decrease pancreatic stimulation (by decreasing HCl in stomach: Tagamet, Zantac, Pepcid, Mylanta, nothing by mouth).
- NG suction
- Possible peritoneal lavage
- Whipple procedure (removal of gallbladder, distal portion of stomach, duodenum, and head of pancreas and anastomosis of remaining portion of stomach, pancreas, and common bile duct to jejunum)
- Long term: Insulin dependence
- The most common complication of pancreatitis is respiratory failure/ARDS.

Ranson's Criteria for Predicting Mortality in Pancreatitis

Assessment done on admission and again in 48 hours
<3 predicted mortality 1%
3–4 predicted mortality 15%
5–6 predicted mortality 40%
>6 predicted mortality 100%

On Admission:		48 Hours Postadmission:	
Age >55 years	1 point	Hct drop >10%	1 point
WBC >16	1 point	BUN >5 after IV hydration	1 point
Glucose >200	1 point	Ca <8	1 point
LDH >350	1 point	Arterial PO_2 <60	1 point
AST >250	1 point	Base deficit >4	1 point
		Fluid sequestration >6 L	1 point

PARACENTESIS

Paracentesis is a "tapping" of the abdomen by means of a hollow needle or trocar to draw off fluid. It may be either diagnostic (to obtain abdominal fluid for analysis) or therapeutic (to remove fluid for patient comfort). Generally, only enough fluid is removed to obtain the desired outcome, although taking as much as 11 L may be required. If more than 5 L are drained, salt-poor albumin is often given to counteract the loss. Complications include hypovolemia (fluid shifts rapidly into the peritoneal cavity to replace what was lost) and reduced tissue perfusion (leading to decreased systemic circulation, renal failure or hepatic coma).

PARENTERAL NUTRITION *(see also Enteral Nutrition, p. 227)*

Total parenteral nutrition (TPN), also known as hyperalimentation, is a form of IV therapy used to provide nutrition to those patients who are unable to assimilate nutrients via the GI tract. It may be administered either peripherally or centrally.

TPN solution typically contains:
- Glucose, 5% to 50% (to provide carbohydrates)

REMEMBER:

Patients with pulmonary disease or those on mechanical ventilation require close monitoring of the amount of dextrose in the solution, as excess carbohydrates may increase production of CO_2 and cause a decline in respiratory function. For peripheral administration, the TPN solution is usually limited to 10% glucose to prevent phlebitis.

- Amino acids, 3% to 15% (to provide protein): For peripheral administration, the TPN solution is usually limited to 5% amino acids to prevent phlebitis.
- Essential vitamins, minerals, electrolytes, and trace elements (to support body functions).
- Lipids (a fat emulsion derived from egg yolks and soy or safflower oil): Often ordered in conjunction with TPN. Lipids may be infused through the TPN line.

REMEMBER:

Patients who are allergic to soy or eggs may react to lipids.

ADMINISTRATION PEARLS
- Use an infusion pump for administration at a constant rate. Never try to play "catch up," as blood glucose levels may be altered.
- TPN can be administered peripherally or centrally but must have a DEDICATED line with a filter. Consider it the patient's "life line."
- Since TPN bags typically contain >1,000 mL, it is appropriate to change a bag before it is completely empty. With each new bag, the tubing and filter should be changed.
- Sudden cessation of TPN may result in hypoglycemia (due to continued release of insulin from the pancreas). If replacement TPN is unavailable, hang a bag of $D_{10}W$ at the same rate. (Check institution-specific policy.)
- When discontinuing TPN, reduce the hourly rate as ordered for the last several hours to stabilize the blood glucose.
- The patient should be scheduled for frequent, routine blood glucose monitoring and weighed daily.

COMPLICATIONS
- Infection risk is considerable because the solution offers an excellent growth medium for microorganisms.
- Altered glucose level (diabetics at higher risk), altered potassium level, and possible hypophosphatemia.
- Calcium and phosphorus in solution may precipitate as calcium phosphate and cause pulmonary emboli.
- Phlebitis and other complications associated with central lines in general.

PEPTIC ULCER *(see Ulcers, p. 241)*

PERITONEAL LAVAGE

Peritoneal lavage, a procedure used to assess for bleeding and now rarely practiced, is primarily used for patients with *blunt* abdominal trauma with altered pain response. It has been almost exclusively replaced by computed tomography (CT) and is contraindicated in patients with *penetrating* abdominal trauma.

PERITONITIS

Peritonitis, an inflammatory involvement of the peritoneum, is caused by the leaking of juices (such as bile or pancreatic juices) as a result of trauma, or by rupture of an organ containing bacteria, which then enter the abdominal cavity. Some of the organisms commonly found are *Escherichia coli*, streptococci (both aerobic and anaerobic), staphylococci, and pneumococci.

Massive doses of antibiotics are given to combat infection, and intestinal or gastric tubes are inserted in an attempt to restore intestinal motility. Fluids and electrolytes are replaced. If the peritonitis is caused by a perforation that is releasing irritating or infected material into the abdominal cavity, surgery to close the abnormal opening and remove the accumulated fluid is indicated.

PORTACAVAL SHUNT *(see Shunts, p. 240)*

PROSTATE

The prostate is a fibrous organ in males that surrounds the urethra. As men age, the prostate frequently enlarges, resulting in compression on the urethra and subsequent problems with urination. Depending on the extent of the enlargement, surgery may be indicated.

- **Transurethral resection (TURP):** Not as common as it once was because drugs are currently available to relieve the symptoms of prostate enlargement, this procedure can be used for benign prostatic hypertrophy. A cystoscope is inserted into the penis, and a special cutting instrument is inserted through the scope to remove the prostate piece by piece. After the blood vessels are cauterized, a catheter is placed in the bladder, and continuous irrigation is instituted. Initially, the urine appears bloody but clears in 1 to 2 days, at which time the irrigation is discontinued and the catheter is removed.
- **Radical prostatectomy (open prostatectomy):** A more involved procedure, used when the prostate is larger. An incision is made in the lower abdomen between the navel and penis (retropubic approach), or alternately, a smaller incision is made between the anus and the base of the scrotum (perineal approach). The prostate is then removed from underneath the pubic bone. A nerve-sparing radical prostatectomy may be employed in an attempt to preserve erectile function. The catheter used in this procedure will remain in place for several days to a few weeks, until the bladder has sufficiently healed. A drainage tube may also be placed in the abdominal cavity to drain blood and fluids from the area.
- **Laparoscopic radical prostatectomy (LRP):** A newer technique, with no results from long-term follow-up available. This procedure is minimally invasive, has less blood loss, and faster recovery than the radical procedure. Five small incisions are made on the abdomen, most of which are no longer than 5 mm. The laparoscope is introduced in the subumbilical site and is used to guide the operation. The surgeon and assistants each use the other four sites for the introduction of instruments. The entire prostate

(continued)

is removed. Like the radical procedure, LRP requires reconstruction of the bladder/urethra connection. A catheter is left in the urethra and is connected to a drainage bag. In the immediate postop period, there is also a drain that goes through the abdominal wall, but this is usually removed the morning following surgery.

- **Transurethral incision of the prostate (TUIP):** In this procedure, no prostate tissue is removed. One or two small cuts or grooves are made in the prostate gland, where it meets the bladder, to help enlarge the diameter of the urethra and to make it easier to urinate. It is typically an outpatient procedure, requiring the patient to wear a catheter for 1 to 2 weeks after surgery. Subsequent retreatment is more likely with TUIP than with any other treatment option.

PROSTATECTOMY *(see Prostate, p. 239)*

PSOAS SIGN

To elicit psoas sign, the patient is asked to raise the right leg while the examiner's hand provides resistance just above the right knee. Alternately, the patient is turned to the left side, and the right leg is extended at the hip by the examiner. Increased abdominal pain with either maneuver indicates a positive result, suggesting irritation of the psoas muscle by an inflamed appendix.

RANSON'S CRITERIA *(see Pancreatitis, p. 236)*

ROUX-EN-Y GASTRIC BYPASS *(see Bariatrics, p. 220)*

SHUNTS

- **Mesocaval shunt:** Anastomosis of superior mesenteric vein to inferior vena cava.
- **Splenorenal (Warren) shunt:** Anastomosis of splenic vein to left renal vein. Some hepatic flow is preserved, but thrombosis of shunt is common.
- **Portacaval shunt:** Rarely used; anastomosis of portal vein to inferior vena cava. Problems arise because the liver is then unable to detoxify, and encephalopathy usually develops.
- **TIPS (transjugular intrahepatic portosystemic shunt):** Has largely replaced previous shunts. Total portal decompression is accomplished through the means of a functional H graft contained within the liver parenchyma, producing a side-to-side portosystemic shunt. Portal hypertension is reduced and bleeding esophageal varices are eliminated when flow is diverted from portal vein into inferior vena cava.

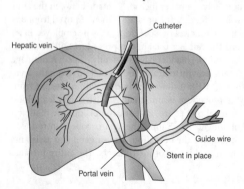

■ Transjugular intrahepatic portosystemic shunt (TIPS). A stent is inserted through a catheter to the portal vein to divert blood flow and reduce portal hypertension.

SMALL BOWEL FEEDING TUBES *(see Enteral Nutrition, p. 228)*

SPLENORENAL SHUNT *(see Shunts, p. 240)*

STENTS, URINARY

A ureteral stent is used to bypass a blockage in the kidney or ureter. It is a soft plastic tube, usually 6 to 10 F that connects the renal pelvis to the urinary bladder. An internal ureteral stent has side holes in it, as well as a hole at each end. If placed through a cystoscope, it is termed a retrograde stent because placement is in the opposite direction of urine flow. If placed by a transrenal approach, it is termed an antegrade stent because it is in the direction of normal urine flow. Usually stents are removed after blockage has been eliminated or the ureter has healed. If, however, they are required for an extended time, they should be changed every 3 to 6 months.

THORACENTESIS *(see also Effusion in Part 3, p. 182)*

Thoracentesis (pleural tap) is removal of excess fluid in the pleural space (space between the chest wall and lung) and is performed either as a diagnostic tool or to alleviate dyspnea. The pleural fluid collection, known as a pleural effusion, may be caused by a number of etiologies: CHF, pulmonary infections, pulmonary emboli, cancer, cirrhosis, pancreatitis, kidney disease, or tumors. A thin needle is inserted into the pleural space posteriorly, with the patient in a sitting or side lying position, and the excess fluid is aspirated into a vacuum tube. Chest x-ray following the procedure is utilized to confirm that no pneumothorax is present.

TIPS *(see Shunts, p. 240)*

TPN *(see Parenteral Nutrition, p. 238)*

TRANSURETHRAL INCISION *(see Prostate, p. 239)*

TRANSURETHRAL RESECTION *(see Prostate, p. 239)*

TUBE FEEDINGS *(see Enteral Nutrition, p. 229)*

ULCERATIVE COLITIS *(see Inflammatory Bowel Disease, p. 235)*

ULCERS

PEPTIC ULCERS

Peptic ulcers are acute or chronic ulcerations in a portion of the digestive tract that is in contact with gastric secretions. The main cause is a bacterial infection (usually *Helicobacter pylori*); however, some ulcers are caused by long-term use of NSAIDs or by cancerous tumors in the stomach or pancreas.

REMEMBER:

Ulcers are *not* caused by stress or spicy food.

(continued)

H. pylori infection is common in the United States. About 20% of people younger than 40 years and 50% of people older than 60 years are infected with it, but without the development of ulcers; the reason is unknown. How people become infected in the first place is also unknown, although there is a theory that it is via food or water. *H. pylori* has been found in the saliva of infected people, so it is also postulated that the bacteria may spread by mouth-to-mouth contact, such as kissing. At this time, the most proven effective treatment is a 2-week course of treatment called triple therapy. Two antibiotics are given to kill the bacteria, and either an acid suppressor or a stomach lining shield is given. Two-week triple therapy is effective for 90% of patients.

Peptic ulcers are divided into two categories:

Duodenal Ulcers

H. pylori accounts for 90% of duodenal ulcers. The remaining 10% are related to an increased quantity or increased level of acidity of the gastric juice. Although the ulcers do not become malignant, perforation is common. Surgical measures are indicated only after all other avenues are exhausted. Current practice is to perform gastric resection with vagotomy to eliminate the acid-secreting stimulus to gastric cells. Branches of the vagus nerve are severed; the number depends on how much reduction in secretory ability is desired. If an insufficient number are cut, however, the ability of the stomach to secrete regenerates with time, and further intervention is required.

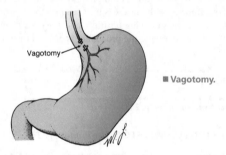

Vagotomy

■ Vagotomy.

Gastric Ulcers

H. pylori causes 80% of gastric ulcers. The remaining 20% of ulcers reabsorb the excess acid secreted through the mucous membrane by abnormal diffusion of H^+. This results in a damaged mucous barrier and renders the ulcer likely to bleed. Treatment is usually aggressive because about 10% of gastric ulcers are malignant. Resection is performed via a Billroth I procedure (partial gastrectomy with gastroduodenoscopy, which is excision of distal one third to one half of the stomach, and anastomosis of remaining portion of stomach to duodenum) or a Billroth II procedure (partial gastrectomy with gastrojejunostomy, which is removal of distal segment of the stomach and antrum, anastomoses of the remainder to the jejunum, and closing of the duodenal stump).

(continued)

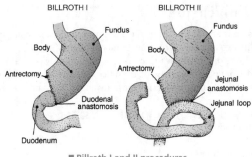

BILLROTH I   BILLROTH II

■ Billroth I and II procedures.

URETERAL STENTS *(see Stents, Urinary, p. 241)*

URETEROSTOMY *(see Urinary Diversions, p. 244)*

URINARY CATHETERS

Catheters may be self-retaining (able to maintain themselves in cavities) or non–self-retaining (must be secured with tape if left indwelling). They come in various sizes, graded from 14 F (smallest) to 22 F (largest), and in various shapes; the curved tip is frequently used for male patients and the straight tip for female patients. The self-retaining protuberance at the tip of the Malecot and de Pezzer catheters must be elongated with a stylet, which is passed through the lumen before insertion. After insertion, the stylet is removed, and the protuberance secures the catheter in place. Straight catheters may have a single eye or many eyes, and they may have a round tip or a whistle tip.

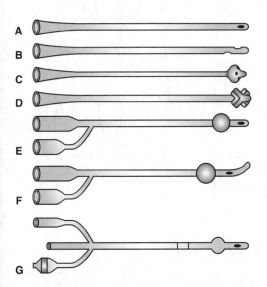

■ Different types of commonly used catheters. A, B, Simple urethral catheters. C, Mushroom or de Pezzer. D, Winged-tip or Malecot. E, Foley with inflated retention bag. F, Foley with Coude tip. G, Three-way catheter (in this illustration the third lumen opens into the urethra to permit irrigation; usually opens at tip for irrigation of the bladder).

URINARY DIVERSIONS

A urinary diversion is any one of several surgical procedures that change the way urine exits the body. The two types are incontinent and continent.

Incontinent diversions result in urine flowing continuously, and a bag or collection device is required. Continent diversions, on the other hand, are a newer type of surgical procedure that allows urine to be stored inside the body until it is drained by catheterization.

TYPES OF OSTOMIES IN THE URINARY SYSTEM

1. Incontinent diversions
   - Cystostomy
   - Ileal conduit (urostomy)
   - Nephrostomy
   - Ureterostomy

2. Continent diversions
   - Indiana pouch
   - Ileocecal pouch
   - Kock pouch
   - Neobladder

CYSTOSTOMY

A cystostomy is created by diverting the flow of urine from the bladder to the abdominal wall. This procedure requires the placement of a tube through the abdominal wall into the bladder. It is usually done because of blockage or stricture of the urethra and can be temporary or permanent.

ILEAL CONDUIT (UROSTOMY)

An ileal conduit is so called because the surgeon converts 6 to 8 inches of ileum into a conduit or "pipeline" for urinary drainage. The ureters are spliced into one end of the conduit and brought out the other side through the abdominal wall to form a stoma. The bowel is then rejoined and continues to function normally. Elimination through the stoma is urine. The patient has no voluntary control; a few drops of urine are discharged every 10 to 20 seconds.

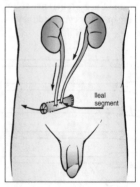

■ Ileal conduit (urostomy).

NEPHROSTOMY

A nephrostomy is created by diverting the flow of urine directly from the kidneys to the abdominal wall. Tubes are placed within the kidney to collect the urine as it is produced, and it drains continuously. This type of diversion is usually created because of obstruction of the ureters, and it is only temporary. However, if cancer is present, it can be permanent.

(continued)

URETEROSTOMY

In this type of diversion, the ureters are disengaged from the bladder and brought out through the abdominal wall at waist level. Sometimes there are two stomas (one on each side). Alternatively, one ureter undergoes anastomosis to the other and is brought to the skin surface to form a single stoma. Elimination is continuous.

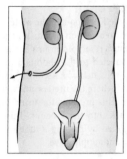

■ Ureterostomy.

INDIANA POUCH

The Indiana pouch uses about 1 foot of large intestine as a storage area for urine. In addition, a 6- to 8-inch piece of small intestine is used to create the stoma. The area of small intestine between the stoma and the reservoir is narrowed during surgery, and this narrowing prevents urine from leaking out the stoma. The ureters are tunneled into the reservoir wall, preventing urine from flowing back into the kidneys.

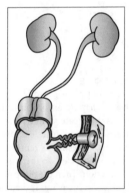

■ Indiana pouch.

ILEOCECAL POUCH

The ileocecal pouch is made using the same procedure as the Indiana pouch, the difference being that a nipple valve is created behind the stoma to make the stoma continent, as opposed to narrowing the small intestine during surgery.

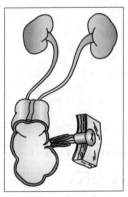

■ Ileocecal pouch.

(*continued*)

KOCK POUCH

With the Kock pouch, the ureters are connected to a section of small intestine used to create a reservoir for urine. The reservoir is connected to the abdomen by a nipple valve and a stoma. A second nipple valve is created where the ureters attach to the reservoir. This prevents the urine from flowing back into the kidneys. This reservoir is emptied by passing a tube through the stoma and nipple valve.

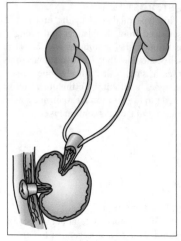

■ Kock pouch.

NEOBLADDER

The orthoptic neobladder procedure involves reshaping a portion of the small intestines to create a new receptacle to replace a diseased bladder. First, a section of small intestine is removed and the bowel is reconnected, so there is no loss of bowel function. Then the piece of removed intestine is cut open and reshaped to form a "pouch" and the ureters are connected to one end, while the urethra is connected to the other. This allows the urine to drain normally. However, although the new bladder has the capacity to stretch and store urine, it does *not* have the ability to contract, meaning urination must occur in a slightly different way. The "new" bladder is emptied by relaxing the sphincter muscle and contracting the abdominal muscles. When the abdominal muscles are contracted, pressure is put on the bladder, causing urine to flow.

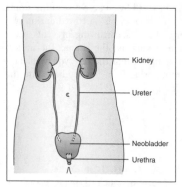

■ Neobladder.

UROSTOMY *(see Urinary Diversions, p. 244)*

VAGOTOMY *(see Ulcers, Duodenal, p. 242)*

WHIPPLE PROCEDURE *(see Pancreatitis, p. 236)*

PART 5

Renal System

ACUTE RENAL FAILURE

Acute renal failure is the rapid deterioration of renal function with a high blood concentration of nitrogen waste products. There are three major categories:

PRERENAL (Hypoperfused Kidney)

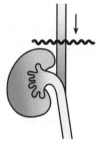

Prerenal events occur before blood reaches the kidney, leading to renal hypoperfusion and resulting in decrease of glomerular perfusion, CHF, and low blood pressure (BP). This is the most common cause of acute renal failure.

■ Prerenal failure.

INTRARENAL (Diseased Kidney)

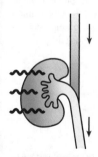

Intrarenal failure is due to intrinsic damage to the kidney. There are two types:

1. Glomerulonephritis has an immunologic basis and causes change in the glomerular membrane and/or cellular structure. The glomerulus loses its ability to be semipermeable, and protein and red blood cells (RBCs) pass through into the urine, resulting in hematuria and proteinuria.
2. Acute tubular necrosis has two origins:
   - **Ischemic (oliguric) necrosis** is related to catastrophic hypotension from many sources, for example, surgery, cardiac or septic shock, trauma, hemorrhage. It is more serious than nephrotoxic necrosis because cells are destroyed in a layer that cannot regenerate (the "basement membrane").

■ Intrarenal failure.

(continued)

- **Nephrotoxic (nonoliguric) necrosis** is related to environmental or occupational insults to the kidney, for example, large doses of iatrogenic agents such as gentamicin, amikacin, or carbenicillin. It has a good prognosis for recovery because the damage involves only the tubuleís layer of epithelial cells, which can regenerate.

Use of Laboratory Values in Differentiating Acute Tubular Necrosis from Decreased Renal Perfusion

	Acute Tubular Necrosis	Reduced Renal Blood Flow
Urine Volume	<400 mL/24 hr	<400 mL/24 hr
Sodium	>40 mEq/L	<20 mEq/L
Specific gravity	1.01	Usually >1.020
Osmolality	250–350 mOsm/L	Usually >400 mOsm/L
Urea	200–300 mg/100 mL	Usually >600 mg/100 mL
Creatinine clearance	<60 mg/100 mL	Usually >150 mg/100 mL
Fe_{Na}	>3.0%	<1.0%
Blood BUN/Cr ratio	10:1	Usually >20:1
Responses to Mannitol	None	None or flow increases to >40 mL/hr
Furosemide	None	Flow increases to >40 mL/hr

POSTRENAL (Obstructed Kidney)

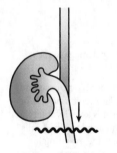

Postrenal failure is caused by blockage of flow in the urinary tract. Treatment of acute renal failure in the first 24 to 48 hours includes correcting hypotension or fluid deficits, administering furosemide (Lasix) (80–320 mg initial dose) or mannitol (12.5–25 g), and/or giving a trial of low-dose dopamine (1–3μg/kg/min) plus Lasix.

■ Postrenal failure.

ACUTE TUBULAR NECROSIS *(see Acute Renal Failure, Intrarenal, p. 247)*

ADH *(see also Aldosterone, p. 249; Renin-Angiotensin System, p. 261)*

Antidiuretic hormone (ADH) is controlled by osmoreceptors (sensitive to osmolar change) and baroreceptors (sensitive to pressure change). Normally, osmoreceptors in the hypothalamus stimulate the posterior pituitary to release ADH in response to a rise in serum osmolality (i.e., when water is lost). ADH then acts on the renal tubule to increase water permeability, and water is reabsorbed. The reverse is true: When serum osmolality falls (water is retained), excess water is excreted by the kidney.

Baroreceptors influence release of ADH in pathologic states. When blood volume is down about 10% or blood pressure falls, these receptors in the heart and various blood vessels contract and initiate a stimulus for ADH release. Water is then retained by the kidney. The reverse is true when baroreceptors are stretched more than normal (i.e., when blood volume rises).

Baroreceptors override osmoreceptors. For example, if blood volume is low, water is retained even though osmolality drops. This is a protective mechanism whereby the body attempts to maintain blood volume even though hemodilution results.

ALDOSTERONE *(see also ADH, p. 249; Renin-Angiotensin System, p. 261)*

Aldosterone is released by the adrenal cortex in response to angiotensin II, causing sodium and water to be reabsorbed and potassium and hydrogen to be excreted.

REMEMBER:

Because aldosterone causes sodium and water to be saved, the actual concentration of sodium does not change, only the extracellular volume.

Aldosterone is released for:
- Increased potassium (to decrease the K^+ level)
- Decreased sodium (to save Na^+)
- Hypovolemia (to save H_2O)

No aldosterone is released in cases of:
- Increased sodium (to decrease the Na^+ level)
- Decreased potassium (to save K^+)

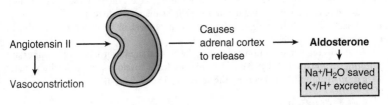

■ Aldosterone release.

ANATOMY, RENAL

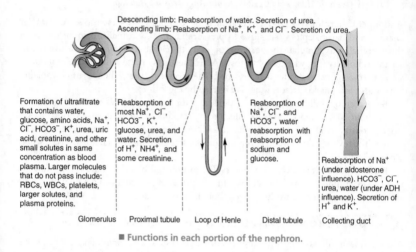

Descending limb: Reabsorption of water. Secretion of urea.
Ascending limb: Reabsorption of Na$^+$, K$^+$, and Cl$^-$. Secretion of urea.

Formation of ultrafiltrate that contains water, glucose, amino acids, Na$^+$, Cl$^-$, HCO3$^-$, K$^+$, urea, uric acid, creatinine, and other small solutes in same concentration as blood plasma. Larger molecules that do not pass include: RBCs, WBCs, platelets, larger solutes, and plasma proteins.

Reabsorption of most Na$^+$, Cl$^-$, HCO3$^-$, K$^+$, glucose, urea, and water. Secretion of H$^+$, NH4$^+$, and some creatinine.

Reabsorption of Na$^+$, Cl$^-$, and HCO3$^-$, water reabsorption with reabsorption of sodium and glucose.

Reabsorption of Na$^+$ (under aldosterone influence). HCO3$^-$, Cl$^-$, urea, water (under ADH influence). Secretion of H$^+$ and K$^+$.

Glomerulus   Proximal tubule   Loop of Henle   Distal tubule   Collecting duct

■ Functions in each portion of the nephron.

ANION GAP

The anion gap is a formula used to signal the presence of a metabolic acidosis, differentiate the cause, and confirm other findings. In maintaining chemical neutrality, the total concentrations of cations and anions in the blood (and other body fluids) are equivalent. Sodium accounts for 95% of all cations, and chloride and bicarbonate account for 85% of all anions. The concept of an anion "gap" developed when blood chemistries began to be reported as a "panel." Since only the major anions and cations are reported on these panels, it is **normal for a "gap" of 8 to 16 mEq/L to exist** (reflecting the absence of the anions/cations not accounted for). The formula to calculate the anion gap is:

$$Na^+ - (Cl^- + HCO_3^-)$$

An anion gap of >16 mEq/L indicates an increase in the number of unmeasured anions. Because most of these unmeasured anions are acids, the increase always reflects a metabolic acidosis. Differential diagnosis includes diabetic ketoacidosis; uremia (renal failure); lactic acidosis from sepsis; shock; ischemic bowel; or intoxication with aspirin, ethanol, antifreeze, or INH.

While a decrease in the anion gap is rare, the clinical significance is equally important, indicating hyponatremia, hypermagnesemia, multiple myeloma, or hypoalbuminemia (a 1-g drop in albumin will decrease the anion gap by 2.5–3 mEq).

REMEMBER:

An actual high anion gap (acidotic) in a patient with a low albumin level may appear as a false normal.

CAVH, CAVHD (see Continuous Renal Replacement Therapy, p. 253)

CONTINUOUS RENAL REPLACEMENT THERAPY
(see also Hemodialysis, p. 256; Peritoneal Dialysis, p. 259)

Continuous renal replacement therapy (CRRT) encompasses "out of body" blood purification methods intended to replace kidney function for extended periods of time, done continuously (24 hours/day). The general principles include blood flowing from a vascular access point, being purified in some manner outside the body by use of filters, creation of an "effluent" (urine), and returning the purified blood to the body via another vascular access. Depending on the mode used, access can be either venovenous or arteriovenous.

Treatment goals include promoting hemodynamic stability, allowing for nutritional support, maintaining fluid and electrolyte balance, maintaining pH balance, and promoting healing and renal recovery.

Modes: SCUF, CVVH, CVVHD, CVVHDF, CAVH, CAVHD

INDICATIONS FOR CRRT
- Oliguria (output <200 mL/12 hr)
- Hyperkalemia (K^+ >6.5 and rising)
- Acidemia (pH <7.1)
- Pulmonary edema
- Azotemia
- Uremic encephalopathy
- Uremic pericarditis
- Severe sodium alteration (<115 or >160 mEq/L)
- Hyperthermia
- Drug overdose (lithium, vancomycin, procainamide)
- Anasarca (accumulation of serum in subcutaneous connective tissue and serous cavities of body)
- Diuretic-resistant cardiac failure

IN SUMMARY, All of the above fall into four categories:
1. Volume overload
2. Acid-base imbalance
3. Uremic syndromes (and their sequelae)
4. Drug/toxin overdose

The contraindications for CRRT are all relative. In general, they include severe vascular disease and bleeding/clotting disorders.

CRRT TERMINOLOGY
- **Ultrafiltration:** The process of removing excess H_2O by creating a pressure differential between the blood and fluid compartments. The addition of positive pressure in the blood path and negative pressure in the dialysate path causes excess H_2O to move from the patient (high pressure) to an area of lower pressure (the dialysate). The negative pressure is an actual suctioning force applied to the membrane.
- **Convection:** Movement of solutes (solids) through a membrane via a "sweeping" action called a solvent drag
- **Diffusion:** Spontaneous movement of solutes from an area of higher concentration to one of lower concentration

(continued)

- **Osmosis:** Spontaneous movement of water from an area of lower concentration to one of higher concentration
- **Hemofiltration:** Movement of large volumes of fluid via ultrafiltration, and some movement of solutes via convection
- **Replacement fluid:** Approximates normal plasma, flexible to meet patient needs (Ringer's lactate, normal saline, albumin, bicarbonate, electrolytes)
- **Dialysate:** Solution that surrounds the patient's blood, separated by a filter, and allows solutes to cross from one side to the other

CRRT methods can be either arteriovenous (AV) or venovenous (VV). The differences are listed in the table.

CRRT: Arteriovenous (AV) Versus Venovenous (VV)	
Arteriovenous	**Venovenous**
Vein and artery are cannulated	Only vein is cannulated
MAP must be >70 (Patient's heart drives therapy)	MAP can be <70 (Therapy is pump driven)
More difficult to manage fluids, electrolytes	Blood movement is monitored via the pump

SCUF (Slow Continuous Ultrafiltration)
- Requires a blood pump
- Blood flow 10 to 180 mL/min
- No dialysate fluids or replacement fluids used
- Removes large amount of fluid (up to 2,000 mL/hr) via ultrafiltration
- Removes limited amount of solutes (via convection)

CVVH (Continuous Venovenous Hemofiltration)
- Requires a blood pump
- Removes fluid via ultrafiltration, if desired (maximum 1,000 mL/hr)
- Removes solutes via convection (does a better job at this than SCUF)
- Uses a porous, semipermeable membrane
- No dialysate; uses replacement fluid instead, which can be given either before filtration (predilution) or after filtration (postdilution)

CVVHD (Continuous Venovenous Hemodialysis)
- Requires a blood pump
- Ultrafiltration rate up to 1 L/hr
- Blood flow 10 to 180 mL/min
- Dialysate flow rate 15 to 45 mL/min
- Provides fluid removal, if desired, up to 1,000 mL/hr
- Clears solutes via diffusion
- No replacement fluid; dialysate used instead

CVVHDF (Continuous Venovenous Hemodiafiltration)
- Requires a blood pump
- The "deluxe" method in that it includes "everything"
- Blood flow 10 to 180 mL/min
- Fluid removed via high-volume ultrafiltration, if desired (maximum 1,000 mL/hr)

(continued)

- Solutes removed via convection and diffusion simultaneously
- Both dialysate and replacement fluids are used. (This is the only difference between this and CVVHD. CVVHDF uses replacement fluid, and CVVHD does not.)

CAVH (Continuous Arteriovenous Hemofiltration)
- Blood is circulated by patient's own arterial pressure (no pump).
- Fluid replacement is infused into the venous port to approximate fluid removal or to maintain weight balance.
- Heparin is infused into the arterial line at approximately 100 U/kg/hr.
- No concentration gradient; therefore, only filtration of fluid occurs.
- Electrolytes are eliminated only as they are pulled along with fluid.
- Advantage: Ease of hourly replacement and virtually no risk of air embolism.
- Disadvantage: Only minimal amount of protein can be removed. Does not use diffusion; therefore, any removal of blood urea nitrogen (BUN) is accomplished by convective transport. Accordingly, the removal of BUN is slow and very dependent on good blood flow through the filter.

CAVHD (Continuous Arteriovenous Hemodialysis)
- Blood is circulated by patient's own arterial pressure (no pump).
- Combines advantages of CAVH with the filtering properties of dialysis, providing a better clearance of urea
- A dialysate solution is infused along with the hemofiltered blood.
- Advantages: No rapid fluid shifts
- Disadvantage: A pressure gradient is necessary for optimal filtration.

(*continued*)

NOTES

- **SCUF**
  No dialysate
  No fluid replacement
  Removes large amount of fluid
  Removes limited solutes
  Requires pump

Access Return

FILTER

Effluent

- **CVVH**
  No dialysate
  Fluid replacement
  Removes fluids
  Removes some solutes
    (more than SCUF)
  Requires pump

Access Return

FILTER ← Fluid replacement

Effluent

- **CVVHD**
  Uses dialysate
  No fluid replacement
  Moves fluid and solutes
    across filter
  Moves more particles
  Requires pump

Access Return

Dialysate → FILTER

Effluent

- **CVVHDF**
  Uses dialysate
  Fluid replacement
  Removes fluid
  Removes solutes
  Requires pump

Access Return

Dialysate → FILTER ← Fluid replacement

Effluent

- **CAVH**
  No dialysate
  Fluid replacement
  Only filtration of fluid occurs
  Limited amount of protein
    removed
  No pump—uses patient's
    own pressure

Venous access Arterial return
Fluid replacement → ← Heparin

FILTER

Effluent

- **CAVHD**
  Uses dialysate
  Fluid replacement
  Rapid clearance of urea
  No pump—uses patient's
    own pressure

Venous access Arterial return
Fluid replacement → ← Heparin
Dialysate → FILTER

Effluent

■ CRRT comparison.

(*continued*)

COMPLICATIONS OF CRRT

Hypotension

Inadequate replacement fluid, incorrect intake/output calculations, extreme fluid shifts, sepsis, fluid balance already achieved.

Electrolyte, pH Imbalances

Inadequate trending and monitoring, incorrect choice of replacement solution or dialysate, citrate anticoagulation (calcium, sodium, and pH shifts).

Hypothermia

Exposure to large amount of room-temperature replacement fluid or dialysate, extracorporeal circuit problems.

Hyperglycemia

High dextrose in dialysate solution, incorrect nutrition, underlying diabetes, calories will be lost if dialysate is dextrose free.

Clogged Filters

Effluent pressures become more negative, filter pressures increase, return pressures become more positive, visual color changes, blood in return line is cooler, visible clots in system.

REMEMBER:

It is important to know which medications will be cleared by dialysis.

- Acetaminophen
- ACE inhibitors (dangerous in patients with ARF, anyway)
- Aminoglycosides
- Aspirin
- Atenolol
- Aztreonam
- Bretylium
- Cephalosporins
- Cimetidine
- Esmolol
- Nipride
- Most penicillins
- Ranitidine

NOTES

CRRT, CVVH, CVVHD, CVVHDV
(see Continuous Renal Replacement Therapy, p. 251)

CREATININE CLEARANCE

Creatinine clearance measures the efficiency of the glomerular filtration of plasma.

$$\text{Creatinine clearance} = \frac{140 - \text{age in years} \times \text{body weight (kg)}}{72 \times \text{serum creatinine}}$$

For women, multiply the result by 0.85.

Normal:
Males: 107 to 139 mL/min
Females: 87 to 107 mL/min

DIALYSIS *(see Continuous Renal Replacement Therapy, p. 251; Hemodialysis, p. 256; Peritoneal Dialysis, p. 259)*

ERYTHROPOIETIN

Erythropoietin stimulates the production of RBCs in bone marrow and prolongs the life of the RBC. Kidneys either produce erythropoietin or synthesize an enzyme that catalyzes its formation. The stimulation for production is believed to be decreased oxygen delivery to the kidney. Erythropoietin deficiency is the primary cause of anemia in chronic renal failure. A deficiency is usually treated with intravenous or subcutaneous epogen, a recombinant human erythropoietin, at 50 to 100 units/kg, three times weekly.

GLOMERULAR FILTRATION RATE

A clinical assessment tool, the glomerular filtration rate (GFR) is used to determine renal function. The glomerulus (a capillary bed) filters about 120 to 125 mL/min through its membrane, or about 180 L daily. The resulting filtrate forms the main component of urine. Normal urine volume is approximately 1 L per day; this indicates >99% reabsorption of filtrate. The glomerular filtration rate helps measure the degree of renal function. It is inversely related to creatinine level.

Glomerular Filtration Rate	
Normal	125 mL/min
Renal insufficiency	<100 mL/min
Signs and symptoms of renal failure	<20 mL/min
Life-threatening renal failure	<10 mL/min

GLOMERULONEPHRITIS *(see Acute Renal Failure, p. 247)*

HEMODIALYSIS *(see also Continuous Renal Replacement Therapy, p. 251; Peritoneal Dialysis, p. 259)*

Hemodialysis is an extracorporeal technique for removing waste products or toxic substances from systemic circulation using a fistula, graft, or shunt.
Fistula: Anastomosis of an artery and a vein.

(continued)

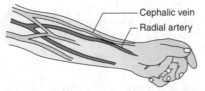

■ An internal arteriovenous fistula is created by a side-to-side anastomosis of the artery and vein.

Graft: The connection of an artery and a vein from an autogenous vein (usually the saphenous) or a bovine or Gore-Tex graft.

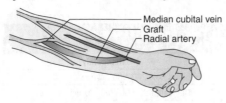

■ A graft can be established between the artery and vein.

Shunt: An older form of the graft. It is an external connection of an artery and vein by means of a silicone Teflon connector. The main disadvantage (and danger) is disconnection of the shunt, resulting in hemorrhage. Therefore, it is rarely used any more.

GRAFT OR FISTULA CARE

1. Auscultate bruit or palpate thrill to assess patency.
2. Do not perform venipuncture, start IV, give injections, or take blood pressure with cuff on access arm.

QUINTON CATHETER

A large-bore two-lumen catheter, providing 350 to 400 mL/min flow, used for temporary access during fistula maturation or long-term access for hemodialysis, apheresis, or medication administration when peripheral IV access is not possible.

Catheter care:*

- The catheter is to be treated with strict aseptic technique and meticulous prep.
- Dressing changes will not precede any other treatment and will not be done at the same time as a wound dressing change.
- The dressing must provide a 1- to 2-inch seal around the entire access site.
- Catheter lumens are color coded: the red lumen (arterial) is for dialysis access, the blue lumen (venous) is for return.
- When not in use, the lumen(s) are blocked with heparin (5,000 units per 1 cc of volume) in an amount that is equal to the lumen of the catheter (printed on the catheter).
- Ports are not routinely flushed unless used.
- Lumens should be wrapped in gauze, secured with tape, and tagged to indicate that they are blocked with heparin.
- The heparin is removed before the catheter is used.
- Usually used for IV fluid therapy and medication **only** with a written order from the nephrologist.
- If accessing for IV use (blue port only), under aseptic technique, the lumen should be scrubbed with an iodophor prep pad, and wrapped with a second iodophor prep pad. After 5 minutes, the port can be exposed and laid on a sterile 4 × 4 before aspirating heparin and proceeding with infusion.

Catheter care is institution specific; it is suggested that individual hospital policy be reviewed.

(continued)

HEPARINIZATION

Before dialysis, "regional" heparinization is usually done to keep blood anticoagulated in the dialysis machine. Heparin rebound may occur for up to 10 hours after heparin has stopped. Monitor patient closely for bleeding.

HEMODIALYSIS VERSUS CRRT

While hemodialysis and CRRT operate on the same principles, they differ in that CRRT is continuous, whereas hemodialysis is done intermittently (usually 4 hours daily, three or four times per week). Refer to chart that follows.

Continuous Renal Replacement Therapy (CRRT) Compared with Hemodialysis	
CRRT	**Hemodialysis**
Blood flow 10–180 mL/min	Blood flow 200–500 mL/min
Dialysate flow 15–45 mL/min	Dialysate flow 500–800 mL/min
MAP <70 acceptable	MAP >70 required
Uses a small hemofilter	Uses large surface dialyzers
Slow fluid shifts	Fast fluid shifts
Hemodynamic stability	Hemodynamic instability
Slow, gentle clearance of waste	Radical, quick clearance of waste

HEMOFILTRATION *(see Continuous Renal Replacement Therapy, p. 252)*

OSMOLALITY

Osmolality is used in clinical practice more often than osmolarity. It is expressed in milliosmoles per kg of water (mOsm/kg). It reflects the measurement of solute concentration per kilogram in blood and urine, and it is usually used when referring to fluids inside the body.
Normal: 280 to 295 mOsm/kg
Fluid overload: <275 mOsm/kg
Dehydration: >295 mOsm/kg

   Serum osmolality is essentially what keeps the fluids in their appropriate compartments, and it measures the "pulling power" of water. Na^+ accounts for at least half of this pulling power; each milliequivalent of Na^+ equals 1 milliosmole. Therefore, $\frac{1}{2} \times 300 = 150$, and Na^+ normal is 135 to 145 mEq/L.

REMEMBER:

Because sodium accounts for nearly half of the osmolality value, a quick way to do a rough guesstimate is to multiply the Na^+ value by 2. The longer and more exact equation is

$$Na^+ \times 2 + \frac{serum\ glucose}{18} + \frac{BUN}{1.8}$$

280 to 300 is normal

<280 = water or intracellular fluid excess.
>300 = water or intracellular fluid deficit.

(continued)

Other factors that account for osmolality:

- Amount of urea in plasma
- Amount of glucose in plasma
- Amount of plasma proteins in plasma (fibrinogen, albumin, globulins)

Osmolality depends on the mechanism of osmosis, causing water to be drawn into the solution of high concentration (the cell) until the concentration of particles is equalized. Intracellular and extracellular osmolalities are always equal. Their measurement indicates overall body hydration or how concentrated body fluids are.

OSMOLARITY

Osmolarity is expressed in milliosmoles per liter of solution (mOsm/L) and is used to describe the number of dissolved particles within a solution. It is generally used to describe fluids outside the body; however, because 1 L of H_2O weighs 1 kg, the term "osmolarity" is often used interchangeably with osmolality.

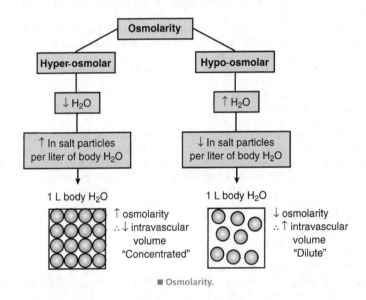

■ Osmolarity.

PERITONEAL DIALYSIS

In peritoneal dialysis, the dialyzing fluid is instilled into the peritoneal cavity, and the peritoneum serves as the dialyzing membrane. It is not as rapid as hemodialysis for volume removal, nor does it provide as much plasma clearance. The major detriments to its use are protein wasting and elevation of the diaphragm affecting ventilation, but its simplicity makes it useful in a small number of patients. Dialysis can be done either manually (with fill/dwell/drain self-timed cycles) or via the use of a mechanized PD cycler (precise fill/dwell/drain times accomplished automatically). The advantage of cyclers is that they provide accurate totals of net gain or loss and therapy can be modified from the typical night hours only to a continuous 24-hour dialysis, if needed. While cyclers are less labor

(continued)

intensive than manual PD, the major disadvantage is that the patient is connected to the cycler for the entire duration of therapy, thereby decreasing mobilization.

PROCEDURE
- Always use sterile technique.
- Bladder should be empty.
- Warm dialysate solution to body temperature. (Cyclers do this automatically.) A solution too cool causes abdominal pain and cramping, whereas one too warm may cause injury to the abdominal organs.
- Weigh patient before and after the procedure. Mark midpoint of abdomen with a pen, and also measure abdominal girth daily, using the same mark.
- Purge all air from the system by running the dialysate through the tubing. (A 1.5% solution is the most common choice, and 4.25% solution is the second choice. Sometimes these two fluids are alternated during exchanges.)
- Add medication to the dialysate as prescribed (heparin, KCl, antibiotics, lidocaine). Infuse the dialysate as fast as tolerated, usually about 2 L in 6 to 15 minutes. (Cycler set to do this automatically.)
- The first exchange must be drained immediately to make sure the catheter is patent. All subsequent exchanges dwell according to physician orders, usually 20 to 45 minutes. (Cycler set to do this automatically.)
- Drain passively at end of dwell time, observing amount and characteristics of drainage:
    Normal = clear, pale yellow
    Cloudy = infection, peritonitis
    Brown = bowel perforation
    Amber = bladder perforation
    Bloody = common in first to fourth exchange; if it continues, may be abdominal bleeding
- After each exchange, record the infused volume, the dwell time, the total drainage, whether patient is in negative balance (patient giving up fluid) or positive balance (patient retaining fluid), and cumulative balance. (Cycler set to do this automatically.)

DIANEAL FLUID
- **REMEMBER:** The higher the percentage of the dianeal fluid, the more water you will pull.
    1.5% (lowest) = Pulls no water
    2.5% = Moderate
    4.25% (max) = Pulls the most water
- **REMEMBER:** The more fluid put into the cavity, the greater the diffusion. (Sending more soldiers into battle.)

TROUBLESHOOTING
- **If outflow stops or slows,** be sure clamp is open. Check tubing for kinks, turn patient side to side, or apply gentle pressure on abdomen to help start flow.
- **If there is a sudden BP drop or tachycardia,** stop dialysis and notify physician.
- **Leakage at exit site** can be caused by kinks in tubing. If tubing is OK, change dressing and wait for next exchange. If leak continues, be sure to weigh fluid loss on dressing, and notify physician. Catheter may have slipped.
- **Sudden acute abdominal pain or back pain** may be related to the temperature of the solution. Also check for air in the system, and monitor the rate of infusion.
- **Scrotal swelling** is most likely caused by a dislodged catheter. Notify the physician.

(continued)

- **Muscle cramps and increased weakness** can be caused by electrolyte imbalances. Send specimen to lab for electrolyte analysis.

QUINTON CATHETER *(see Hemodialysis, p. 257)*

RENIN-ANGIOTENSIN SYSTEM *(see also Aldosterone, p. 249; ADH, p. 249)*

Baroreceptors are the primary influence on sodium regulation. Located in the renal cortex, they control the release of renin from the adjacent cells (juxtaglomerular apparatus) in response to decreased blood pressure or decreased extracellular fluid. The renin converts angiotensin I to angiotensin II, a potent vasoconstrictor, which results in increased blood pressure and increased GFR (glomerular filtration rate). Angiotensin II also triggers the release of aldosterone, causing an increase in renal sodium and water retention, thus increasing extracellular fluid volume, increasing blood pressure, and inhibiting further renin secretion. Any increase in Na^+ intake or increase in blood volume also suppresses renin and aldosterone release, permitting increased Na^+ excretion.

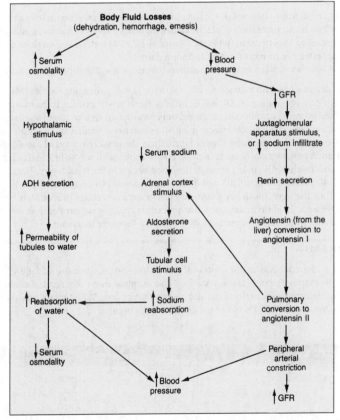

■ Relationship of antidiuretic hormone, renin, and aldosterone to fluid regulation by the kidneys.

RHABDOMYOLYSIS

Rhabdomyolysis occurs after skeletal muscle injury that allows the release of muscle cell contents (CK, lactate dehydrogenase, myoglobin, uric acid, K^+, PO_4, organic acids, and creatinine) into extracellular fluid. Many of these contents are toxic at high levels, literally occluding the kidneys and causing renal failure. Trauma is the number one cause, although rhabdomyolysis is often seen in patients with status epilepticus or burns or is self-induced by healthy individuals who exceed their capacity for exercise endurance or use cocaine. Lab tests reveal elevated serum CK, Hematest-positive urine, and few or no RBCs on urinalysis. Treatment involves first flushing the kidneys with massive volume replacement and sometimes giving mannitol and Lasix concurrently for diuresis and to increase serum osmolality. The most significant problem during the 4 hours after administration is hyperkalemia.

SCUF *(see Continuous Renal Replacement Therapy, p. 252)*

STENTS, RENAL

Although renal artery stenosis (RAS) has multiple causes, it is most commonly a result of atherosclerosis. Accumulation of plaque causes the renal arteries to narrow, leading to:
- Uncontrolled hypertension (typically defined as BP >140 systolic and on three or more antihypertensive medications that include a diuretic);
- Renal insufficiency (an estimated creatinine clearance less than institutional normal).

The diagnosis of RAS is based on clinical exam as well as imaging studies (MRA, CT scan, duplex, angiography), CXR, EKG, and labs. Renal artery stenting is the most widely performed procedure to alleviate this condition; however, in view of recent studies showing no advantage over medical management, its popularity is waning and it is now viewed as controversial by many. To be eligible for stenting, the renal artery vessel should ideally be >4 mm. A puncture site or small incision is established to either the brachial or femoral artery, and a catheter is guided through the blood vessels to the renal artery. The catheter carries a tiny balloon that inflates and deflates to compress plaque against the walls of the artery. Then the stent, much like a coronary artery stent (see Stents in Part 2), is inserted and deployed to hold the artery open. The procedure typically requires only an overnight hospital stay, with routine physician follow up every 3 months thereafter.

UREMIA

Uremia is the retention in the blood of urinary constituents because of failure of the kidney to excrete them. Nausea, vomiting, and eventual coma can result. In addition, bleeding abnormalities, pericarditis, and pleuritis may occur. With today's availability of dialysis, the clinical features of uremia do not usually occur.

NOTES

PART 6

Endocrine System

ADDISON'S DISEASE *(see also Aldosterone in Part 5, p. 249)*

Addison's disease results from hypofunction of the adrenal cortex of the kidney, causing a severe decrease in levels of aldosterone and cortisol with resultant fluid and electrolyte imbalances; protein, fat, and carbohydrate disturbances; and ultimately circulatory collapse. Although abrupt withdrawal of steroids is a common cause, approximately 70% of cases are idiopathic. Addison's disease is the "opposite" of Cushing's disease, in which there is an oversecretion of glucocorticoid hormones.

The pituitary gland secretes adrenocorticotropic hormone (ACTH), which stimulates the adrenal cortex to secrete its own hormones. Addison's disease is diagnosed by stimulating ACTH with drug therapy and evaluating the response of the adrenal cortex. Normally, the excretion of hydroxycorticoids and ketosteroids increases, whereas patients with Addison's disease show little or no increase. Also, eosinophils in the patient's blood are measured. A drop of 60% to 90% in the count after ACTH is given is normal, but there is little drop in the count in a patient with Addison's disease.

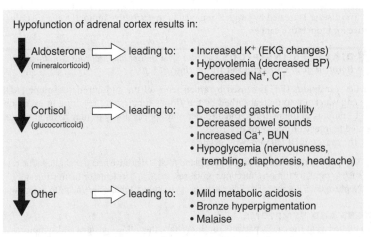

Hypofunction of adrenal cortex results in:

▼ Aldosterone (mineralcorticoid)	⟹ leading to:	• Increased K⁺ (EKG changes) • Hypovolemia (decreased BP) • Decreased Na⁺, Cl⁻
▼ Cortisol (glucocorticoid)	⟹ leading to:	• Decreased gastric motility • Decreased bowel sounds • Increased Ca⁺, BUN • Hypoglycemia (nervousness, trembling, diaphoresis, headache)
▼ Other	⟹ leading to:	• Mild metabolic acidosis • Bronze hyperpigmentation • Malaise

■ Signs and symptoms of Addison's disease.

Addisonian crisis is a life-threatening exacerbation of the disease with severe hypotension, shock, coma, and vasomotor collapse.

Treatment is based on fluid replacement with 5% dextrose in normal saline and the IV administration of corticosteroids.

(continued)

REMEMBER:

No patient with Addison's disease should ever receive insulin. The patient may die of the resultant hypoglycemia.

ADRENAL INSUFFICIENCY
(see Addison's Disease, p. 263; Cushing's Disease, p. 264)

CUSHING'S DISEASE

Cushing's disease results from oversecretion of ACTH by a pituitary or adrenal basophilic tumor, although many times it is caused by steroids, which are given for a variety of conditions, ranging from asthma to lupus, rheumatoid arthritis, other inflammatory conditions, or immune suppression following a transplant.

It is diagnosed by the presence of high-glucocorticoid metabolites in urine and plasma, indicating that adrenal hyperactivity exists. It is the "opposite" of Addison's disease, in which there is a severe decrease in the levels of aldosterone and cortisol.

SIGNS AND SYMPTOMS
- Persistent hyperglycemia
- Protein tissue wasting (weakness, osteoporosis)
- K^+ depletion (dysrhythmias, renal disorders)
- Na^+ and H_2O retention (edema, hypertension, congestive heart failure)
- Abnormal fat distribution (moon face; buffalo hump; striae on breasts, axilla, legs)
- Increased susceptibility to infection
- Mood swings

The disease is treated by surgical removal of the causative tumor. Drugs are only palliative for inoperable cancer.

DIABETES INSIPIDUS *(see also Syndrome of Inappropriate Antidiuretic Hormone, p. 273; Cerebral Salt Wasting in Part 1, p. 14)*

Diabetes insipidus (DI) is caused by a deficiency of the antidiuretic hormone (ADH), causing water not to be reabsorbed by the kidney tubules and resulting in excretion of large amounts of dilute urine. The disorder may appear slowly or may develop suddenly, related to injury or infectious disease.

The causes of DI fall into two categories:

1. **Vasopressin deficiency:** The pituitary gland itself is defective because of idiopathic causes such as pituitary tumors, infectious processes, vascular accidents, or neurosurgery.
2. **Nephrogenic:** Because of an inherited defect, the kidney tubules are unable to absorb water.

SIGNS AND SYMPTOMS
No matter what the cause, patients routinely have the following signs and symptoms:
- Polydipsia and polyuria (may drink 5–40 L per day and excrete the same 5–40 L per day). Unless the patient drinks almost continuously, there is always a danger of dehydration and hypovolemic shock.
- Decreased urine osmolality
- Decreased urine specific gravity (<1.005)
- Increased serum osmolality
- Increased serum Na^+

(continued)

Comparison of DI and SIADH ("Opposites")		
	DI	**SIADH**
Serum Osmolality (285–295)	⬆ ("High and Dry")	⬇ ("Waterlogged")
Urine Osmolality (50–1,200)	⬇	⬆
Sodium (135–145)	⬆	⬇
Specific Gravity (1.010–1.030)	⬇	⬆

TREATMENT

DI is treated with replacement ADH. Desmopressin acetate (DDAVP) is a synthetic ADH and is given IV on an emergent basis or as a nasal spray for long-term therapy.

Aqueous vasopressin (Pitressin), given IV or subcutaneously, is sometimes used for transient or severe DI. It is short acting and may cause angina or hypertension. Dehydration and electrolyte imbalances must also be attended to, and replacement IV therapy with hypotonic solutions (0.5 normal saline) is administered, often to match the urine output on an hour-to-hour basis.

DIABETES MELLITUS (see also Insulin in Part 8, Drugs, p. 318)

There are basically two types of diabetes mellitus: Type 1 and Type 2. They vary in their causes and their treatment.

TYPE 1 DIABETES MELLITUS

Type 1 diabetes is thought to develop because of an autoimmune response causing the β cells within the islet tissue of the pancreas to be destroyed. Because insulin is not available, the blood glucose level rises above what is safe for the body. **REMEMBER:** Insulin is the "key" that unlocks the cells, allowing the glucose to enter. No insulin = no key = glucose is "locked out" of cells and remains in blood = high blood glucose levels. Over time, these high glucose levels damage blood vessels and nerves throughout the body and increase the risk of eye, heart, blood vessel, nerve, and kidney disease. Patients with Type 1 diabetes are dependent on insulin to survive. For this reason, Type 1 diabetes was once known as insulin-dependent diabetes mellitus (IDDM) and was also once known as juvenile-onset diabetes, because it usually develops during childhood or the teen years. Symptoms include increased urination, increased thirst, increased appetite, and weight loss.

TYPE 2 DIABETES MELLITUS

Type 2 diabetes is the most common, occurring in about 90% to 95% of all patients with diabetes. It occurs when the pancreas still makes insulin, but not enough to meet the body's needs. In some cases, enough insulin is made, but the body is unable to use it. Type 2 diabetes is often affected by obesity and can sometimes be controlled by maintenance of proper body weight, proper diet, and exercise. It was once known as non–insulin-dependent diabetes

(continued)

mellitus (NIDDM). Whereas Type 2 diabetes does not always require medication, it is not the milder form of the disease: It can cause the same harmful effects as Type 1 diabetes.

Because the high glucose levels develop gradually in Type 2 diabetes, there are often no symptoms early in the disease, or the specific symptoms for diabetes (listed above) are easily overlooked.

Optimum serum glucose levels before meals should be below 100 mg/dL. The glycosylated hemoglobin (HgAlc) test tells how well blood glucose levels have been controlled over the previous 2 to 3 months. For most people, a good HgAlc level is 6% to 7%.

PRE-DIABETES

Defined by a blood glucose higher than normal, but not high enough to be diagnosed as diabetes mellitus, *pre-diabetes* has been proven to put people at an increased risk for progression to Type 2 diabetes (usually within 10 years). There are no symptoms, although the person is frequently overweight or obese. The cornerstone of therapy is diet and exercise, with a goal of reducing total body weight by 5% to 10%. Diagnosis is confirmed in one of two ways:

Fasting glucose test: No food is eaten overnight, and a blood glucose level is checked in the morning before eating.

> Normal = <100 mg/dL; Pre-diabetic = 100 to 125 mg/dL; Diabetic = >126 mg/dL

Oral glucose tolerance test: No food is eaten overnight, after which a glucose-rich drink is consumed. Two hours later a blood glucose test is taken.

> Normal = <140 mg/dL; Pre-diabetic = 140 to 199 mg/dL; Diabetic = >200 mg/dL

Although several drugs have been shown to reduce diabetes risk to varying degrees, none has been approved by the FDA. The American Diabetes Association recommends that metformin is the only drug that should be considered for use in diabetes prevention, and then only in cases of very high-risk individuals, with a body mass index of at least 35, and those who are younger than 60 years.

DIABETIC KETOACIDOSIS *(see also Hyperglycemic Hyperosmolar Nonketotic Coma, p. 270)*

Diabetic ketoacidosis (DKA) is a life-threatening medical emergency, seen most often in patients with Type 1 diabetes mellitus (insulin dependent). It occurs when there is insufficient insulin to metabolize glucose, resulting in a cascade of events leading to hyperglycemia, ketosis, and acidosis.

(continued)

NOTES

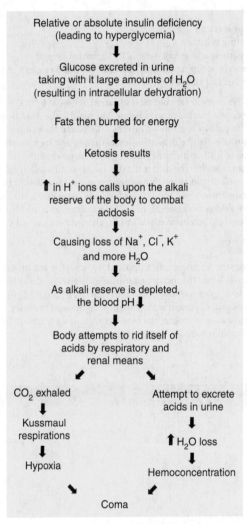

Relative or absolute insulin deficiency
(leading to hyperglycemia)

Glucose excreted in urine
taking with it large amounts of H_2O
(resulting in intracellular dehydration)

Fats then burned for energy

Ketosis results

↑ in H^+ ions calls upon the alkali
reserve of the body to combat
acidosis

Causing loss of Na^+, Cl^-, K^+
and more H_2O

As alkali reserve is depleted,
the blood pH ↓

Body attempts to rid itself of
acids by respiratory and
renal means

CO_2 exhaled

Kussmaul
respirations

Hypoxia

Attempt to excrete
acids in urine

↑ H_2O loss

Hemoconcentration

Coma

■ Diabetic ketoacidosis (DKA).

SIGNS AND SYMPTOMS

The signs and symptoms of DKA can be directly linked to three factors:

1. **Severe dehydration** resulting in dry mucous membranes, thirst, loss of skin turgor, and increased serum osmolarity
2. **Loss of essential electrolytes,** resulting in a glucose level of >250 mg/dL (usually in the 600 range)
3. **Acidosis** resulting in Kussmaul's respirations, acetone breath, and a positive anion gap

(*continued*)

THERAPY

The goal of therapy is to:

1. Restore circulating volume
2. Return blood glucose and serum osmolality to normal ranges
3. Resolve acidosis (by stopping the breakdown of fats into ketones)
4. Correct electrolyte imbalances

Initially 0.9% NS is given for volume restoration, followed by 0.45% NS with KCl for maintenance. Once the glucose level is below 250 mg/dL, the fluid is changed to D_5W. Concomitantly, the patient is given an insulin drip. (Until the potassium level is determined, however, this is withheld to avoid exacerbating any hypokalemia.) When instituted, an IV bolus of 0.15 units/kg of regular insulin is given, followed by an IV drip of at the rate of 0.1 units/kg/hr. The drip is titrated hourly until a fall in the glucose of 50 to 70 mg/dL is achieved. Rapid correction of the hyperglycemia should be avoided due to the risk of cerebral edema. Once the glucose level has normalized, the therapy cannot be discontinued until acidosis is resolved, the pH normalizes, and the HCO_3 is >18 mEq/L. IV therapy can then be discontinued and insulin given subcutaneously.

REMEMBER:

Monitor closely for the Somogyi effect (a paradox), whereby the insulin actually causes a *high* blood glucose level. This occurs after insulin is given and the blood glucose level decreases. If the level goes too low, stress hormones are produced, which promote the breakdown of glycogen. Glycogen is the chemical compound the body uses to store glucose, and with the loss of glycogen, the blood glucose level will rise. The end result is a "rebound" or an "insulin-induced" hyperglycemia.

(*continued*)

NOTES

Comparison of Hyperglycemic Hyperosmolar Nonketotic Coma and Diabetic Ketoacidosis

Hyperglycemic Coma	Diabetic Ketoacidosis
Patient has Type 2 diabetes and may be treated by diet alone, diet and an oral hypoglycemic agent, or diet and insulin therapy	Patient has Type 1, insulin-dependent diabetes
Patient usually older than 40 years	Patient usually younger than 40 years
Insidious onset	Usually rapid onset
Symptoms include:	Symptoms include:
1. Slight drowsiness, insidious stupor, or frequent coma	1. Drowsiness, stupor, coma
2. Polyuria for 2 days to 2 weeks before clinical presentation	2. Polyuria for 1–3 days before clinical presentation
3. Absence of hyperventilation, no breath odor	3. Hyperventilation with possible Kussmaul's respiration pattern, "fruity" breath odor
4. Extreme volume depletion (dehydration, hypovolemia)	4. Extreme volume depletion (dehydration, hypovolemia)
5. Serum glucose 600–2,400 mg/dL	5. Serum glucose 300–1,000 mg/dL
6. Occasional gastrointestinal symptoms	6. Abdominal pain, nausea, vomiting, and diarrhea
7. Hypernatremia	7. Mild hyponatremia
8. Failure of thirst mechanism, leading to inadequate water ingestion	8. Polydipsia for 1–3 days
9. High serum osmolality with minimal CNS symptoms (disorientation, focal seizures)	9. High serum osmolality
10. Impaired renal function	10. Impaired renal function
11. HCO_3 level >16 mEq/L	11. HCO_3 level <10 mEq/L
12. CO_2 level normal	12. CO_2 level <10 mEq/L
13. Anion gap <7 mEq/L	13. Anion gap >7 mEq/L
14. Usually normal serum potassium	14. Extreme hypokalemia
15. Ketonemia absent	15. Ketonemia present
16. Lack of acidosis	16. Moderate to severe acidosis
17. High mortality rate	17. High recovery rate

DKA *(see Diabetic Ketoacidosis, p. 266)*

GRAVES' DISEASE *(see also Thyrotoxicosis, p. 274)*

In Graves' disease, excessive quantities of thyroid hormone are released in relation to heightened sensitivity to adrenergic stimuli. This causes all bodily processes to be literally "speeded up." Diagnosis is made by the basal metabolic rate determination test (BMRD), the protein-bound iodine test (PBI), serum T_3 and T_4 determinations, and the ^{131}I urine excretion test (requires a 24-hour sample). Although it may not be necessary (since characteristic clinical manifestations will already be evident), a TSI (thyroid-stimulating immunoglobin) value of >130% will provide a definitive diagnosis. The greater the value, the higher the degree of disease.

(continued)

The patient experiences diaphoresis, tachycardia, and heat intolerance. Emotions are usually adversely affected, for example, extreme fatigue followed by episodes of overactivity. Characteristically, the eyes bulge (exophthalmos), and there may be a goiter caused by hyperplasia and hypertrophy of the thyroid cells.

Treatment is with antithyroid drugs (propylthiouracil, methimazole) or radioiodine therapy. Occasionally, surgery is required if the patient's condition is unresponsive to drugs, and a subtotal thyroidectomy (removal of 5/6 of the gland) is performed.

HHNK (see Hyperglycemic Hyperosmolar Nonketotic Coma, p. 270)

HYPERGLYCEMIC HYPEROSMOLAR NONKETOTIC COMA
(see also Diabetic Ketoacidosis, p. 266)

Hyperglycemic hyperosmolar nonketotic coma (HHNK) is due to a relative (not total) insulin deficiency causing hyperosmolality of extracellular fluid and cellular dehydration. It is frequently seen in patients with Type 2 diabetes (non–insulin dependent). Enough insulin remains to prevent ketone body formation. The causes are related to mild diabetes, acute illness, trauma, diuretics, and steroids. The risk factors include pancreatitis, thiazide or steroid management, total parenteral nutrition or high-caloric feedings, and diet-controlled diabetes (see Comparison of Hyperglycemic Coma and Diabetic Ketoacidosis Table, p. 269).

Relative insulin deficiency

⬇

Hyperosmolality of ECF ➡ cellular dehydration ➡ diuresis

⬇

Hyperglycemia increases ➡ insulin remains sufficient to prevent
ketone body formation

⬇

Osmotic gradient develops between brain and plasma

⬇

Loss of brain H_2O

⬇

CNS dysfunction (coma)

■ Evolution of hyperglycemic hyperosmolar nonketonic coma (HHNK).

SIGNS AND SYMPTOMS
- Serum glucose >650 mg/dL, usually >1,000 mg/dL
- Serum osmolality >350 mOsm/kg
- Severe dehydration (especially of brain)
- No ketones
- No Kussmaul's respirations (shallow breathing only)
- No metabolic acidosis; normal anion gap

TREATMENT
Little if any insulin is needed. The main focus is on replacing the volume deficit; patient's volume may be depleted as much as 12 L. The goal is to replace half of the fluid shortage in the first 24 hours. Normal saline, 2 or 3 L over 2 hours, is initially given until vital signs recover, and then changed to ½ NS with KCl.

HYPERTHYROID *(see Graves' Disease, p. 269; Thyrotoxicosis, p. 274)*

HYPOALDOSTERONISM
(see Addison's Disease, p. 263; Aldosterone in Part 5, p. 249)

HYPOPARATHYROID *(see also Hypocalcemia in Part 9, p. 352)*

Hypoparathyroid is a clinical state resulting from the inadequate secretion of parathormone by the parathyroid gland, causing decreased levels of calcium and increased levels of phosphate. It is related to surgery of the thyroid gland, radiation injury to the thyroid, or pancreatitis.

SIGNS AND SYMPTOMS
These are related to a low calcium level (usually <8.5 mg/dL) and an increased phosphate level:

- Numbness, tingling in fingers, toes
- Positive Chvostek's sign
- Positive Trousseau's sign
- Laryngeal stridor, dyspnea, cyanosis
- Confusion, seizures
- Prolonged QT on electrocardiogram

TREATMENT
The goal is to replete the calcium with supplements: 1 to 5 g orally three times daily, or 5 to 20 mL of a 10% IV solution at a rate not to exceed 0.5 mL/min. Do not mix in normal saline, because it causes calcium excretion. Vitamin D supplements are given concomitantly to increase calcium absorption.

HYPOTHYROID *(see Myxedema, p. 271)*

MYXEDEMA

Myxedema is a severe deficiency of the thyroid to secrete sufficient hormones to meet the requirements of the tissues that normally respond to the hormones. Levels of T_3 and T_4, ^{131}I uptake, and thyroid-stimulating hormone (TSH) are all decreased, as evidenced by the slowing of all body activities (decrease in metabolic rate, physical acuity, and mental acuity).

REMEMBER:

"Myxedema madness" refers to the pronounced personality changes, such as paranoia and delusions.

There can be enlargement of the heart because of pericardial effusion and an increased tendency toward atherosclerosis and heart strain. Anemia may also be present, along with a host of other symptoms ranging from cold, dry skin and weight gain to periorbital edema.

Treatment is based on thyroid hormone replacement with thyroxine, triiodothyronine, or combinations of these hormones.

PHEOCHROMOCYTOMA

A benign tumor of the adrenal medulla, pheochromocytoma causes increased secretion of epinephrine and norepinephrine, resulting in proximal or sustained hypertension. It is often accompanied by severe headaches and the signs and symptoms of sympathetic activity (e.g., sweating, anxiety, palpitations). The patient is at risk for cerebral vascular accident (CVA), cardiovascular damage, or sudden blindness. Severe symptoms can result in death.

DIAGNOSIS

Diagnostics used should be based on the clinical degree of suspicion of a pheochromocytoma. Patients at lower risk should be screened with a 24-hour urine collection for catecholamines and metanephrines. High-risk patients (i.e., those who have a syndrome that may predispose them to pheochromocytoma) should be screened with plasma metanephrine testing.

In addition to blood and urine collection, the use of the phentolamine (Regitine) test is sometimes employed. After baseline blood pressure is recorded, an antipressor agent such as Regitine is administered IV. Blood pressure readings are taken at prescribed intervals until the pressure returns to its baseline level. A hypotensive effect lasting 10 to 15 minutes is diagnostic for pheochromocytoma, but a negative response does not rule it out.

If biochemical studies rule in favor of pheochromocytoma, imaging is then used to determine the exact location of the tumor. MRI is preferred over CT, and MIBG scans (metaiodobenzylguanidine) are reserved for cases where biochemical studies are positive but MRI and CT are negative. More recently, PET scans have shown promising results in the detection and localization of pheochromocytoma, but further study results are awaited.

TREATMENT

Initial therapy is aimed at returning the blood pressure to safe levels, usually with Nipride. Thereafter, treatment is laparoscopic surgical removal of the tumor. There is a high probability of profound shock 24 to 48 hours postoperatively because catecholamine blood levels drop dramatically. There is also a high risk of hemorrhage because adrenal glands are highly vascular. The prognosis for removal of a benign tumor is good, however, and blood pressure usually returns to a normal level by the second or third postoperative day.

NOTES

PITUITARY GLAND: PHYSIOLOGY

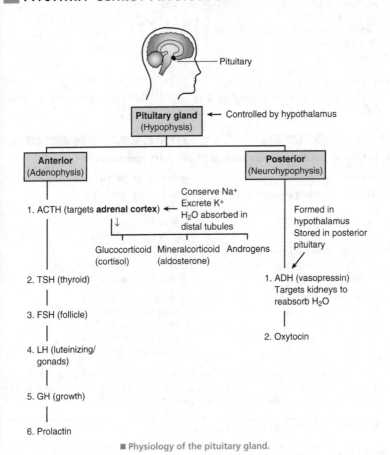

- Pituitary

Pituitary gland (Hypophysis) ← Controlled by hypothalamus

Anterior (Adenophysis)

Posterior (Neurohypophysis)

1. ACTH (targets **adrenal cortex**) ←

Conserve Na⁺
Excrete K⁺
H_2O absorbed in
distal tubules
↓

Formed in
hypothalamus
Stored in posterior
pituitary

Glucocorticoid   Mineralcorticoid   Androgens
(cortisol)   (aldosterone)

1. ADH (vasopressin)
   Targets kidneys to
   reabsorb H_2O

2. TSH (thyroid)

3. FSH (follicle)

2. Oxytocin

4. LH (luteinizing/
   gonads)

5. GH (growth)

6. Prolactin

■ **Physiology of the pituitary gland.**

SIADH (see Syndrome of Inappropriate Antidiuretic Hormone, p. 273)

SYNDROME OF INAPPROPRIATE ANTIDIURETIC HORMONE

The syndrome of inappropriate antidiuretic hormone (SIADH) is a disease of the posterior pituitary characterized by sustained secretion of ADH, in spite of subnormal serum osmolality, resulting in water intoxication and hyponatremia. The patient is literally "waterlogged" (remember "<u>S</u>wimming <u>In</u> <u>ADH</u>") though edema may not be present. To positively diagnose SIADH, other causes of hyponatremia must be excluded, and renal, adrenal, and thyroid function must be normal (see p. 265, Comparison of DI and SIADH Table).

(continued)

CAUSES
- Malignancy (especially oat cell cancer of the lung)
- Pulmonary disease
- Neurologic disorders (e.g., CVA, head trauma)
- Hypothyroidism
- Drugs

SIGNS AND SYMPTOMS
A syndrome denotes a collection of signs and symptoms, which therefore can be subdivided according to origin.

Origin of SIADH and Associated Signs and Symptoms	
Origin	**Signs and Symptoms**
Those due to **water intoxication**	Dilutional hyponatremia Decreased serum osmolality Increased urine osmolality Increased urine sodium
Those due to **hyponatremia** (dependent on severity and length of onset)	Fatigue, malaise Headache, confusion, neurologic damage Abdominal cramping
Those due to **other** causes	Weight gain without edema Increased urine osmolality Increased urine specific gravity Inappropriate urine Na^+ loss Increased circulating volume

The cornerstone of treatment is fluid restriction and is aimed at prevention of water intoxication and correction of electrolyte disturbances. Hypertonic saline, usually 3% (see Hot Salt in Part 8, Drugs, Doses, Tables), and IV furosemide (Lasix) are given for an acute episode.

THYROID STORM *(see Thyrotoxicosis, p. 274)*

THYROTOXICOSIS *(see also Graves' Disease, p. 269)*

Thyrotoxicosis is a rapidly developing, life-threatening emergency characterized by greatly accentuated signs and symptoms of hyperthyroidism. Increased amounts of thyroid hormones are inappropriately released into the bloodstream, and metabolism is greatly exaggerated. Also known as thyroid storm, it is fatal without intervention and has a 10% mortality rate.

SIGNS AND SYMPTOMS
The signs and symptoms are related to the increase in the metabolic process:
- High fever, heat intolerance, diaphoresis
- Tachycardia (out of proportion to fever) with dysrhythmias (especially atrial)
- Tremors, muscle weakness
- Low TSH
- Elevated free T_4

(continued)

TREATMENT

Treatment depends on the severity of the symptoms. It centers on suppressing hormonal release with iodides and giving propylthiouracil to block conversion of T_4 to T_3.

REMEMBER:

Always give propylthiouracil (PTU) at least 1 hour before the iodides. Methimazole and propranolol (Inderal) may also be used, and plasmapheresis may ultimately be required.

REMEMBER:

Never give aspirin to these patients, because the drug increases the free T3.

NOTES

PART 7

Hematologic and Immune Systems

AIDS

AIDS is an infectious disease caused by human T-cell lymphotrophic Type III virus (HTLV-III). It is an acquired deficiency of the body's immune system. The immune system continually produces cells and antibodies that attack and destroy germs that otherwise would render a patient ill. The AIDS virus zeros in on certain T lymphocytes and breaks down the immunity, thus removing any natural resistance and leaving the patient vulnerable to a variety of viruses, bacteria, yeasts, fungi, and parasites. The virus is carried in the blood and transmitted through the blood.

A phase of infection with HIV, described clinically but no longer commonly diagnosed in practice, is AIDS-related complex (ARC). Patients with ARC usually experience fatigue, weight loss, and night sweats, along with superficial fungal infections of the mouth (oral thrush) and fingernails and toenails. They do, however, lack the opportunistic infections and neoplasms that define AIDS. It is uncommon for HIV-infected persons to die at the stage of ARC.

Pneumonia is the major cause of death, usually caused by the protozoa *Pneumocystis carinii* or by the cytomegalovirus (CMV). The most characteristic cancer that develops is Kaposi's sarcoma. It spreads rapidly and is usually fatal. It initially may be limited to skin (red-brown lesions) but quickly spreads internally. Another cancer that often develops is lymphoma, a cancer of the lymphatic system, which eventually causes death.

The screening tests for AIDS are (1) the enzyme-linked immunosorbent assay (ELISA) and (2) the Western blot test. Both identify antibodies produced by the immune system after infection by the virus and are therefore not accurate until a person has been infected for 4 to 12 weeks.

AIDS PROFILE
- Lymphocytopenia, thrombocytopenia
- Low T_4:T_8 ratio
- Brain dementia (30%–40%)
- Unexplained weight loss
- Night sweats
- Red-brown spots on skin or mucous membranes
- Swollen lymph nodes lasting more than 1 month
- Persistent white spots or unusual blemishes in the mouth
- Fever >99°F for more than 10 days
- Persistent cough and shortness of breath
- Persistent diarrhea

(continued)

TREATMENT

The recommended therapy for HIV infection is the HAART regime (highly active anti-retroviral therapy). It combines three or more anti-HIV medications in a daily dosing program. While the therapy does not cure the HIV infection (and the individual can still transmit HIV to others), the goal is to control the reproduction of the virus and slow the progression of the disease.

There are multiple categories of anti-HIV medications currently approved by the FDA with countless clinical trials underway investigating new agents. Classes of anti-HIV medications known thus far include:

1. **Nucleotide reverse transcriptase inhibitors (NRTIs):** These drugs are used to prevent healthy T cells in the body from becoming infected with HIV and are sometimes referred to as "nukes." They are, in effect, "faulty" versions of building blocks that HIV needs to make more copies of itself. When HIV uses an NRTI instead of a normal building block, reproduction of the virus is stalled.

2. **Nonnucleoside reverse transcriptase inhibitors (NNRTIs):** Sometimes called "non-nukes," these drugs attach themselves to reverse transcriptase and prevent the enzyme from converting RNA to DNA. In turn, the genetic material of HIV cannot be incorporated into the healthy genetic material of the cell, and this prevents the cell from producing new virus. A new NNRTI, the first in over a decade, has recently been approved, Intelence (etravirine).

3. **Protease inhibitors (PIs):** These inhibitors are designed to attack HIV by blocking the protease enzyme. When new viral particles break off from an infected cell, protease cuts long protein strands into the sections needed to assemble a mature virus. When the protease enzyme is blocked, the new viral particles cannot mature. PIs, when used in conjunction with other AIDS drugs, have been noted to cause the HIV levels in the blood to decrease dramatically and the numbers of WBCs to rise. Rapid resistance to this class of drug has been noted. As a consequence, several firms are researching the development of a new PI that will not be cross-resistant with existing drugs. A new PI drug, Prezista (darunavir) is now available.

4. **Vaginal HIV Microbicides:** Clinical trials are now underway to evaluate the safety and efficacy of this agent. Research has demonstrated that although called "microbicides," most do not actually kill the virus, but instead impede its ability to infect the host cells.

5. **Entry Inhibitors:** This is a new generation of antiviral compounds, presently undergoing active preclinical and clinical development as potential therapies for HIV-1 infection.

6. **Attachment and Fusion Inhibitors:** This is a new class of anti-HIV drug that is intended to protect host cells from HIV infection by preventing attachment of the virus to a new cell and breaking through the cell membrane. Preventing attachment blocks HIV entry into the cell. Digestive acids break this drug down, so most are given by IV infusion.

7. **CCR5 Antagonists:** A new class of antiretroviral drugs that could provide an alternative to HIV positive patients with resistance to multiple drugs. An example of a drug in this class, Selzentry (maraviroc), works by blocking a protein, CCR5, on the immune cells that HIV uses as a portal to enter and thereby infect the cell. Maraviroc carries a warning as it poses an increased risk of heart attack.

8. **Other categories:** Gene Therapy, Integrase Inhibitors, Maturation Inhibitors, Zinc Finger Inhibitors, Viral Decay Accelerator.

There are currently no HIV/AIDS vaccines approved for use, although many are in current clinical studies.

ALBUMIN

Albumin is used as a blood volume expander in the treatment of hypovolemic shock, hemorrhage, trauma, acute hemodilution, or acute vasodilation. It improves "third space" fluid loss, including that occurring in acute peritonitis, mediastinitis, burns, and after radical surgery. It is used to reduce cerebral edema caused by neurosurgery or anoxia. It is also used in the treatment of hypoproteinemia, hepatic cirrhosis, and nephrosis.

VOLUME
- **5%** (isotonic and isosmotic; 95% NS + 5% albumin) 250 to 500 mL bottles
- **25%** (salt poor; 75% NS + 25% albumin) 50 mL (12.5 g) or 100 mL (25 g)

INFUSION RATE
- Tubing accompanies albumin. No filter is necessary. No saline needed. May piggyback into mainline IV.
- 5% albumin:
    For shock: Initial dose of 500 mL given as rapidly as possible. Additional 500 mL may be given in 30 minutes.
    For patients with low blood volume: Administer at 2–4 mL/min.
- 25% albumin:
    Therapy based on clinical response. Administer as rapidly as tolerated.
    For patients with low blood volume: 1 mL/min.

SPECIAL CONSIDERATIONS
No ABO blood group antibodies are present; therefore, compatibility is not a factor.

ANAPHYLACTIC SHOCK *(see Shock, Anaphylactic, p. 293)*

ANEMIA

Hemolytic: Excessive erythrocyte destruction
Iron deficiency: Nutritional deficiency ($\downarrow$MCV, $\downarrow$MCH, $\downarrow$MCHC)
Pernicious (aplastic):   Bone marrow failure ($\downarrow$RBCs)

NOTES

APHERESIS *(see Apheresis in Part 2, p. 76)*

BLOOD COMPATIBILITY *(see Transfusions: Compatibility, p. 294)*

BLOOD, COMPOSITION OF *(see also Body Fluid Compartments, p. 280)*

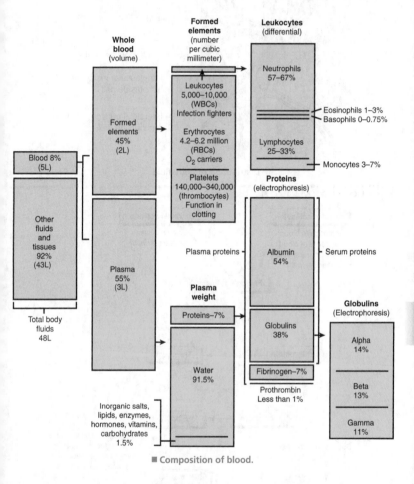

■ Composition of blood.

A person's actual amount of blood varies with height and weight, but an average man has 12 pints and an average woman has 9 pints (or an average person has 4.5–6.0 L). Approximately 8% of body weight is accounted for by blood.

BODY FLUID COMPARTMENTS *(see also Blood, Composition of, p. 279)*

Body fluid averages about 70% of total body weight, divided as follows:

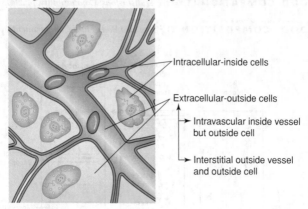

Intracellular-inside cells

Extracellular-outside cells

→ Intravascular inside vessel but outside cell

→ Interstitial outside vessel and outside cell

■ Distribution of body fluid.

CLOT FORMATION

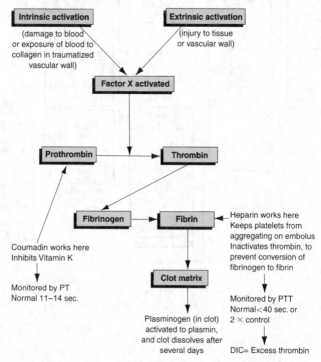

Intrinsic activation
(damage to blood or exposure of blood to collagen in traumatized vascular wall)

Extrinsic activation
(injury to tissue or vascular wall)

Factor X activated

Prothrombin → **Thrombin**

Fibrinogen → **Fibrin** ← Heparin works here
Keeps platelets from aggregating on embolus
Inactivates thrombin, to prevent conversion of fibrinogen to fibrin

Coumadin works here
Inhibits Vitamin K

Monitored by PT
Normal 11–14 sec.

Clot matrix

Plasminogen (in clot) activated to plasmin, and clot dissolves after several days

Monitored by PTT
Normal <40 sec. or 2 × control

DIC= Excess thrombin

■ Clot formation. (Adapted from Bullock, B. L. [1996]. *Pathophysiology: Adaptations and alterations in function* [4th ed.]. Philadelphia: Lippincott-Raven.)

CLOTTING CASCADE

Intrinsic pathway—works slowly (2–6 min) (inside vessel)–contact collagen damaged endothelium blood injury

Extrinsic pathway—works rapidly (15 sec.) (outside vessel)–tissue injury

Intrinsic activator enzymatic complex formed

Hageman factor (XIIa)
Prekallekrein
High–molecular weight kininogen

XI ———→ XIa

IX ———→ Ca^{++} IXa

Factor X activation complex

IXa, VIII, phospholipids

Tissue factor and tissue phospholipids released

Enzyme complex formed

Tissue factor
Factor VII
Phospholipids

Ca^{++}

X ——Ca^{++}——→ Xa ◄——————— X

Prothrombin activator complex

Xa, V, phospholipids

Prothrombin ——Ca^{++}——→ Thrombin

Fibrinogen ——Ca^{++}——→ Fibrin (unstable)

Fibrin stabilizing XIII ———→ XIIIa ———→ Ca^{++}

Fibrin (stable), cross-linkage bonds formed

■ Blood coagulation sequence. a, activated enzyme, Ca^{++} calcium is necessary in several reactions. Final common pathway begins with the activation of factor X.

CLOTTING FACTORS

Clotting Factors

Official Number	Synonym	Contemporary Version	
I	Fibrinogen	I	(fibrinogen)
II	Prothrombin	II	(prothrombin)
III	Tissue thromboplastin	III	(tissue factor)
IV	Calcium	IV	(calcium)
V	Labile factor	V	(labile factor)
		VI	PF₃ (platelet coagulant activities)
		VI	PF4
VII	Stable factor	VII	(stable factor)
VIII	Antihemophilic factor	VIII	AHF (antihemophilic factor)
		VIII	VWF (von Willebrand's factor)
		VIII	RAg (related antigen)
IX	Christmas factor	IX	(Christmas factor)
X	Stuart-Prower factor	X	(Stuart-Prower factor)
XI	Plasma thromboplastin (antecedent)	XI	(plasma thromboplastin antecedent)
XII	Hageman factor	XII	HF (Hageman factor)
		XII	PK (prekallikrein, Fletcher)
		XII	HMWK (high–molecular-weight kininogen)
XIII	Fibrin stabilizing factor	XII	Fibrin stabilizing factor

The Roman numerals and synonyms designating each clotting factor accepted by the International Committee on blood clotting factors are located in the left-hand columns. Note the absence of factor VI. The version in the right-hand column incorporates more recently recognized clotting factors but is not officially recognized. (Green, D. General considerations of coagulation proteins. Ann Clin Lab Sci 8[2]: 95–105. Copyright 1987 by the Institute for Clinical Science, Inc. Reprinted with permission.)

COLD AGGLUTININS

Cold agglutinins are reported as a critical value on an antibody screen. Agglutinins are antibodies that cause RBCs to clump together. Since cold agglutinins are active at cold temperatures, any patient with a positive cold agglutinin screen will need to have the blood warmer used when transfusing red blood cells. (See Hotline Fluid Warner; Ranger Fluid Warmer; Level 1 Volume Infuser in Part 2)

COLLOIDS

Colloids are also known as plasma expanders. These substances contain large insoluble molecules and result in an increase in osmotic pressure. This osmotic pressure will draw fluid from the interstitial compartment into the intravascular space and will cause an increase in the total vascular blood volume. (See Figure on page 280.) Colloids cause an increase in plasma volume, while crystalloids cause an increase in interstitial volume. Colloids made from blood products include albumin and plasmanate, while artificial colloids are dextran and hespan.

REMEMBER:

Even though colloids are called plasma expanders, they do not carry oxygen like red blood cells and are not the same thing. Also, the effect of colloids is limited, lasting only 24 to 48 hours.

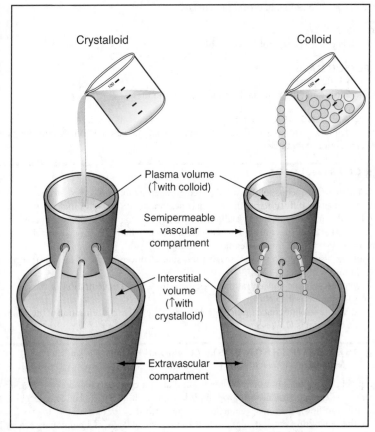

Crystalloid

Colloid

Plasma volume (↑with colloid)

Semipermeable vascular compartment

Interstitial volume (↑with crystalloid)

Extravascular compartment

■ Colloid vs. crystalloid. (Adapted from Marino, P. L. [2007]. *The ICU book* [3rd ed.]. Philadelphia: Lippincott Williams & Wilkins.)

CONSUMPTIVE COAGULOPATHY
(see also Disseminated Intravascular Coagulation, p. 286)

A group of disorders characterized by the abnormally regulated activation of "procoagulant" pathways, resulting in decreased levels of hemostatic components. The prototype in this category is disseminated intravascular coagulation (DIC).

Types of consumptive coagulopathy include:
- Type I   DIC plus secondary fibrinolysis—acute DIC
- Type II   DIC (circulating thrombin)—compensated/chronic DIC
- Type III   Primary fibrinolysis (circulating plasmin)

CRYOPRECIPITATE

Cryoprecipitate is a component of blood obtained by freezing and thawing plasma. It is used to correct deficiencies of factor VIII, factor XIII, and fibrinogen and occasionally used to control bleeding in uremia, and in DIC.

VOLUME
- Usually given as a pool of 10 to 20 units

INFUSION RATE
- Use Y infusion set
- 1 to 2 mL/min (10 mL diluted component per minute)

SPECIAL CONSIDERATIONS
Cryoprecipitate contains a small volume of plasma and no RBCs. Plasma compatibility is preferred but not required.

CRYSTALLOIDS

Crystalloids are aqueous solutions composed of water-soluble molecules (electrolytes and water) that easily diffuse across the vascular membrane *into the interstitial spaces* (resulting in only 10%–25% of the crystalloid solution remaining in the vascular space). (See figure on page 283.) They are used to maintain or replenish body fluids, or correct electrolyte imbalances. There are three types of this solution:
- Isotonic—solute concentration *equals* the solute concentration of the plasma; most common is LR.
- Hypotonic—solute concentration is *less than* the solute concentration of the plasma; most common is 0.45 NS.
- Hypertonic—solute concentration is *greater than* the solute concentration of the plasma; most common is D_5 ½ NS.

DEEP VEIN THROMBOSIS *(see also Anti-embolism Stockings in Part 11, p. 369; Pulmonary Embolism in Part 3, p. 200)*

Deep vein thrombosis is a medical condition that occurs when a blood clot (thrombus) forms in a deep vein, usually of a lower limb, leading to either a partial or complete blockage of blood flow. Pulmonary embolism can occur if the clot of the DVT breaks loose from the wall of the vein and migrates to the lungs where it blocks a pulmonary artery. If the clot is large, it can cause sudden death. The syndrome of DVT and PE is referred to by the collective term venous thromboembolism.

(continued)

It is characterized by three factors, known as **Virchow's Triad:** (1) decreased flow rate of blood; (2) vein injury; and (3) increased tendency of blood to clot. Since most DVTs occur within 48 hours of surgery, prophylaxis with range of motion, anti-embolism stockings, and sequential compression devices is paramount. Each improves venous return and reduces venous stasis in the leg veins. There are several documented factors that increase risk for DVT and the Autar DVT Scale was developed as a predictive index. Classic symptoms of DVT include pain, swelling and redness of the leg, and dilation of the surface veins. Ultrasound is frequently used for diagnosis, as well as D-dimer levels. Anticoagulation is the usual treatment, although thrombolysis is employed in the case of an extensive clot.

Autar DVT Risk Assessment Scale

SCORING		
	6 or less	No risk
	7–10	Low risk (<10%)
	11–14	Moderate risk (11%–40%)
	15 or greater	High risk (>41%)

AGE SPECIFIC		SURGICAL INTERVENTIONS (Score only one item)	
10–30 years	0	Minor surgery (<30 minutes)	1
31–40 years	1	Major surgery	2
41–50 years	2	Emergency major surgery	3
51–60 years	3	Thoracic	3
61+ years	4	Abdominal	3
		Urological	3
		Neurosurgical	3
		Orthopedic	4

MOBILITY		HIGH-RISK DISEASES	
Ambulatory	0	Ulcerative colitis	1
Limited (uses aid self)	1	Anemia	2
Very limited (needs help)	2	Chronic heart disease	2
Chair bound	3		
Complete bed rest	4		

BODY MASS INDEX		TRAUMA (Score preoperative only)	
Underweight BMI 16–19	0	Head	1
Average BMI 20–25	1	Chest	1
Overweight BMI 26–30	2	Spinal	2
		Pelvic	3
		Lower limb	4

SPECIAL RISK: Oral Contraceptives			
20–35 years	1		
35+	2		

DIC *(see Disseminated Intravascular Coagulation, p. 286)*

DISSEMINATED INTRAVASCULAR COAGULATION
(see also Consumptive Coagulopathy, p. 284)

DIC is associated with thrombocytopenia secondary to intravascular consumption of platelets and clotting factors. It is a secondary process due to an underlying condition. The prognosis depends on the severity of the triggering event, rather than the presence of DIC itself.

STEP 1 (EARLY)
Clotting: Excessive activation of platelets, diffuse fibrin generation and deposition, with resultant microvascular thrombi (clots) in various organs, contributing to multi-organ ischemia and failure.

STEP 2 (LATE)
Bleeding: Systemic hemorrhage due to constant activation and "consumption" of clotting proteins/factors and platelets. Clot deposition in the early stage of DIC leads to secondary fibrinolysis and contributes to bleeding.

The process of clotting and bleeding may result in symptoms such as tissue ischemia, shock, altered mental status, dyspnea, and oliguria.

DIC is secondary to triggering mechanisms such as:
- Infection/sepsis
- Trauma/burns
- Extensive surgery
- Malignancy: leukemias, solid organ tumors, etc.
- Obstetric complications such as HELLP syndrome, eclampsia, retained placenta, etc.
- Transplant rejection
- Anaphylaxis
- Sickle cell crisis
- Acute hemolytic transfusion reaction (i.e., ABO incompatibility)
- Pulmonary and/or fat embolism
- Snake bites
- Rhabdomyolysis
- Hyperthermia/hypothermia
- Acute pancreatitis/shock

(continued)

NOTES

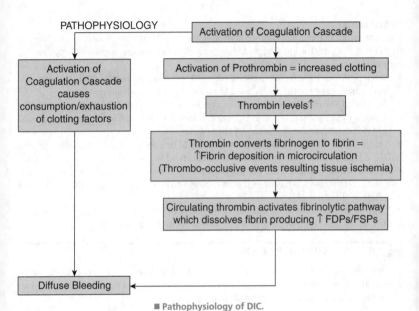

PATHOPHYSIOLOGY

Activation of Coagulation Cascade

Activation of Coagulation Cascade causes consumption/exhaustion of clotting factors

Activation of Prothrombin = increased clotting

Thrombin levels↑

Thrombin converts fibrinogen to fibrin = ↑Fibrin deposition in microcirculation (Thrombo-occlusive events resulting tissue ischemia)

Circulating thrombin activates fibrinolytic pathway which dissolves fibrin producing ↑ FDPs/FSPs

Diffuse Bleeding

■ Pathophysiology of DIC.

Acute DIC/Expected Lab Values

Laboratory Test	Expected Result	Rationale
Platelet Count	Decreased	Generalized hyperactivation of the clotting system resulting in a "consumption" of clotting factors and platelets
Prothrombin Time (PT)	Increased/Prolonged	Inadequate clotting cascade/consumption of clotting factors
Activated Partial Thromboplastin Time (PTT)	Increased/Prolonged	Inadequate clotting cascade/consumption of clotting factors
Thrombin Time (TT)	Increased/Prolonged	Measures the time required to convert fibrogen to fibrin
Fibrogen	Decreased	Inadequate clotting cascade/consumption of clotting factors
Antithrombin III	Decreased	Protein that prevents blood coagulation
Fibrin Degradation Products/ Fibrin Split Products	Increased	Measures the degradation products of fibrin/clot. Elevated levels indicate fibrin lysis. High sensitivity for identifying thrombosis. FDPs/FSPs and D-dimers are abundant in DIC and frequently clump together. Bleeding is caused by failure of the coagulation cascade, which results in the systemic release of fibrinogen and FDPs/FSPs
D-Dimer Assay	Increased	
Schistocytes	Present	End result of blood cell fragmentation

(*continued*)

TREATMENT

The cornerstone of treatment is aimed at treating the underlying disorder and eliminating the trigger mechanism. The clotting problems generally resolve when the underlying cause is corrected.

- Platelets and clotting factors may be administered to stop bleeding and/or if invasive procedures are required, which place the patient at risk for bleeding.
- The role of standard heparin remains controversial in acute DIC, with the majority of studies suggesting that it is NOT helpful. However, low molecular weight heparins (LMWHs) are frequently used as an alternative.
- Antithrombin III (AT III) replacement appears to be effective in decreasing the signs of DIC if high doses are administered, but the effects on survival at this time are uncertain.
- Restoration of anticoagulant pathways may be achieved with administration of activated protein C, which has been shown to be effective in reducing mortality with organ failure in clinical trials.
- Xigris is indicated for the reduction of mortality in patients with severe sepsis associated with acute organ dysfunction and who are at high risk of death.

FRESH FROZEN PLASMA

Fresh frozen plasma (FFP) is used to increase the level of clotting factors in patients with a demonstrated deficiency. It is not used for volume expansion, as a nutritional supplement, or prophylactically with massive blood transfusions.

VOLUME

- 200 to 250 mL (amount usually written on unit)

INFUSION RATE

- Use Y infusion set with 0.9 NS flush.
- 200 mL/hr or more slowly if circulatory overload is a potential problem.

SPECIAL CONSIDERATIONS

- Plasma contains no RBCs, and crossmatching is not required; however, ABO-compatible plasma should be administered.
- One unit should be thawed at a time because FFP must be used within 24 hours of thawing, and using it later results in the loss of the labile clotting factors V and VIII.
- Infuse using a blood filter or a component filter.

HESPAN

Hespan (6% hetastarch in saline) is a synthetic colloid made from corn. It is indicated for use as a plasma volume expanding agent in cases of shock resulting from hemorrhage, trauma, sepsis, or burns. Expansion after infusion is equal to or greater than that produced by dextran 70 or 5% albumin.

VOLUME

- 500 mL

INFUSION RATE

- Tubing accompanies dose. No saline needed. May piggyback into mainline IV.
- Usual dose is 20 mL/kg/day, but this is not an absolute.
- Total volume may be infused over 1 hour if the clinical situation demands.

(continued)

SPECIAL CONSIDERATIONS

- Serum amylase values can be approximately $2 \times$ normal after the Hespan infusion and does not indicate pancreatitis.
- Much lower risk of an allergic reaction than dextran.
- May prolong coagulation profile and decrease platelets.

HEXTEND

A new formulation of 6% hetastarch in Lactated Ringer's solution, shown to be effective for plasma volume expansion. When compared with Hespan or 5% albumin, it has proven equally safe and effective but with a better side effect profile.

VOLUME

- 500 mL

INFUSION RATE

- Tubing accompanies dose. No saline needed. May piggyback into mainline IV.
- In general, dose should not exceed 1,500 mL/day; however, higher doses have been safely given.
- In acute hemorrhagic shock, up to 20 mL/kg/hr has been reported.

SPECIAL CONSIDERATIONS

- Incompatible with sodium bicarbonate and calcium products (blood).
- Avoid with patients in renal failure, oliguria or anuria (not related to hypovolemia), and hyperkalemia because solution contains potassium. For the same reason, use caution if the patient is on digoxin.
- Avoid use in lactic acidosis, as the solution contains lactate.

HIV (see AIDS, p. 276)

HODGKIN'S DISEASE

Hodgkin's disease (HD) is a chronic, progressive neoplastic disorder of unknown cause characterized by enlargement of lymph glands, spleen, and liver. Proliferating cells are abnormal histiocyte called Reed-Sternberg cells.

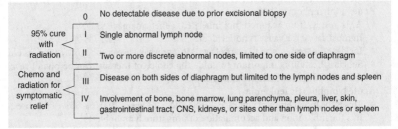

	0	No detectable disease due to prior excisional biopsy
95% cure with radiation	I	Single abnormal lymph node
	II	Two or more discrete abnormal nodes, limited to one side of diaphragm
Chemo and radiation for symptomatic relief	III	Disease on both sides of diaphragm but limited to the lymph nodes and spleen
	IV	Involvement of bone, bone marrow, lung parenchyma, pleura, liver, skin, gastrointestinal tract, CNS, kidneys, or sites other than lymph nodes or spleen

■ Staging.

Non-Hodgkin's Lymphoma (NHL) is five times more common than Hodgkin's disease. It is still a hematologic cancer, but involves different lymphocytes than HD, and microscopic examination of biopsy shows no Reed-Sternberg cells. NHL has 10 subtypes

(*continued*)

and 20 disease entities. It is further divided by grade: low grade (slow growing) and high grade (rapid progression), as well as by cell type, either T or B. Treatment varies according to severity, but includes either chemotherapy, radiation, immunotherapy, bone marrow transplant, or sometimes a "watch and wait" approach if the cancer is slow growing.

IDIOPATHIC THROMBOCYTOPENIC PURPURA

ITP is a bleeding disorder caused by low numbers of circulating platelets (thrombocytes). It is an autoimmune condition caused by the immune system producing antibodies against the patient's own platelet cells. These antibodies attach to the platelets, are circulated through the spleen, and for some reason (idiopathic) destroyed. Platelet counts in patients are usually less than 50,000 (sometimes lower than 10,000) and there is no sign of bleeding. Splenectomy, immunosuppressive therapies, gamma globulin infusions, and plasmapheresis may be recommended. Platelet transfusions are usually not used, since the platelets will only survive a few hours, no longer than the patient's own platelets.

ITP (see Idiopathic Thrombocytopenic Purpura, p. 290)

LEUKEMIA

Leukemia is a group of malignancies caused by abnormal reproduction of white blood cells that create useless, immature cells called blasts. The blasts overpopulate bone marrow and spill into the bloodstream and lymph system. The patient has an elevated leukocyte count with a shift to the left (see Lab Values: Hematology in Part 9, p. 348 to define this shift).

The major forms of leukemia fall into four categories, first dividing the disease by the type of cell involved (either myelogenous or lymphocytic) and then by disease course (acute or chronic). The categories can then be further divided into subsets by measuring specific features of the cells involved. The subsets allow for optimal treatment and a better determination of disease course.

1. **Acute myelogenous leukemia (AML)** is also known as:
   Acute myelocytic leukemia
   Acute myeloblastic leukemia
   Acute granulocytic leukemia
   Acute nonlymphocytic leukemia
   - AML results from acquired (not inherited) genetic damage to DNA.
   - In most cases, the cause is not evident.
   - Incidence increases over 40 years of age. Most prevalent age group is 60 to 90 years old.
   - Subclassification is important to guide the choice of therapy; can be one of seven different patterns of cell involvement.
2. **Acute lymphocytic leukemia**
   - This is the most common type of leukemia under the age of 19 (80%–85% of the cases).
   - It is the infiltration and accumulation of immature lymphoblasts.
3. **Chronic myelogenous leukemia** is also known as:
   Chronic granulocytic leukemia
   Chronic myelocytic leukemia
   Chronic myeloid leukemia

(continued)

- This type results from an acquired (not inherited) injury to the DNA of a stem cell in the bone marrow.
- The injury is not present at birth, and what causes the change is not yet understood.
- Most cases occur in adults.
- Ninety-five percent of cases show the presence of a "Philadelphia chromosome."
- The onset is associated with symptoms that usually develop gradually.

4. **Chronic lymphocytic leukemia (CLL)**
   - CLL is a disease of the elderly: 95% of the patients are over the age of 50.
   - It is the gradual accumulation of abnormal lymphocytes.
   - The patient usually is asymptomatic. CLL is frequently diagnosed during a routine examination when an enlarged lymph node or enlarged spleen is detected or a routine blood test shows an elevated number of lymphocytes.

Treatment for all the leukemias is based on chemotherapy. For acute leukemia, the regimen includes three phases: *Induction* (to achieve remission); *consolidation* (to further decrease cells); and *maintenance* (moderate doses over a prolonged time). For chronic leukemias, chemotherapy is usually oral, with minimal toxicity progressing to aggressive as the disease progresses. Sometimes radiation is used for lymph nodes or large masses. Bone marrow transplantation, after old marrow has been ablated with chemotherapy and radiation, is an option if a donor match can be found.

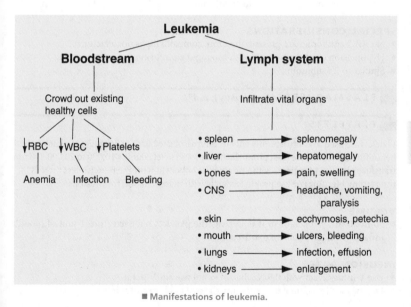

■ Manifestations of leukemia.

LYMPHOSARCOMA

Lymphosarcoma is a malignant condition of unknown cause, primarily involving lymphatic tissue. The earliest sign is painless enlarged lymph nodes. Eventually, lymphosarcoma invades bone marrow. The prognosis is poor, and treatment is palliative, with radiation and chemotherapy.

MULTIPLE MYELOMA

Multiple myeloma is a neoplasm of the bone marrow that is rapidly fatal (from the Greek *myelo*, marrow; *oma*, tumor). The patient has backache and bone pain; hyperglobuline-mia; and a disruption of erythrocytes, leukocytes, and thrombocytes. The urine contains Bence Jones protein. Treatment is palliative by amputation of the affected bone.

PLASMA PROTEIN FRACTION

Plasma protein fraction (PPF) is a blood volume supporter used in the emergency treatment of hypovolemic shock caused by burns, trauma, surgery, and infections. It is also used as a temporary measure in the treatment of blood loss when whole blood is not available. It is used to replenish plasma protein in patients with hypoproteinemia (if sodium restriction is not a problem).

VOLUME
- 250 or 500 mL

INFUSION RATE
- Tubing accompanies dose. No saline needed. May piggyback into mainline IV.
- Up to 15 mL/min, usual rate 1 to 10 mL/min.

SPECIAL CONSIDERATIONS
- No ABO antibodies are present; therefore compatibility is not a factor.
- Hypotension can be associated with too rapid an infusion.
- Similar to 5% albumin.

PLASMAPHERESIS *(see Part 1, p. 49)*

PLATELETS

Platelets are used to control or prevent bleeding associated with deficiencies in platelet number or function. They are used prophylactically for platelet counts <10,000 to 20,000. Do **not** transfuse platelets to patients with immune thrombocytopenic purpura (unless there is life-threatening bleeding) or use prophylactically with massive blood transfusions.

VOLUME
- 50 to 70 mL (1 pack or unit represents the platelets removed from 1 unit of blood); usually given in "pools" of 6 to 10 units.

INFUSION RATE
- Use Y infusion set with 0.9 NS flush. Do not use an IV pump.
- Determined by volume tolerance, usually one pool over 10 minutes.

SPECIAL CONSIDERATIONS
- Because platelets are stored at room temperature (to preserve function), bacterial growth is a constant possibility. In order to minimize this risk, platelets are often "given a sunburn" and irradiated with UV light to minimize the microbial contamination.
- Platelets are stored with gentle agitation for a maximum of 5 days. Once bag is entered for pooling, platelets must be transfused within 4 hours.

(continued)

- Platelet concentrates contain few RBCs; therefore, ABO compatibility is not required. Patients who are Rh⁻, however, generally receive Rh⁻ platelets. Under certain circumstances, it may be necessary to give these individuals Rh⁺ platelets.
- Use a special component filter.
- One unit of platelets should increase the platelet count by 6,000.

RED BLOOD CELLS (Packed) *(see also Transfusions, p. 294)*

Packed RBCs are used to increase the oxygen-carrying capacity in anemic patients without a need for volume expansion. They are also used to replace acute or chronic blood loss. They are essentially whole blood with 80% of the plasma removed; they lack clotting factors and platelets.

VOLUME
- 250 to 350 mL per unit

INFUSION RATE
- Use Y infusion set with 0.9 NS flush.
- Depends on patient's volume status, usually 2 to 3 hours per unit (not to exceed 4 hours); more rapid if the clinical situation demands.

SPECIAL CONSIDERATIONS
- Can cause the hemoglobin and hematocrit to rise faster than whole blood.
- Hemoglobin up 1 g/dL and hematocrit up 2% to 3% per unit RBCs given.
- Blood filter required.

SHOCK, ANAPHYLACTIC
(see also Transfusions: Adverse Reactions, p. 295; Shock Parameters in Part 2, p. 147)

Anaphylactic shock is most commonly precipitated by a hypersensitivity reaction to an antigen (i.e., iodine, penicillin). B lymphocytes secrete specific IgE antibodies in response to the causative substance, resulting in a stimulation of mediator (i.e., histamines) secretion. Histamine, in turn, causes systemic reactions: Wheezing, laryngeal edema with bronchospasm, vasodilation, urticaria (macular eruptions on head and arms before spreading in a symmetrical pattern), and ultimately shock. The vasodilation causes increased capillary permeability, fluid loss resulting in hypovolemia, hypotension, and low cardiac output.

Epinephrine is the drug of choice for treatment (reverses bronchospasm, hypotension), along with diphenhydramine (Benadryl) (decreases action of histamines). Albumin is given to draw fluid back into the intravascular space, and vasopressors are added to the regimen if needed (no dobutamine).

THIRD SPACING

Third spacing refers to fluid (in addition to extracellular and intracellular fluid) that should be in the vascular system but is accumulating in a potential space, or "third space," where it is not supposed to be. It is unavailable to support the circulation, yet remains inside the body. This phenomenon is frequently seen in ascites, burns, massive bleeding into a joint or body cavity, or postoperatively after a large amount of fluid has been administered. An early clue to third spacing is decreased urine output despite adequate fluid therapy. Urine output decreases because fluid shifts out of the intravascular space. The kidneys then

(continued)

receive less blood flow and attempt to compensate by decreasing urine output. Other signs include increased heart rate, decreased blood pressure, decreased central venous pressure, edema, increased body weight, and skewed intake/output ratio. Albumin or colloids are often administered (large protein molecules) to help keep the fluid intravascular.

TRALI

Transfusion-related acute lung injury (TRALI) is a complication of a blood transfusion (typically fresh frozen plasma but can be related to packed red blood cells as well) that occurs during or within 6 hours of the transfusion. The etiology of the condition is unclear. It is a process that is typically underdiagnosed and underreported, yet it is the leading cause of transfusion-related deaths. The patient will present with noncardiogenic pulmonary edema, along with dyspnea, cyanosis, hypotension, fever and chills, and mild to severe hypoxia. Diagnosis is based upon:

- PCWP <18 mm Hg with absent JVD
- No murmurs or gallops
- Normal cardiac silhouette
- No evidence of MI by EKG and enzyme testing
- Bilateral infiltrates
- O_2 saturation <90% on room air
- No preexisting acute lung injury prior to transfusion

Treatment is focused on respiratory and circulatory support. Since TRALI is not related to fluid overload or cardiac dysfunction (but rather to altered vascular permeability in the lungs), maintenance of circulating volume may be beneficial. Since pulmonary congestion is due to capillary leak syndrome, diuretics may be harmful and are contraindicated. The role of corticosteroids remains controversial.

TRANSFUSIONS *(see also specific blood component)*

Points to remember:

- Use only 0.9 NS for infusions. Lactated Ringer's solution causes agglutination, and dextrose causes hemolysis.
- Temperature of blood warmer should never be above 98.6°F, or hemolysis can occur.
- After multiple units of blood, Ca^+ should be given to prevent hypocalcemia. (Do not mix Ca^+ in normal saline.)

COMPATIBILITY

Summary of Blood Compatibility						
			Can Receive			
% Pop.	Patient Type	Whole Blood	RBCs	FFP	Platelets	Cryoprecipitate
44	O	O	O	Any ABO type	Any ABO type	Any ABO type
43	A	A	A or O	A or AB	A or AB preferred	A or AB
9	B	B	B or O	B or AB	B or AB preferred	B or AB
4	AB	AB	Any ABO type	AB	AB preferred	AB
85	Rh$^+$		NEGATIVE OR POSITIVE ACCEPTABLE			
15	Rh$^-$	Rh$^-$	Rh$^-$	Rh$^+$ or Rh$^-$	Rh$^-$ preferred	Rh$^+$ or Rh$^-$

(continued)

ADVERSE REACTIONS

Transfusion reactions range from self-limiting febrile responses to life-threatening intravascular hemodialysis (see also TRALI, p. 294).

Nonhemolytic Transfusion Reactions

Nonhemolytic transfusion reactions are the most common, occurring in 3% to 4% of all transfusions. They are the result of recipient antibodies forming against donor cells. These reactions seldom proceed to hypotension or respiratory distress and are commonly manifested by fever, chills, headache, and general malaise.

Hemolytic Transfusion Reactions

Hemolytic transfusion reactions are more rare, but more serious, occurring in 1 per 40,000 transfused units of RBCs and resulting in death in 1 per 100,000 units transfused. The reaction is directly related to incompatibility of a blood group, often because of a clerical error. Symptoms usually occur after a small amount of blood has been transfused, and almost always before the unit is transfused completely. The patient may have fever (sometimes >104°F), chills, flushing, nausea, burning at the IV site, chest tightness, restlessness, joint pain, and back pain. The reaction may progress to shock. Treatment is with fluids and diuretics.

When this type of transfusion reaction is suspected, the donor blood should be sent back to the blood bank to determine whether the correct unit of blood was administered to the intended patient. Typing, crossmatch, antibody screen, and direct and indirect Coombs tests should be repeated.

- Free serum hemoglobin appears as a pink color of the serum in a clotted centrifuged specimen. This may be observed with as little as 5 to 10 mL of hemolyzed blood.
- Serum bilirubin peaks in 3 to 6 hours as the free hemoglobin is metabolized.
- Haptoglobin binds to hemoglobin and the serum hemoglobin level falls, reaching its nadir in 1 to 2 days.
- Examine urine for hemoglobinuria.
- If intravascular or extravascular hemolysis is developing, a repeat complete blood count will not show the expected rise in hematocrit.
- For the patient undergoing a massive transfusion, serially measure the PT, PTT, fibrinogen, potassium level, pH, and calcium level.

Delayed Hemolytic Transfusion Reactions

Delayed hemolytic transfusion reactions occur anywhere from days to months after transfusion and are usually clinically benign, requiring no treatment. Symptoms vary but typically include: fever, an unexplained drop in hematocrit, increased bilirubin (jaundice), and/or dark urine. There are two types:

1. *Primary Immune Response* occurs when the patient generates a new antibody in response to the recipient. It may take several weeks to months before the level is even detectable in an antibody screen. Because of this, there is no clinical evidence of hemolysis. The donor cells are slowly coated and slowly removed from the body. Once produced, the antibody may be detectable for the life of the patient, although it is possible that it may fall below the level of detectability.

(continued)

2. *Anamnestic Response* occurs when an antibody that was produced in response to a previous transfusion falls below the level of detectability. When a new transfusion is initiated, the antibody screen will appear negative and the units will appear compatible.
   However, within days to weeks, a secondary immune response triggers the production
   of huge quantities of IgG antibody. This large quantity of antibodies (along with the
   large quantities of transfused cells) <u>results in hemolysis</u>. If an additional transfusion is
   ordered within the appropriate time frame, a positive antibody screen will be present.

Anaphylactic Reactions

Anaphylactic reactions (see also Shock, Anaphylactic, p. 293) are most often observed
in patients with a hereditary IgA deficiency. These reactions occur in 1 per 20,000 transfused units. Symptoms usually occur with less than 10 mL of blood transfused, and only
rarely occur more insidiously. The reaction is associated with rapid development of chills,
abdominal cramping, dyspnea, vomiting, and diarrhea.

- Risk of transfusion-related hepatitis B is 1 per 50,000 units transfused.
- Risk of transfusion-related hepatitis C is 1 per 3,000 to 4,000 units transfused. This re-
  action is known to cause chronic hepatitis and occurs in 50% of all infected recipients.
- Risk of transfusion-related HIV infection is 1 per 150,000 units transfused.

VIRCHOW'S TRIAD *(see Deep Vein Thrombosis, p. 285)*

WHOLE BLOOD

Whole blood is used to treat acute, massive blood loss requiring the oxygen-carrying
properties of RBCs along with the volume expansion provided by plasma. However,
if the whole blood is >24 hours old, the platelets and clotting factors are no longer
functional.

VOLUME

- 400 to 500 mL blood plus 60 mL anticoagulant per unit.

INFUSION RATE

- Use Y infusion set with 0.9 NS flush. Use micropore filter.
- As rapidly as necessary to stabilize the hemodynamic status.

SPECIAL CONSIDERATIONS

- Acute blood loss of as much as one third of a patient's total blood volume can often be
  treated with crystalloid and/or colloid solutions. Advances in the use of blood components have made whole blood transfusions rare; therefore, whole blood is not routinely
  used because of the excessive volume it affords.
- Twenty-four hours may elapse before a rise in the hemoglobin and hematocrit can be seen.

NOTES

PART 8

Drugs, Doses, Tables

ABCIXIMAB (REOPRO)

ABCIXIMAB is a GP IIb/IIIa inhibitor, used as an adjunct to PTCA or atherectomy to prevent acute cardiac ischemia complications in patients at high risk for abrupt closure of the treated coronary vessel. It is intended to be used with aspirin and heparin therapy. ABCIXIMAB is FDA approved for patients with non–Q-wave MI or unstable angina with planned PCI within 24 hours.

DOSAGE
0.25 mg/kg as an IV bolus, given 10 to 60 minutes before start of PTCA or atherectomy, followed by a continuous infusion of 10 μg/min for 12 hours. (Continuous infusion is sometimes ordered at 0.125 μg/kg/min for 12 hours.)

PRECAUTIONS
- Use a dedicated IV line with an in-line filter.
- May cause bradycardia, thrombocytopenia, increased risk of bleeding.

ACE INHIBITORS

Angiotensin converting enzyme (ACE) inhibitors prevent the production of angiotensin II, a potent vasoconstrictor that stimulates the production of aldosterone by blocking its conversion to the active form. The result is systemic vasodilation.

Primary therapeutic effects include:
- Treatment of high blood pressures (acts as an arterial and venous dilator)
- Decreased preload and afterload in patients with CHF (arterial vasodilation reduces the pressure the heart must pump against, making it easier to eject blood)
- Prolonging survival in patients who have had a heart attack and now have a weak heart muscle
- Prevention of heart attack and stroke in patients with vascular disease and in those who have diabetes with other vascular risk factors

REMEMBER:

ACE inhibitors end in "pril." Some common ones are captopril, lisinopril, and ramipril.

ACETADOTE

Acetadote is the only FDA-approved IV formulation of acetylcysteine (Mucomyst), developed specifically for use after ingestion of a hepatotoxic dose of acetaminophen.

DOSAGE
- Load: 150 mg/kg in 250 cc D_5W, infuse over 15 minutes
- Maintenance: 50 mg/kg in 500 cc D_5W over 4 hours, followed by 100 mg/kg in 1 L D_5W over 16 hours

(continued)

CONSIDERATIONS
- Serum sample should be drawn at least 4 hours after ingestion.
- Drug should be administered within 8 hours of ingestion for maximal protection against hepatic injury.
- If time of ingestion is unknown, the drug level is unknown or cannot be interpreted, or is not available within the 8 hour time interval, the drug should be administered immediately if 24 hours or less have elapsed from the reported time of ingestion, regardless of the quantity reported to have been ingested.

ACTIVASE *(see Alteplase, p. 298)*

ADENOSINE

Adenosine is a first-line antiarrhythmic used to treat PSVT and WPW. It has an unusually rapid onset, and its half-life is less than 10 seconds.

DOSAGE
6 mg IV rapid push over 1 to 3 seconds. After 1 to 2 minutes, if no resolution, give 12 mg IV rapid push over 1 to 3 seconds. May repeat once in 1 to 2 minutes.

PRECAUTIONS
Immediately after administration, there is usually a distinct change in the electrocardiographic rhythm, such as PVCs, SB, or more commonly a short run of asystole. This usually resolves in seconds.

ADRENALINE *(see Epinephrine, p. 312)*

AGGRASTAT *(see Tirofiban, p. 336)*

ALTEPLASE *(see also Reteplase, p. 333; Tenecteplase, p. 334)*

Alteplase (Activase, t-PA, rt-PA, Cathflo) is a tissue plasminogen activator that binds to fibrin, converting plasminogen to plasmin. This conversion allows the drug to dissolve the clot causing the blockage and restores blood flow and oxygen to the affected area.

INDICATIONS (FURTHER DEFINED WITHIN EACH CATEGORY)
1. Acute myocardial infarction
2. Acute ischemic stroke
3. Acute massive pulmonary embolism
4. Catheter clearance

CONTRAINDICATIONS TO USE
Absolute
- Severe uncontrolled hypertension
- Active internal bleeding
- History of CVA
- Recent (within 2 months) intracranial or intraspinal surgery or trauma
- Past or present bleeding disorder
- Seizure at onset of stroke

(continued)

Relative
- Recent (within 10 days) major surgery
- Recent (within 10 days) GI or GU bleeding
- Recent trauma
- Puncture of noncompressible vessel within 10 days
- Diabetic or other hemorrhagic retinopathy
- Traumatic CPR
- Advanced age (>75 years)
- Pregnancy
- Current use of oral anticoagulants
- History of uncontrolled hypertension (systolic >180 mm Hg, diastolic >110 mm Hg)

1. ALTEPLASE FOR ACUTE MYOCARDIAL INFARCTION

Indications
- Patient must be symptomatic with chest pain, typical of MI, for <6 hours, preferably <4 hours.
- Chest pain longer than 6 hours, if intermittent with ongoing signs of ischemia.
- A 1-mm ST segment elevation in two or more leads.

Dosing
There are two dosage regimens used in the management of acute MI; no studies have compared the success of the outcomes of either. The recommended total dose in both is based on patient weight, *not to exceed 100 mg of the drug*, because larger doses may cause intracranial bleeding.

Accelerated Infusion (90 Minutes)			
Patient Weight	**IV Bolus Over 1 to 2 Minutes**	**IV Infusion Over Next 30 Minutes**	**IV Over Next 60 Minutes**
Less than 67 kg	15 mg	0.75 mg/kg (not to exceed 50 mg)	0.50 mg/kg (not to exceed 35 mg)
More than 67 kg	15 mg	50 mg	35 mg

Three-Hour Infusion Recommended Dose is 100 mg*		
First Hour (60%)	**Second Hour (20%)**	**Third Hour (20%)**
10 mg IV bolus push, then 50 mg over remaining time	20 mg	20 mg

For patients who weigh less than 67 kg, a dosage of 1.25 mg/kg administered over 3 hours as described above may be given.

Concomitant Heparin Therapy
Although the value of anticoagulants during and after administration of Activase has not been fully studied, heparin has been administered concomitantly for 24 hours or longer in more than 90% of patients.

2. ALTEPLASE FOR ACUTE ISCHEMIC STROKE

Indications
Treatment should begin within 3 hours after the onset of stroke symptoms, and after exclusion of intracranial hemorrhage by CT scan.

(*continued*)

Dosing

The recommended dosage is 0.9 mg/kg infused over 60 minutes, with 10% of the total dose administered as an initial IV bolus.

- Do NOT use the cardiac dose!
- Do not exceed 90 mg maximum dose.
- Do NOT give aspirin, heparin, or Coumadin for 24 hours.

3. ALTEPLASE FOR ACUTE PULMONARY EMBOLISM

Dosing

The recommended dose is 100 mg IV over 2 hours. Heparin therapy should be given near the end of the alteplase infusion, or immediately after it, when the partial thromboplastin time (PTT) or prothrombin time (PT) returns to twice normal or less.

4. Alteplase for Catheter Clearance

58% of catheter occlusions are thrombotic, occurring as a result of a thrombus within, surrounding, or at the tip of the catheter. The occlusions can be either:

- Complete (infusion or aspiration is not possible);
- Partial (can infuse, but unable to aspirate fluids).

REMEMBER:

Both types of occlusion should be treated.

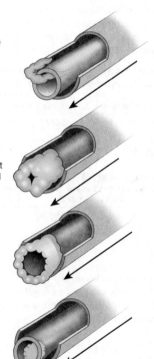

A **fibrin tail, or flap**, results from a deposit resting on the tip of the catheter. Fluids can be infused (the force of forward flow is able to "push" the fibrin tail away from the catheter tip) but aspiration is unsuccessful (the fibrin tail is "sucked into" the catheter lumen and causes the occlusion.) Although this is termed a partial occlusion, it should be treated since it will continue to progress and ultimately result in a total occlusion.

A **fibrin sheath** occurs when a deposit sticks to the circumference of the catheter (similar to a sock encasing an ankle). Initially there may be flow, but it will be sluggish and sporadic. This condition should be treated, as it will eventually progress to a point where the deposit "caps off" the catheter tip entirely.

A **mural thrombus** forms because the catheter is touching the vein wall and rubbing against it. This deposit can occur anywhere along the length of the catheter, but it most commonly occurs at the entry site and at the catheter tip.

An **intraluminal thrombus** arises from inadequate flushing after blood draws or after checking for blood return from the line. Blood "ebbs" back inside the catheter lumen, causing a thrombus to form, and results in a partial line occlusion.

■ Thrombotic catheter occlusions.

(*continued*)

Dosing and Procedure

1. Withdraw 2 mL of reconstituted solution from vial.
2. Instill as much volume of the drug solution as possible into occluded catheter.
3. After <u>30 minutes of dwell time,</u> assess catheter function by attempting to aspirate. *Vigorous suction and excessive compression of catheter should be avoided during procedure!* Excessive pressure could rupture catheter or cause expulsion of clot into the circulation. If the catheter is functional, gently aspirate 4 to 5 mL of blood to remove the drug and residual clot. Follow with an irrigation of sodium chloride. Never irrigate unless the alteplase has been aspirated. If the catheter is NOT patent, continue to Step 4.
4. After <u>2 hours of dwell time,</u> reassess catheter function. If functional, gently aspirate 4 to 5 mL of blood to remove drug and residual clot. Follow with an irrigation of sodium chloride. If the catheter is NOT patent, continue to Step 5.
5. A second dose of alteplase may be instilled. (Depending on the institution, may require a physician order.) Repeat procedure beginning with Step 1.
6. If after a second attempt the catheter is not patent, stop procedure, recap line, and notify physician. No further attempts should be made without further investigation (e.g., chest x-ray, flow study).

CONSIDERATIONS IN THE USE OF ALTEPLASE

- Observe for reperfusion arrhythmias, hypotension (acute MI).
- Monitor for hypertension (acute stroke). Treat with NTG paste, labetalol, and/or Nipride.
- Monitor lab results, especially coagulation profile. Watch for ecchymotic areas on patient, especially at flank.
- Avoid intramuscular injection or arterial punctures.
- Observe for bleeding, either internally or at external puncture sites.
- Use a dedicated, nonfiltered line for infusion.
- Acetaminophen may be ordered to control fever.

AMIKACIN *(see Therapeutic Drug Levels in Part 9, p. 357)*

AMINOPHYLLINE

A smooth muscle relaxant, aminophylline is sometimes useful in asthma and bronchospasms.

Mix: 500 mg in 500 mL D_5W or 0.9 NS.

Infuse: If patient does not receive long-term maintenance theophylline, an IV loading dose of 5.6 mg/kg over 30 minutes is required. Maintenance IV dose ranges from 0.2 to 0.9 mg/kg/hr. Titrate infusion to therapeutic drug level of 10 to 20 mcg/mL.

Maintenance Dose of Aminophylline

Adult, heavy smoker, 16–50 years	0.7 mg/kg/hr (max 0.9 mg/kg/hr)
Adult, nonsmoker >16 years	0.4 mg/kg/hr
Adult with cardiac decompensation, cor pulmonale, or liver dysfunction	0.2 mg/kg/hr

AMIODARONE (CORDARONE)

Amiodarone is a class III antiarrhythmic agent used for a wide variety of atrial and ventricular tachyarrhythmias, and for rate control of rapid atrial arrhythmias in patients with impaired LV function when digoxin has proven ineffective.

REMEMBER:

Use a 0.22 micron in-line filter for administration.

Dosage for stable wide complex tachycardia:

- RAPID LOAD OVER 10 MINUTES
  150 mg at 15 mg/min

  Mix: 1 ampule (3 cc) amiodarone (150 mg)
       with 100 cc D$_5$W
       Concentration 1.5 mg/mL

  Infuse: **Set pump at 600 mL/hr for 10 minutes**
       (100 cc total volume infusion)

- FOLLOW BY SLOW LOAD OVER NEXT 6 HOURS
  360 mg at 1 mg/min

  Mix: 6 ampules (18 cc) amiodarone (900 mg)
       with 500 cc D$_5$W
       Concentration 1.8 mg/mL

  Infuse: **Set pump at 33 mL/hr for 6 hours**
       (Approximately 200 cc total volume infusion)

- COMPLETE WITH MAINTENANCE OVER NEXT 18 HOURS
  540 mg at 0.5 mg/min

  No Mix: Use fluid remaining from previous bag

  Infuse: **Set pump at 17 mL for remaining 18 hours**
       (Approximately 300 cc total volume infusion)

Dosage for cardiac arrest:

300 mg (dilute to 20–30 mL with D$_5$W) IV push.
Consider additional 150 mg IV push in 3 to 5 minutes.
Maximum cumulative dose should be 2.2 g IV/24 hours.

■ Amiodarone administration.

PRECAUTIONS
- May produce vasodilation and hypotension (most common).
- May have negative inotropic effects.
- May prolong QT interval.
- Stable for 5 days when stored in glass bottles. A substantial loss of drug (40% over 120 hours) occurs from solutions stored in PVC bags or infused through PVC IV administration sets.
- Terminal elimination is extremely long (half-life lasts up to 40 days).

ANGIOMAX (BIVALIRUDIN)

Intended for use with aspirin, Angiomax is a direct thrombin inhibitor with a naturally reversible mechanism of action. It is used as an anticoagulant (and as an alternative to unfractionated heparin) in patients undergoing percutaneous transluminal angioplasty. More recently, it has been approved for use in patients with or at risk of heparin-induced thrombocytopenia and thrombosis syndrome, who are undergoing percutaneous coronary intervention.

DOSAGE
- 1 mg/kg IV bolus, then 2.5 mg/kg/hr IV infusion over 4 hours, beginning just prior to PCTA procedure.
- May give 0.2 mg/kg/hr IV infusion for up to 20 hours if necessary.

PRECAUTIONS
- Reduce dose with renal dysfunction.
- Monitor for excessive bleeding, which would indicate the need to discontinue the drug.

ANTIDYSRHYTHMIC DRUGS

- **Class Ia (sodium blockade)**
  Depresses sodium conduction into the cell, prolongs action potential duration, and increases refractory period. Effective in suppressing both atrial and ventricular dysrhythmias. The use of these agents is gradually on the decline, primarily as a result of the unfavorable risk-to-benefit ratio.
  Examples: quinidine, procainamide
- **Class Ib**
  Decreases action potential duration and automaticity and increases fibrillation threshold in ventricles. Used widely in the acute treatment of ventricular tachycardia. (More recently, however, alternate drugs are increasingly being considered as first-line agents.)
  Examples: lidocaine, phenytoin, Mexitil, tocainide
- **Class Ic**
  Depresses sinus node automaticity and prolongs conduction in atria, AV node, and ventricles. Used only for patients with life-threatening ventricular dysrhythmias. Contraindicated for use in patients with structural cardiac abnormalities and limited usefulness in the management of dysrhythmias.
  Examples: flecainide (Tambocor), propafenone (Rythmol)
- **Class II (See also Beta Blockers, p. 305)**
  Blocks beta receptors, resulting in slowed heart rate and reduced automaticity in Purkinje fibers and increases effective refractory period of AV node. Used to slow ventricular rate of supraventricular tachycardias and may also help to control ventricular arrhythmias.
- **Class III (potassium blockade)**
  These drugs have a variety of pharmacokinetic and electrophysiologic properties. Prolongs duration of action potential.
  Examples: amiodarone (Cordarone), ibutilide (Corvert), sotalol (Betapace), dofetilide (Tikosyn)

(continued)

- **Class IV (See also Calcium Channel Blockers, p. 306)**

  Blocks calcium entry into the "slow" channels of the SA and AV nodes, thereby increasing the refractory period of the AV node and decreasing the ventricular rate. Their use in tachydysrhythmias is limited. Also relaxes smooth muscle and dilates coronary arteries.

- **Unclassed**

  Slows the AV node conduction and used primarily to treat paroxysmal supraventricular tachycardia.

  Example: adenosine (Adenocard), digoxin

ARGATROBAN *(see also HIT/HITT in Part 9, p. 350)*

An anticoagulant that is a direct thrombin inhibitor, used primarily in patients diagnosed with HIT (heparin induced thrombocytopenia).

Mix: 250 mg in 250 cc 0.9 NS to make a 1 mg/1 mL concentration.

Infuse: Initial adult dosage at 2 mcg/kg/min continuous IV infusion. After initial dose, dose may be adjusted (not to exceed 10 mcg/kg/min) until PTT is 1.5 to 3 times the initial baseline (but not to exceed 100 seconds). Dose modification required for hepatic impairment, but not for renal impairment.

Considerations: Monitored by PTT.

ATIVAN (LORAZEPAM) *(see also Moderate Sedation, p. 323)*

An antianxiety and amnestic, Ativan is used frequently in the ICU setting for sedation.

Mix: Best solubility is in concentrations of 0.1 mg/mL or 0.2 mg/mL. Dilute in D_5W or NS.

Load (for sedation):   2 mg IV (may not be necessary if patient is receiving intermittent benzodiazepines, e.g., diazepam or midazolam).

Maintain: Continuous infusion of 0.5 to 1 mg/hr (0.25 mg/hr if patient is less agitated or has cardiorespiratory problems). Titrate to achieve sedation. Increase in 1-mg increments. Up to 5 to 10 mg/hr has been used. When sedation is adequate, wean to lowest amount needed.

PRECAUTIONS

- Very viscous; mix well and observe for crystallization (may occur more frequently if diluted in NS rather than D_5W, and with 4 mg/mL vials rather than 2 mg vials). Frequent IV tubing changes may be necessary.
- Refrigerate before dilution; protect from light.
- Stable at room temperature for 12 hours in plastic, 24 hours in glass.
- Continuous long-term use is not recommended. Withdrawal symptoms (i.e., rebound insomnia) can occur following cessation after as little as 1 week of therapy.
- If long-term therapy is prescribed, abrupt discontinuation should be avoided and a gradual weaning schedule should be followed.

BANANA BAG

Also known as a "rally bag," this IV mixture (most commonly used for chronic alcoholics) contains vitamins and minerals to replenish nutritional deficiencies.

Mix: 1 L 0.9 NS with

- 10 mL MVI
- 100 mg thiamine
- 1 mg folic acid
- Some institutions routinely add 1 to 3 g of magnesium sulfate.

Infuse: Typically infused over 4 to 8 hours.

BETA BLOCKERS

Beta receptors are found in a number of places in the body: heart, lung, arteries, brain, and uterus, to name a few. Like a key in a lock, beta blocker drugs (also known as beta adrenergic blocking agents) fit into the beta receptor sites and prevent epinephrine and other catecholamines from binding to the receptors that cause a response.

The body has two main beta receptors:

- Beta 1, responsible for heart rate and contractility.
- Beta 2, responsible for function of muscles that control body functions but that you do not have control of (such as bronchial smooth muscle).

REMEMBER:

Beta 1 works primarily on the heart (you have ONE heart).
Beta 2 works primarily on the lungs (you have TWO lungs).

Beta blocker drugs can be selective or nonselective.

- *Selective beta blocker drugs* block beta 1 receptors more than they block beta 2 receptors, which means that they act primarily on the heart and will decrease heart rate and contractility. Some examples of selective beta blockers are metoprolol (Lopressor, Toprol XL), atenolol (Tenormin), esmolol (Brevibloc), and bisoprolol (Zebeta). Selective beta blocker drugs should be chosen when possible.
- *Nonselective beta blocker drugs* block both beta 1 and beta 2 receptors, resulting in cardiac *and* pulmonary effects. These drugs are typically not given to patients with pulmonary disease because they may cause bronchoconstriction. Some examples of nonselective beta blockers are propranolol (Inderal), carvedilol (Coreg), labetalol (Normodyne, Trandate), and sotalol (Betapace).

IMPORTANT POINTS

- Avoid use in patients with bradycardia or heart blocks greater than first degree.
- Use with caution when given concurrently with calcium channel blockers because of intensified cardiosuppression.
- Beta blockers may mask signs of hypoglycemia in diabetic patients.
- Most common side effects are bradycardia and hypotension (these resolve when medication is withdrawn), weakness, drowsiness, reduced peripheral circulation, constipation, and GI upset.

BIVALIRUDIN *(see Angiomax, p. 303)*

BREVIBLOC *(see Esmolol, p. 313)*

BUMEX (BUMETANIDE)

Bumex is a potent loop diuretic with rapid onset and short duration. It is indicated for treatment of edema associated with CHF and hepatic or renal dysfunction. Usual dose is 0.5 mg to 2 mg IV or PO daily, but use of a continuous drip in the ICU is not uncommon. Since 1 mg of Bumex has the potency equivalent of 40 mg of furosemide, a drip rate of 0.1 to 1 mg/hr is standard, though higher doses are sometimes seen. In a small number of patients, IV infusion may result in severe muscle cramps or stiffness. This complication appears to be dose related, and generally subsides when the drug is discontinued. Patients who experience this reaction may need to be diuresed with equivalent doses of furosemide (Lasix) instead.

CALCIUM *(see also Calcium in Part 9, p. 341; Hypocalcemia in Part 9, p. 352; Hypercalcemia in Part 9, p. 350)*

Calcium is an electrolyte that helps maintain the function of the nervous and muscular systems. It is also important in blood coagulation.

CALCIUM CHLORIDE (10%)
- Each ampule (10 mL) contains 272 mg Ca (13.6 mEq) and is three times stronger than calcium gluconate.
- Infuse IV push at a maximum rate of 1 mL/min (1.4 mEq/min).
- Infuse IVPB at a maximum rate of 100 mg/min.

CALCIUM GLUCONATE (10%)
- Each ampule (10 mL) contains 90 mg Ca (4.5 mEq) and is one third the strength of calcium chloride.
- Infuse IV push at a maximum rate of 1.5 mL/min (7.7 mEq/min).
- Infuse IVPB at a maximum rate of 200 mg/min.

CALCIUM CHANNEL BLOCKERS

Calcium channel blockers inhibit calcium influx across cardiac and smooth muscle cells, resulting in decreased myocardial contractility and decreased oxygen demand while dilating coronary arteries and peripheral arterioles.

Primary therapeutic effects include:
- Treatment of hypertension.
- Control of angina.
- Management of certain types of abnormal heart rhythms (e.g., atrial fibrillation).
- Use after a heart attack when beta blockers cannot be tolerated.
- Management of cardiomyopathy.
- Prevention of vascular spasm after subarachnoid hemorrhage (nimodipine only).

There are many calcium channel blockers on the market, and their differences vary widely. For example, amlodipine (Norvasc) has very little effect on heart rate and contraction, so it is a good choice for use in individuals who have heart failure or bradycardia. Conversely, drugs like diltiazem (Cardizem) have their greatest effect on the heart and in reducing the strength of contraction, so they are best utilized for tachycardias.

REMEMBER:
- Do not give calcium channel blockers to patients with sick sinus syndrome or heart blocks greater than first degree.
- Risk of AV block is increased with concurrent use of digoxin.
- Calcium channel blockers should be administered several hours apart from beta blockers to minimize cardiosuppression.
- Diltiazem and verapamil have the most interactions with other drugs. They may increase blood levels of Tegretol, Zocor, Lipitor, and Mevacor, leading to toxicity.

CARDENE *(see Nicardipine, p. 327)*

CARDIZEM *(see Diltiazem, p. 309)*

CATHFLO *(see Alteplase, p. 298)*

CEREBYX (FOSPHENYTOIN)

Cerebyx is indicated for short-term parenteral administration when other means of phenytoin administration are unavailable, inappropriate, or deemed less advantageous. It is used for control of generalized convulsive status epilepticus and prevention and treatment of seizures occurring during neurosurgery. *Cerebyx should always be prescribed in phenytoin sodium equivalent (PE) units.*

Dosage: Before IV administration, Cerebyx should be diluted in D_5W or 0.9% NS for injection to a concentration ranging from 1.5 to 25 mg PE/mL.

Load: 10 to 20 mg PE/kg given IV or intramuscularly. If administered IV, infuse at a rate no greater than 150 mg PE/min.

Maintenance: 4 to 6 mg PE/kg/day

PRECAUTIONS
- High risk of hypotension; be sure to administer IV slowly.
- Observe patient throughout the period when maximal drug concentrations occur (10–20 minutes after completion of infusion).

CHOLINERGIC AGENTS

Also known as parasympathomimetics, cholinergic drugs produce the same effects as the body's parasympathetic nervous system (the part of the peripheral nervous system responsible for dealing with everyday activities such as digestion, sphincter muscle relaxation, salivation, and reducing heart rate and blood pressure). Nerve impulses in the parasympathetic nervous system are transmitted from one nerve junction to another with the help of acetylcholine, and cholinergic agents work by either mimicking the effect of acetylcholine or blocking the effects of acetylcholinesterase (giving acetylcholine a longer life). Cholinergic drugs are frequently used in the diagnosis of myasthenia gravis and are widely used in surgery to reduce urinary retention and to counteract the effects of some muscle relaxants given.

Conversely, *anti*cholinergic drugs are used to *inhibit* parasympathetic nerve impulses by *blocking* the binding of acetylcholinergic to receptor sites in the nerve cells. Anticholinergics are used to treat a variety of disorders such as gastrointestinal cramps, urinary bladder spasm, asthma, motion sickness, muscular spasms, and as an aid to anesthesia.

CHRONOTROPIC AGENTS

Chronotropic agents affect the heart rate. Positive chronotropes (e.g., epinephrine and Isuprel) will increase the heart rate, while negative chronotropes (e.g., beta blockers, calcium channel blockers, such as diltiazem) will decrease the heart rate.

CISATRACURIUM *(see Nimbex, p. 328)*

CORDARONE *(see Amiodarone, p. 302)*

CORLOPAM (FENOLDOPAM)

A rapid-acting vasodilator used for short-term management (up to 48 hours) of severe hypertension, including malignant hypertension with deteriorating end organ function. **Mix:** In 0.9% NS or D_5W as directed in the following table:

Corlopam Concentration		
mL of Concentrate (mg of Drug)	**Added to**	**Final Concentration**
4 mL (40 mg)	1,000 mL	40 μg/mL
2 mL (20 mg)	500 mL	40 μg/mL
1 mL (10 mg)	250 mL	40 μg/mL

Infuse: Start dosage at 0.03 to 0.1 μg/kg/min, and titrate every 15 minutes by 0.05 to 0.1 μg/kg/min until desired blood pressure is achieved. No bolus is required.

Corlopam Maintenance (Concentration 40 μg/mL)									
Dose (μg/ kg/min)	**0.25**	**0.05**	**0.1**	**0.2**	**0.3**	**0.4**	**0.5**	**0.6**	**0.7**	**0.8**
Weight (kg)	Infusion Rate mL/hr									
40	1.5	3	6	12	18	24	30	36	42	48
50	1.8	3.7	7.5	15	22.5	30	37.5	45	52.5	60
60	2.2	4.5	9	18	27	36	45	54	63	72
70	2.6	5.2	10.5	21	31.5	42	52.5	63	73.5	84
80	3	6	12	24	36	48	60	72	84	96
90	3.3	6.7	13.5	27	40.5	54	67.5	81	94.5	108
100	3.7	7.5	15	30	45	60	75	90	105	120
110	4.1	8.2	16.5	33	49.5	66	82.5	99	115.5	132
120	4.5	9	18	36	54	72	90	108	126	144

CONSIDERATIONS

- Infusion can be abruptly discontinued without adverse effect, or may be tapered gradually.
- There are no known contraindications to Corlopam.
- Adverse reactions include allergic-type reactions (anaphylactic symptoms), tachycardia, hypotension, hypokalemia (monitor potassium levels every six hours after initiating a bolus), or an increase in intraocular pressure.
- Avoid concomitant use of β-blockers.

CORVERT *(see Ibutilide, p. 318)*

COUMADIN

Coumadin (warfarin) is an anticoagulant that inhibits vitamin K and directly interferes with clotting factors II, VII, IX, and X.
Dosage: 2 to 10 mg PO daily, based on PT ratio (1.5–2.5 × control) or INR of 2 to 3.

(continued)

The half-life of Coumadin is 36 to 42 hours; therefore, an increase in the INR is not seen until 2 days after the first dose is administered.

PRECAUTIONS

Anticoagulant effect can be reversed by 5 to 25 mg of vitamin K given IM or SQ.

DALTEPARIN *(see Fragmin, p. 315)*

DEXMEDETOMIDINE *(see Precedex, p. 331)*

DILTIAZEM (CARDIZEM)

Diltiazem is a calcium channel blocker used in SVT, atrial fibrillation, angina, and hypertension.

Dosage: 0.25 mg/kg IV push over 2 minutes (average 20 mg IV). If no response, may repeat in 15 minutes at 0.35 mg/kg over 2 minutes.

Mix: 250 mg in 250 mL D_5W

Infuse: 10 to 15 mg/hr; titrate to heart rate.

PRECAUTIONS

May cause bradycardia, headache, weakness, GI disturbances, dizziness. Concurrent IV administration with beta blockers can cause severe hypotension. Avoid in patients receiving oral beta blockers.

DIPRIVAN *(see Propofol, p. 332)*

DOBUTAMINE (DOBUTREX)

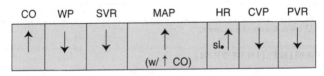

CO	WP	SVR	MAP	HR	CVP	PVR
↑	↓	↓	↑ (w/ ↑ CO)	sl.↑	↓	↓

■ Dobutrex at a glance.

Dobutamine is a synthetic sympathomimetic catecholamine with inotropic, chronotropic, and vasodilator effects. It is useful in treating heart failure (especially with an increase in SVR and PVR by increasing contractility with no significant increase in heart rate.) The blood pressure is increased because of the increased cardiac output. The vasodilatory effects of the drug, however, are more pronounced in some patients, and may actually cause a decrease in the blood pressure.

Infuse: 2 to 10 μg/kg/min (can go up to 40 μg/kg/min with physician approval)

(continued)

Mix: 250 mg in 250 mL D_5W or 0.9% NS

$$\frac{16.67 \times cc/min}{wt\ (kg)} = \mu g/kg/min$$

Dobutamine Maintenance (250 mg in 250 mL)				
Dose (µg/kg/min)	2	3	4	5
Weight (kg)	Infusion Rate (mL/hr)			
50	6	9	12	15
60	7	10	14	18
70	8	12	17	21
80	9	14	20	24
90	11	16	22	27
100	12	18	24	30

Or mix: 500 mg in 250 mL D_5W or 0.9% NS

$$\frac{3.33 \times cc/min}{wt\ (kg)} = \mu g/kg/min$$

Dobutamine Maintenance (500 mg in 250 mL)				
Dose (µg/kg/min)	2	3	4	5
Weight (kg)	Infusion Rate (mL/hr)			
50	3	4.5	6	7.5
60	4	5	7	9
70	4	6	8.5	10.5
80	5	7	10	12
90	5	8	11	13.5
100	6	9	12	15

DOBUTREX *(see Dobutamine, p. 309)*

DOPAMINE (INTROPIN)

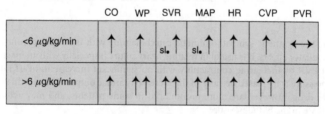

■ Dopamine at a glance.

Dopamine is a natural catecholamine that is the immediate precursor of norepinephrine. It is used to raise low blood pressure that is refractory to fluid therapy, to treat heart failure, and to correct hemodynamic imbalance in shock syndrome. Onset of the drug is rapid, usually 5 minutes, with duration lasting about 10 minutes.

(continued)

Infuse:

- Low dosage (renal perfusion): 1 to 3 μg/kg/min (generally accepted but institution specific)
- Medium dosage (increases contractility): 3 to 10 μg/kg/min
- Medium dosage (produces vasoconstriction): >10 μg/kg/min
- High dosage (works like Levophed): >20 μg/kg/min

Mix: 400 mg in 250 mL D$_5$W or 0.9% NS

$$\frac{26.67 \times \text{cc/min}}{\text{wt (kg)}} = \mu\text{g/kg/min}$$

Dopamine Maintenance (400 mg in 250 mL)

Dose (μg/kg/min)	2	3	4	5
Weight (kg)	Infusion Rate (mL/hr)			
50	4	6	7.5	9
60	4.5	7	9	11
70	5	8	10.5	13
80	6	9	12	15
90	7	10	13.5	17
100	7.5	11	15	19

Or mix: 400 mg in 500 mL D$_5$W or 0.9% NS

$$\frac{13.25 \times \text{cc/min}}{\text{wt (kg)}} = \mu\text{g/kg/min}$$

Dopamine Maintenance (400 mg in 500 mL)

Dose (μg/kg/min)	2	3	4	5
Weight (kg)	Infusion Rate (mL/hr)			
50	8	11	15	19
60	9	14	18	23
70	11	16	22	26
80	12	18	24	30
90	14	20	27	34

Or mix: 800 mg in 250 mL D$_5$W or 0.9% NS

$$\frac{53.33 \times \text{cc/min}}{\text{wt (kg)}} = \mu\text{g/kg/min}$$

Dopamine Maintenance (800 mg in 250 mL)

Dose (μg/kg/min)	2	3	4	5
Weight (kg)	Infusion Rate (mL/hr)			
50	2	3	4	5
60	2	3	4.5	6
70	3	4	5	6.5
80	3	4.5	6	7.5
90	3	5	7	8.5
100	4	5.5	7.5	9

(continued)

PRECAUTIONS
- Renal ischemia occurs at high doses.
- Causes tissue sloughing if IV infiltrates (use Regitine).

DROMOTROPIC AGENTS

Dromotropic agents affect atrial-ventricular (AV) nodal conduction. A positive dromotrope will increase the conduction (e.g., atropine sulfate), and a negative dromotrope will slow conduction (e.g., Lanoxin).

DROTRECOGIN ALFA (see Xigris, p. 338)

ENOXAPARIN (see Lovenox, p. 321)

EPINEPHRINE (ADRENALINE)

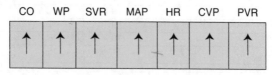

| CO | WP | SVR | MAP | HR | CVP | PVR |
| ↑ | ↑ | ↑ | ↑ | ↑ | ↑ | ↑ |

■ Epinephrine at a glance.

Epinephrine is a potent catecholamine used to increase cardiac output by increasing heart rate, resulting in an increase in cerebral and coronary blood flow and an increase in SVR.

It is a first-line drug for any pulseless rhythm. Give 1 mg IV push every 3 to 5 minutes.

Mix: 1 mg in 250 mL D_5W or 0.9% NS

Epinephrine Maintenance	
Dose (μg/min)	Infusion Rate (mL/hr)
1	15
2	30
3	45
4	60
5	75
6	90
7	105
8	120
9	135
10	150

Infuse: Start at 1 μg/min and titrate up to 10 μg/min for effect.*

*Note: May be ordered in **μg/kg/min**. Start at 0.01 μg/kg/min and titrate up to 0.2 μg/kg/min for effect.*

PRECAUTIONS
- Do not mix with $NaHCO_3$.
- Causes tissue necrosis if IV infiltrates.

EPTIFIBATIDE (INTEGRILIN)

Eptifibatide is a GP IIb/IIIa receptor blocker used to prevent platelet aggregation. It is often seen in combination with aspirin and heparin to provide a comprehensive platelet blockade. Primary indications for use are in unstable angina, non–Q-wave MI, and in the prevention of ischemic complications postpercutaneous cardiac intervention.

DOSAGE IN MANAGEMENT OF UNSTABLE ANGINA

Infuse: Initial dosage of 180 µg/kg IV over 1 to 2 minutes.
Follow by 2 µg/kg/min IV for up to 72 hours.

If percutaneous coronary intervention is performed during eptifibatide therapy, infusion should be continued for 18 to 24 hours after the procedure to a maximum total duration of 96 hours of therapy.

DOSAGE IN PATIENTS UNDERGOING ANGIOPLASTY
(NOT PRESENTING WITH UNSTABLE ANGINA)

Infuse: Initial dosage of 180 µg/kg IV over 1 to 2 minutes, immediately before procedure.
Follow by 2 µg/kg/min IV.
Then a second 180 µg/kg IV injection 10 minutes after the first.

The infusion should be continued until hospital discharge or for up to 18 to 24 hours; a minimum of 12 hours is recommended.

CONSIDERATIONS

- Does not require a dedicated line because the drug is compatible with alteplase, atropine, dobutamine, heparin, lidocaine, meperidine, metoprolol, morphine, NTG, and verapamil. It may be infused in the same line as 0.9 NS or D_5NS. The only **incompatibility** is with Lasix.
- Minimize arterial and venous punctures and intramuscular injections to minimize blood loss.
- Properly care for femoral access site to minimize bleeding. Document a PTT of <45 seconds, and stop heparin 3 to 4 hours before pulling sheath.

ESMOLOL (BREVIBLOC)

A β-adrenergic blocker, esmolol is used to control SVT or hypertension. It has a very short half-life.

Mix: 5 g (20 mL) in 500 mL D_5W or 0.9% NS
Load: 500 µg/kg/min for *1 minute*.

Esmolol Load	
Weight (kg)	**Infusion Rate (mL/hr)**
50	150
60	180
70	210
80	240
90	270
100	300
110	330

(continued)

Following load: Run maintenance infusion for 4 minutes at 50 μg/kg/min.

Esmolol Maintenance						
Dose (μg/kg/min)	50	100	150	200	250	300
Weight (kg)	Infusion Rate (mL/hr)					
50	15	30	45	60	75	90
60	18	36	54	72	90	108
70	21	42	63	84	105	126
80	24	48	72	96	120	144
90	27	54	81	108	135	162
100	30	60	90	120	150	180
110	33	66	99	132	165	198

If therapeutic effect not observed: Repeat loading dose for 1 minute.
After second load: Run maintenance infusion for 4 minutes, increasing to 100 μg/kg/min.
Continue: Titrating, repeating loading infusion over 1 minute and increasing maintenance infusion in increments of 50 μg/kg/min and running for 4 minutes.
End point: When desired effect is reached, omit loading infusion and reduce incremental dosage in maintenance infusion from 50 to 25 μg/kg/min or lower. Usual maintenance dosage is 50 to 300 μg/kg/min. Dosages >200 μg /kg/min do not significantly increase benefits.

FENOLDOPAM *(see Corlopam, p. 308)*

FENTANYL *(see also Moderate Sedation, p. 323)*

Most commonly used as sedation for procedures, fentanyl can also be used as an option for pain control. The drug needs to be dosed frequently (every 1–2 hours) and is comparable to morphine in achieved results.

- **50 mcg of IM fentanyl = 5 mg IM morphine**

  An easier option is **PCA dosing:**
- Usual recommended bolus: 25 to 50 mcg
- Usual start dose after load: 20 mcg
- Usual dose range: 5 to 40 mcg
- Usual lock out: 5 to 8 minutes

  Fentanyl patches are indicated for moderate to severe *chronic* pain and are not intended for use in postoperative pain, short-term pain, or intermittent pain. Patches are available in four strengths:
- 25 mcg
- 50 mcg
- 75 mcg
- 100 mcg

  After a patch is applied, peak effect does not occur until 24 to 72 hours, so dose increases should only be made every 72 hours. A new patch should be applied every 72 hours; however, some patients require a new patch every 48 hours, due to inadequate pain relief on day 3. Do *not* cut the patch, as this alters the release mechanism. When the patch is removed, there is a gradual decline in the drug level (it takes 17 hours to reach a 50% reduction), so patients having an adverse effect need to be monitored closely for at least 24 hours.

FOSPHENYTOIN *(see Cerebyx, p. 308)*

FRAGMIN (DALTEPARIN)

Fragmin is a low–molecular-weight heparin that inhibits thrombus and clot formation by blocking factor Xa and factor IIa. It is used for DVT prophylaxis, which may lead to pulmonary embolism after surgery, and unstable angina and non–Q-wave MI for the prevention of complications in patients taking aspirin.

DOSAGE
- DVT prophylaxis: 2,500 IU SC each day starting 1 to 2 hours before surgery and repeating once daily for 5 to 10 days postoperatively. For high-risk patients, may give 5,000 IU SC starting the evening before surgery, then daily for 5 to 10 days.
- For unstable angina: 120 IU/kg SC every 12 hours with aspirin therapy for 5 to 8 days.
- For systemic anticoagulation: 200 IU/kg SC daily or 100 IU/kg SC twice a day.

PRECAUTIONS
- Be sure to give deep SC; **do not give IM.**
- Treat overdose with protamine sulfate (1% solution). Each mg of protamine neutralizes 1 mg of Fragmin. Give very slowly over 10 minutes.

GENTAMICIN *(see Therapeutic Drug Levels in Part 9, p. 357)*

GP IIb/IIIa INHIBITORS

Glycoprotein IIb/IIIa inhibitors (abciximab, eptifibatide, tirofiban) block a key receptor involved in platelet aggregation and provide a more comprehensive platelet blockade than aspirin and heparin combined. They are primarily used for acute coronary syndromes (unstable angina, non–Q-wave MI) and in the prevention of ischemic complications post-percutaneous cardiac intervention.

HEPARIN

Heparin inhibits the conversion of prothrombin to thrombin and prevents aggregation of platelets. In case of overdose, use protamine sulfate (1 mg protamine sulfate neutralizes 100 units heparin). In October 2009, standardization of the unit dose worldwide, resulted in a heparin potency reduction of approximately 10% for doses destined for the United States. The letter "N" next to the lot number identifies the new doses. IV bolus doses may require adjustment based on this potency reduction.

Mix: 20,000 units/500 mL D_5W or 0.9% NS (40 units/mL); or
25,000 units/500 mL D_5W or 0.9% NS (50 units/mL); or
25,000 units/250 mL D_5W or 0.9% 0.9 NS (100 units/mL)

Infuse: Titrate drip to keep the PTT 1½ to 2 times the pretreatment level. Frequently, a sliding scale protocol is utilized. (Normal PTT = 30–40 seconds, so treatment goal is a PTT of 60–80 seconds.) Lower doses are recommended for patients at high hemorrhagic risk or without active thrombus or with elevated baseline PTT.

(continued)

REMEMBER:

Drip calculation is easy!

Heparin Drip Calculation		
Concentration		**Calculation**
20,000/500	(40 u/mL)	mL/hr × 40 = units/hr
25,000/500	(50 u/mL)	mL/hr × 50 = units/hr
25,000/250	(100 u/mL)	mL/hr × 100 = units/hr

HERB-DRUG INTERACTIONS

Many herbs have drug interactions with other prescription drugs or disease entities. Listed below are a few of the more common ones.

Herb	Herb Specifics	Increases Bleeding and/or Interacts with Anticoagulant	DC Prior to Invasive Procedures	Alters Blood Glucose Levels	Alters Hemodynamics (BP/HR)
Dong Quai	May not be safe if hormone-sensitive breast, uterine, or ovarian cancers. May increase effects of digoxin, beta blockers, calcium channel blockers, and anti-arrhythmic drugs. Interacts with some antibiotics (sulfonamides).	Yes	Yes	Yes`	Yes
Echinacea	Interacts with cyclosporin and other immunosuppressants. Associated with hepatotoxicity, especially if pre-existing liver disease.	–	Yes, as far in advance as possible	–	–
Garlic	Antiplatelet activities that may possibly increase INR. Also may cause fibrinolysis (breakdown of blood clots).	Yes	Yes, at least 7 days before surgery	–	–
Ginkgo Biloba	Ingestion of seeds is potentially deadly. Herb may be additive to SSRI antidepressants such as sertraline (Zoloft®)—increased risk of causing serotonin syndrome. Interacts with digoxin and MAO inhibitors.	Yes	Yes, 36 hours or greater preferred	Yes	Yes, if serotonin syndrome
Ginseng	May cause seizures and cerebral arteritis at high doses. Interacts with some MAO inhibitors causing headache, tremors, mania, or insomnia. Analgesic effect of opioids may be inhibited and interaction with sedatives may occur. Interactions with cholesterol-lowering, anticancer, antiviral, steroid, anti-inflammatory, antipsychotic, erectile dysfunction, immunomodulator, and glucocorticoid drugs, as well as caffeine. Early evidence suggests that ginseng may increase the QTc interval (thereby increasing the risk of abnormal heart rhythms).	Yes, may REDUCE the effect of warfarin (Coumadin®). May increase bleeding if pre-existing bleeding disorder or taking drugs that affect blood clotting.	Yes	Yes-hypo	Yes, if taking drugs for BP. Effect may be increased in patients with heart failure.
Green Leaf Tea	Contains vitamin K, may interfere with warfarin, particularly if green tea is taken in large doses. Contains caffeine.	Yes	–	–	Yes

(continued)

Herb	Herb Specifics	Increases Bleeding and/or Interacts with Anticoagulant	DC Prior to Invasive Procedures	Alters Blood Glucose Levels	Alters Hemodynamics (BP/HR)
Kava	Multiple cases of liver toxicity, including liver failure, have been reported, incidence enhanced if taken with hepatotoxic drugs such as alcohol or acetaminophen (Tylenol®). Chronic use may lead to kidney damage. May add to the effects of MAO-I antidepressants. Contains diuretic properties. Avoid in Parkinson's disease. Kava may cause excessive drowsiness when taken with SSRI antidepressant drugs, or concomitantly with opioid analgesics such as oxycodone and propoxyphene. May increase the effect of antiseizure medications and suicide risk with certain types of depression.	Yes	Yes, at least 2–3 weeks prior. May cause the effects of anesthesia to last longer.	–	–
Licorice	In general, licorice increases the absorption of many drugs, thereby, increasing the activity of the side effects. May cause increased risk of hypokalemia if used in combination with nonpotassium sparing diuretics. May cause pseudoprimary aldosteronism (hypertension, edema, hypokalemia). Licorice may also interact with glucocorticoids, ulcer medications, interferon, or lithium.	Yes	–	–	Yes, increased BP if chronic high doses
Melatonin	Increases cholesterol levels and is associated with arrhythmias. Eye pressures may be affected, use cautiously in glaucoma. Metabolized in the liver. Melatonin may affect the seizure threshold and increase the risk of seizure.	Yes	Yes	Yes-Hyper	Yes, decrease in BP
Omega-3 Fatty Acids	Lowers triglyceride levels but can actually increase (worsen) low-density lipoprotein (LDL/"bad cholesterol") levels by a small amount. May work against the LDL-lowering properties of "statin" drugs like atorvastatin (Lipitor®) and lovastatin (Mevacor®).	Yes	–	Yes-Hypo	Yes, decrease in BP
St. John's Wort	Interferes with metabolism of many drugs, may increase drug levels initially (causing increased effects or potentially serious adverse reactions) and/or decreased levels in the long-term (which can reduce the intended effects). Decreases efficacy of many drugs such as oral contraceptives, carbamazepine, cyclosporin, irinotecan, midazolam, nifedipine, simvastatin, theophylline, warfarin, or HIV drugs such as NNRTIs or PIs. Combination with antidepressants may lead to serotonin syndrome and mania. In general, caution is advised in almost all drug categories.	Yes, antiplatelet effect	Yes	–	Yes, if serotonin syndrome. Severe hypertension if taken in combination with MAOIs

HOT SALT *(see Hyponatremia in Part 9, p. 354)*

IBUTILIDE (CORVERT)

Ibutilide is a class III antiarrhythmic that increases the effective refractory period and prolongs repolarization in both atrial and ventricular tissue. It has no beta blocking activity and is used for treatment of supraventricular arrhythmias, including atrial fibrillation and atrial flutter. Because it has such a short duration of action, ibutilide is most effective for the conversion of atrial fibrillation or atrial flutter of relatively brief duration.

DOSAGE
- Patients >60 kg: Give 1 mg (10 mL) administered IV (diluted or undiluted) over 10 minutes.
- Patients <60 kg: 0.01 mg/kg initial IV dose.
- If the patient does not convert to NSR within minutes after *completion* of the initial dose, a second dose may be infused. The second dose is the same as the first dose.

CONSIDERATIONS
- Ventricular arrhythmias develop in approximately 2% to 5% of patients. Monitor EKG continuously for arrhythmias during administration and for 4 to 6 hours after administration.
- Patients with impaired LV function are at highest risk for arrhythmias.

INHALATION MEDICATIONS *(see Respiratory Inhalation Medications in Part 3, p. 202)*

INSULIN

When insulin errors are made, studies have shown that patient harm occurs at rates almost twice that of other drugs.

REMEMBER:
- If giving two types of insulin, draw up **clear first, then cloudy.**
- Name confusion has been reported with Lantus, Lente, and lispro; with HumALOG and HumULIN; and also with combination products such as HumULIN 70/30, NovOLOG Mix 70/30, and NovoLIN 70/30. Use caution.
- Lantus **cannot be mixed** with any other drug or any other insulin.
- The rapid-acting insulin Apidra (glulisine) and short-acting insulin (Regular) are the only insulins that can be given IV.
- Rapid-onset insulins [HumALOG (lispro) and NovOLOG (aspart)] are given SQ, and typically used for SQ infusion pumps.
- Levemir (insulin detemir) is preferred over other long-acting insulins since **most patients may be managed with once a day dosing.** There is minimal weight gain when starting therapy, and pain at injection site is minimal.
- It is recommended that Levemir (insulin detemir) NOT be mixed with other insulins.
- Rapid-acting and short-acting insulins are often called "meal insulins" because they work to help keep glucose in target range after eating.
- Intermediate and long-acting insulins are known as "basal insulins" because they work for most or all of a day to keep glucose in target range.

(continued)

Insulins

Insulin	Action	Onset*	Peak*	Duration*	Comment
Apidra (glulisine)	Rapid	15 minutes	30–90 minutes	1–2.5 hours	Give within 15 minutes prior to a meal or within 20 minutes after a meal
HumALOG (lispro)	Rapid	15–30 minutes	30–90 minutes	2–5 hours	Must eat within 10 minutes of administration
HumALOG 75/25	Intermediate + Rapid	15 minutes	0.5–1.5 hours	24 hours	Combination insulin
HumULIN N (NPH)	Intermediate	2–4 hours	6–12 hours	10–18 hours	Usually given 1–2 times daily. Can be mixed with other insulins
HumULIN R (Regular)	Short	0.5–1 hours	2–3 hours	3–6 hours	After administration, wait 30 minutes to eat
HumULIN 50/50	Intermediate + Short	0.5–1 hours	2–12 hours	24 hours	Combination insulin
HumULIN 70/30	Intermediate + Short	0.5–1 hours	2–12 hours	24 hours	Combination insulin
Lantus (glargine)	Long	1 hour	No peak, works at full level	24 hours	Cannot be mixed with other drugs or insulins
Lente	Intermediate	2–4 hours	6–12 hours	10–18 hours	Usually given 1–2 times daily. Can be mixed with other insulins
Levemir (detemir)	Long	1–2 hours	3–4 hours (up to 14 hours)	Up to 24 hours	Given once daily. May require BID dosing in some patients
NovoLIN N (NPH)	Intermediate	2–4 hours	6–12 hours	10–18 hours	Usually given 1–2 times daily. Can be mixed with other insulins
NovoLIN R (Regular)	Short	30–60 minutes	2–3 hours	3–6 hours	After administration, wait 30 minutes to eat
NovOLOG (aspart)	Rapid	15–30 minutes	30–90 minutes	2–5 hours	Must eat within 10 minutes of administration
NovoLog 70/30	Intermediate + Rapid	15 minutes	1–3 hours	24 hours	Combination insulin
Ultralente	Long	6–10 hours	8–18 hours	18–24 hours	Given once daily

*Times are approximate as individual response varies

INTEGRILIN (see Eptifibatide, p. 313)

INOTROPIC AGENTS

Inotropic agents increase the force of myocardial contraction, enhance stroke volume, and thereby increase cardiac output. *REMEMBER:* Iron = strength. They are divided into three groups: (1) cardiac glycosides (digitalis and derivatives); (2) sympathomimetics (epinephrine, dopamine, dobutamine, Levophed); and (3) phosphodiesterase inhibitors (Inocor, milrinone).

INTROPIN *(see Dopamine, p. 310)*

LABETALOL (NORMODYNE)

Labetalol is a β-adrenergic blocker used to control blood pressure in severe hypertension. It can be administered by either of two methods.

REPEATED IV INJECTION
Give an initial dose of 20 mg IV slowly over 2 minutes (this corresponds to 0.25 mg/kg for an 80-kg patient). Additional doses of 40 to 80 mg can be given at 10-minute intervals until the desired blood pressure has been reached or a total of 300 mg has been given. Maximum effect usually occurs within 5 minutes of injection.

SLOW CONTINUOUS IV INFUSION
Mix 200 mg (40 mL) in 160 mL D_5W or 0.9% NS (to make a 1 mg/1 mL solution) and infuse at a rate of 2 mL/min to deliver 2 mg/min.

Alternatively, the drip can be mixed by adding 200 mg (40 mL) to 250 mL D_5W or 0.9% NS (to make a 2 mg/3 mL solution) and infused at a rate of 3 mL/min to deliver approximately 2 mg/min.

PRECAUTIONS
- Because the half-life of the drug is 5 to 8 hours, continuous IV infusion should continue only until the desired blood pressure is reached, at which time a scheduled oral dosage regimen of the drug should be started.
- The patient should remain supine during administration, because a substantial decrease in blood pressure is expected.

LEVOPHED (NOREPINEPHRINE)

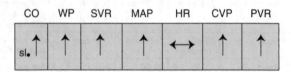

■ Levophed at a glance.

Norepinephrine is a naturally occurring catecholamine that increases contractility and thereby increases blood pressure with only a mild increase in cardiac output. It is used to treat hypotension and decreased SVR and to temporarily maintain organ perfusion. It causes an increase in myocardial oxygen consumption and myocardial ischemia.

Mix: 4 mg in 500 mL D_5W (8 μg/mL). Avoid dilution in 0.9% NS alone.

Depending on patient's fluid status, drip may need to be double concentrated to 4 mg in 250 mL (16 μg/mL) or quadrupled to 8 mg in 250 mL (32 μg/mL). To calculate the micrograms per milliliter infusion, use this formula:

$$\mu g/mL \times rate \div 60$$

Infuse: Start at 0.5 μg/min and titrate to effect. Normal range is 2 to 12 μg/min; maximum is 30 μg/min. Therapeutic range varies widely from patient to patient.

(continued)

PRECAUTIONS

- Needs to be infused via a central access line. In an emergency, a large (preferably antecubital) vein may be used until a central line is placed.
- Monitor urine output. May be reduced initially, but with adequate volume and blood pressure, it should rebound.
- Extravasation: Phentolamine (Regitine) should be infiltrated into the area.

LIDOCAINE *(see also Tocainide, p. 336)*

Lidocaine is an antiarrhythmic agent used to suppress ventricular irritability. It decreases automaticity and elevates the ventricular fibrillation threshold. It has little or no effect on EKG rhythm.

Dosage: Give 1 to 1.5 mg/kg IV push. May repeat in 3 to 5 minutes up to total of 3 mg/kg.
Mix: 2 g in 500 mL D_5W
Infuse: 1 to 4 mg/min

Lidocaine Maintenance	
Dose (mg/min)	Infusion Rate (mL/hr)
1	15
2	30
3	45
4	60

PRECAUTIONS

- Drug can precipitate asystole or PEA.
- Half-life increases after 24 to 48 hours of infusion; therefore, dose should be decreased after 24 hours, and lidocaine levels should be monitored for toxicity.
- Dose should be cut in half initially for patients with decreased hepatic blood flow.

For IV site discomfort (institution specific): 100 mg to 1 L fluid

LORAZEPAM *(see Ativan, p. 304)*

LOVENOX (ENOXAPARIN)

Lovenox is a low–molecular-weight heparin that has antithrombotic properties, used for prophylaxis of DVT and prophylaxis of ischemic complications of unstable angina and non–Q-wave myocardial infarction (administered concurrently with aspirin).

DOSAGE

- **DVT prophylaxis:** 30 mg SC twice a day, initial dose as soon as possible (not more than 24 hours) after surgery. Continues throughout the postoperative period of 7 to 10 days, then 40 mg SC for up to 3 weeks.
- **Prevention of DVT in high-risk medical patients:** 40 mg/daily SC for 6 to 11 days; may use up to 14 days.
- **For patients undergoing abdominal surgery:** 40 mg SC daily, begun within 2 hours preoperatively and continued for 7 to 10 days.
- **For patients with unstable angina or non–Q-wave MI:** 1 mg/kg SC every 12 hours for 2 to 8 days.

(continued)

PRECAUTIONS
- Do not give intramuscularly.
- If platelet count falls below 100,000, discontinue Lovenox.
- Treat overdose with protamine sulfate (1% solution). Up to 60% of Lovenox can be reversed. Each milligram of protamine neutralizes 1 mg of Lovenox. Give very slowly over 10 minutes.

ADMINISTRATION TECHNIQUE
- DO NOT expel bubble from 30 or 40 mg syringes, unless adjusting the dose.
- Make sure bevel is up on the syringe prior to injection.
- Flick residual medication off the needle prior to administration.
- Pick an area on the abdomen between the right or left anterolateral and right or left posterolateral abdominal wall and cleanse. Stay at least 2 inches away from the umbilicus. Gently pinch that area of the abdomen to make a fold in the skin.
- Insert the syringe at a 90-degree angle, using a straight down approach.
- The skin fold should be held throughout the injection. Inject smoothly, then remove the needle.
- DO NOT rub the injection site (will cause ecchymosis).

MAGNESIUM SULFATE

Magnesium sulfate is used as a magnesium replenisher. It is also used to reduce the incidence of postinfarct arrhythmias.

For arrest status, torsades: 1 to 2 g in 10 mL D_5W IV push over 1 to 5 minutes
As a replenisher: *   Mix in 0.9% NaCl or D_5W:

1 g	50 cc	Infuse over 30 minutes
2 g	100 cc	Infuse over 60 minutes
3 g	100 cc	Infuse over 2 hours
4 g	250 cc	Infuse over 3 hours
5 g	250 cc	Infuse over 4 hours

Institution specific; these are general guidelines only.

MIDAZOLAM (see Versed, p. 338)

MILRINONE (PRIMACOR)

Milrinone is an inotropic vasodilating agent with little chronotropic activity. It increases cardiac output without increasing myocardial oxygen demand or heart rate, and it decreases wedge pressure and vascular resistance. If patient starts to require more dopamine and dobutamine, this drug may be indicated. It is used for short-term IV therapy of congestive heart failure or for calcium antagonist intoxication.

Mix: 20 mg in 100 mL 0.9% NS or D_5W (0.2 mg/mL)
Load: 50 μg/kg administered over 10 minutes; response should be seen in 5 to 15 minutes. Patient "pinks up" and diuresis begins.
Infuse: Dose titrated to hemodynamic and clinical response from 0.3 μg/kg/min to maximum of 0.75 μg/kg/min (0.5 μg/kg/min works well for 90% of patients).

(continued)

Milrinone Maintenance			
Dose (µg/kg/min)	0.375	0.50	0.75
Weight (kg)	Infusion Rate (mL/hr)		
50	5.6	7.5	11.2
60	6.7	9.0	13.5
70	7.8	10.5	15.7
80	9.0	12.0	18.0
90	10.1	13.5	20.2
100	11.2	15.0	22.5
110	12.3	16.5	24.7

PRECAUTIONS

- Incompatible with furosemide and procainamide.
- Hypotension should respond to IV fluids and Trendelenburg position; vasopressors may be required.
- Half-life of 3 to 12 hours means effect of drug will remain long after it's turned off.

MODERATE SEDATION (see also Ramsey Scale in Part 1, p. 49; Riker Sedation-Agitation Scale in Part 1, p. 50; Aldrete Scoring System in Part 11, p. 368)

Moderate sedation (previously known as "conscious" sedation) refers to a drug-induced depression of consciousness during which patients respond purposefully to verbal commands, either alone or accompanied by light tactile stimulation. Reflex withdrawal from a painful stimulus is not a purposeful response. No interventions are required to maintain a patent airway, and spontaneous ventilation is adequate. Cardiovascular function is maintained. Patients are evaluated for conscious sedation by using the American Society of Anesthesia (ASA) classification scale and the Mallampati Airway Classification System.

(continued)

NOTES

ASA (American Society of Anesthesia) Classification Scale		
Class I	Normal healthy patient	Appropriate for moderate sedation
Class II	Patient with mild systemic disease • None or only slightly limiting organic heart disease • Mild diabetes controlled with oral medication • Essential hypertension medication • Anemia • Chronic bronchitis	Appropriate for moderate sedation
Class III	Patient with severe systemic disease • Diabetes, well controlled with insulin • Immunosuppressed • Moderate degree of pulmonary • Insufficiency • Stable coronary artery disease • Asthma (under treatment) • Extreme obesity	Requires careful evaluation by a physician regarding the involvement of anesthesia to ensure patient safety
Class IV	Patient with severe systemic disease that is a threat to life • Organic heart disease; cardiac insufficiency • Persistent anginal syndrome • Active myocarditis • Pulmonary, hepatic, endocrine, or renal insufficiency	Requires anesthesia consult
Class V	Moribund patient not expected to survive 24 hours with or without surgery	Requires anesthesia consult

The **Mallampati Airway Classification** system (see figure below) is used prior to moderate sedation to evaluate the patient for a possible difficult intubation by relating tongue size to pharyngeal size. The class is determined with the patient in the sitting position. Ask the patient to look you in the eye and open his mouth as widely as possible. This is the first assessment and should correspond to one of the classes as shown on next page. Next, have the patient phonate (say AH), and once again assess the airway. The class may be the same as the first, but usually improves (i.e., class III to class I). Class I corresponds with the best laryngoscopic view, while class III signals the possibility of a difficult intubation.

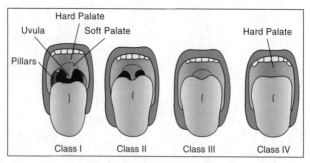

■ Mallampati Airway Classification.

(continued)

MODERATE SEDATION DRUGS

Narcotic Analgesics		
Drug/Dose	**Pharmacodynamics**	**Reversal Agent**
Morphine sulfate 2–10 mg over 4–5 minutes	Onset: IV within 5 minutes Peak: 20 minutes Duration: 3–5 hours	Naloxone (Narcan)
Fentanyl (Sublimaze) 25–100 mcg over 1–2 minutes	Onset: IV = immediate IM = 7--15 minutes Peak: 10 minutes Duration: IV = 1–2 hours IM = 0.5–1 hour	Naloxone (Narcan)
Meperidine hydrochloride (Demerol) 25–150 mg	Onset: PO, IM, SQ = 10–15 minutes IV = within 5 minutes Peak: IV = within 1 hour IM = 90 minutes Duration: 2–4 hours	Naloxone (Narcan)

Benzodiazepines (Antianxiety)		
Drug/Dose	**Pharmacodynamics**	**Reversal Agent**
Midazolam hydrochloride (Versed) 0.5–2 mg	Onset: PO = 20 minutes IV = 5 minutes Peak: IM = 0.5–1 hour IV = 1–5 minutes Duration: 20–30 minutes Up to 6 hours	Flumazenil (Romazicon)
Diazepam (Valium) 2–10 mg	Onset: PO = 20–30 minutes IV = immediate Duration: 20–30 minutes	Flumazenil (Romazicon)
Lorazepam (Ativan) 0.05 mg/kg with max of 2–4 mg IV, IM, PO	Onset: IV = 15 minutes PO = 30–60 minutes Duration: 8–12 hours	Flumazenil (Romazicon)

Sedatives/Hypnotics		
Drug/Dose	**Pharmacodynamics**	**Reversal Agent**
Chloral hydrate 500–1,000 mg	Onset: PO, PR = 20–30 minutes IM = 0.5–1 hour Duration: 4–8 hours	None
Pentobarbital (Nembutal) 100–250 mg	Onset: PO, PR = 15–60 minutes IM = 10–15 minutes IV = within 1 minute Duration: PO, PR = 1–4 hours IV = 15 minutes	None

(continued)

Reversal Agents/Antagonists

Drug/Dose	Pharmacodynamics	Reversal Agent
Naloxone (Narcan) 0.1–0.2 mg every 2–3 minutes prn	Onset: IV within 2 minutes Duration: 45 minutes	Not recommended for reversal of seizures. Large quantity can be given without significant toxicity.
Flumazenil (Romazicon) 0.2 mg IV over 15 seconds. Wait 45 seconds. May repeat 0.2 mg at 1-min intervals. Total max dose: 1 mg.	Onset: IV = almost immediate	Resedation may occur and repeated dosing may be required.

NATRECOR (NESIRITIDE)

Natrecor is an intravenous B-type natriuretic peptide (BNP) indicated for the treatment of patients with acutely decompensated congestive heart failure who have dyspnea at rest or with minimal activity. It has been shown to reduce pulmonary capillary wedge pressure, achieving 95% of its effect in 1 hour.

Reconstitute:
- Add 5 mL diluent from prefilled 250 mL D_5W bag to 1.5 mg vial of Natrecor.
- Do not shake vial, but rock gently. Solution should be clear and colorless.
- Reconstituted concentration = 1.5 mg/5 mL or 0.3 mg/mL (300 μg/mL).

Mix:
- Take reconstituted 5 mL and add to 250 mL D_5W.
- Final concentration = 1.5 mg/255 mL or 0.006 mg/mL (6 μg/mL).

Bolus:
- Recommended starting dose is a bolus of 2 μg/kg given over 1 minute.
- To calculate bolus volume: Patient weight (kg) ÷ 3.
- Withdraw the bolus volume as calculated from the prepared infusion bag, NEVER from the reconstituted vial.

Infusion:
- A continuous infusion of 0.01 μg/kg/min is recommended, never more than 0.03 μg/kg/min.
- To calculate infusion rate: Patient weight (kg) × 0.1.

PRECAUTIONS
- If hypotension occurs, the infusion rate should be immediately decreased or discontinued, and blood pressure supported by IV fluids or changes in body position.
- Natrecor can be restarted at a 30% reduced dosage (no bolus) once blood pressure is stabilized.
- Natrecor binds to heparin and therefore should not be administered through a central heparin-coated catheter.

(*continued*)

Natrecor Weight-Adjusted Bolus Volume and Infusion Flow Rate (2 µg/kg Bolus Followed by a 0.01 µg/kg/min Infusion)					
Patient Weight (kg)	Volume of Bolus (mL)	Rate of Infusion (mL)	Patient Weight (kg)	Volume of Bolus (mL)	Rate of Infusion (mL)
50	16.6	5	80	26.7	8.0
55	18.3	5.5	85	28.3	8.5
60	20	6	90	30	9
65	21.7	6.5	95	31.7	9.5
70	23.3	7	100	33.3	10
75	25	7.5	110	36.7	11

NEMBUTAL *(see Pentobarbital, p. 330)*

NEO-SYNEPHRINE (PHENYLEPHRINE)

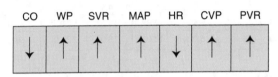

CO	WP	SVR	MAP	HR	CVP	PVR
↓	↑	↑	↑	↓	↑	↑

■ Neo-Synephrine at a glance.

Phenylephrine is a sympathomimetic adrenergic agent that acts by constricting the patient's blood vessels and raising the systolic pressure. This in turn stimulates baroreceptors in the carotid sinus and sets off reflex activity that slows the heart by increasing vagal tone. Phenylephrine resembles epinephrine, with a more prolonged action and less effect on the heart.

Mix: 20 mg in 250 mL D_5W or 0.9% NS
Infuse: (To raise blood pressure rapidly) 100 to 180 µg/min
Maintenance: (When blood pressure is stabilized) 20 to 80 µg/min

NESIRITIDE *(see Natrecor, p. 326)*

NICARDIPINE (CARDENE)

Nicardipine is a calcium channel blocker and potent vasodilator used for chronic stable angina and management of essential hypertension.

Mix: 25 mg (10 mL) in 250 mL D_5W or 0.9% NS (to make a 0.1 mg/mL solution).
Do not mix with lactated Ringer's solution; not compatible with $NaHCO_3$.
Infuse: Initially begin with 5 mg/hr (50 mL/hr) and increase by 2.5 mg/hr (25 mL/hr) every 15 minutes to a maximum of 15 mg/hr (150 mL/hr).

PRECAUTIONS
- Monitor closely for orthostasis and bradycardia.
- If used concomitantly with digitalis, may increase digitalis level.

NIMBEX (CISATRACURIUM)

Cisatracurium (Nimbex) is a neuromuscular blocking agent used to ease endotracheal intubation or relax skeletal muscle during mechanical ventilation.

Mix:
- Withdraw and discard 70 mL from a 250 mL bag of D_5W or 0.9% NS (do not use lactated Ringer's solution).
- Add one 20 mL vial Nimbex (10 mg/mL) to bag.
- Concentration is 200 mg per 200 mL or 1 mg/mL.

Infuse: 0.5 μg/kg/min to 10.2 μg/kg/min (average 3 μg/kg/min)

Nimbex Maintenance

Dose (μg/kg/min)	1	2	3	4	5	6
Weight (kg)	Infusion Rate (mL/hr)					
50	3.0	6.0	9.0	12.0	15.0	18.0
60	3.6	7.2	10.8	14.4	18.0	21.6
70	4.2	8.4	12.6	16.8	21.0	25.2
80	4.8	9.6	14.4	19.2	24.0	28.8
90	5.4	10.8	16.2	21.6	27.0	32.4
100	6.0	12.0	18.0	24.0	30.0	36.0

PRECAUTIONS
- Nimbex does **not** provide pain relief.
- Peripheral nerve stimulator should be used to monitor the neurologic response.
- Onset is rapid (2–3 minutes), with peak effect in 3 to 5 minutes.
- Recovery in 90% of patients is within 25 to 93 minutes (half-life = 22 minutes).

NIPRIDE (NITROPRUSSIDE)

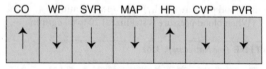

CO	WP	SVR	MAP	HR	CVP	PVR
↑	↓	↓	↓	↑	↓	↓

■ Nipride at a glance.

Nitroprusside is a venous and arterial dilator used to increase cardiac output by decreasing left ventricular afterload, to decrease blood pressure in hypertensive crisis, and to decrease pulmonary hypertension. It is the drug of choice for afterload reduction when ischemia is absent.

Infuse: 0.5 to 10 μg/kg/min (usual dosage is 3.0 μg/kg/min)

(continued)

Mix: 50 mg in 250 mL D$_5$W

$$\frac{3.33 \times cc/min}{wt\ (kg)} = \mu g/kg/min$$

Nipride Maintenance (50 mg in 250 mL)

Dose (µg/kg/min)	2	3	4	5
Weight (kg)	Infusion Rate (mL/hr)			
50	30	44	60	74
60	36	54	72	90
70	42	62	84	104
80	48	72	96	120
90	54	80	108	134

Or mix: 100 mg in 250 mL D$_5$W

$$\frac{6.66 \times cc/min}{wt\ (kg)} = \mu g/kg/min$$

Nipride Maintenance (100 mg in 250 mL)

Dose (µg/kg/min)	2	3	4	5
Weight (kg)	Infusion Rate (mL/hr)			
50	15	22	30	37
60	18	27	36	45
70	21	31	42	52
80	24	36	48	60
90	27	40	54	67

PRECAUTIONS
- Solution is stable for 24 hours only.
- Cover IV bag with opaque shield; solution should not be exposed to light.
- Check thiocyanate level if infusion continues longer than 72 hours or if rate is ≥4 µg/kg/min.

NITROGLYCERIN

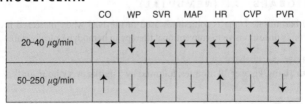

	CO	WP	SVR	MAP	HR	CVP	PVR
20–40 µg/min	↔	↓	↔	↔	↔	↓	↔
50–250 µg/min	↑	↓	↓	↓	↑	↓	↓

■ Nitroglycerin at a glance.

Nitroglycerin is a venous vasodilator used to decrease preload and afterload in left ventricular failure. It is also used for myocardial ischemia and as a dilator for coronary vasculature. Half-life is 5 to 7 minutes, so effects are short lasting.

(continued)

Infuse: No optimum fixed dose; titrate to response. Usual rate is 10 to 100 μg/min, with increments of 5 μg/min every 3 to 5 minutes. (Sometimes ordered in μg/kg/min; usual dosage is 0.1–5.0 μg/kg/min.)

Mix: 25 mg in 250 cc D$_5$W (1.66 × rate = mcg/min)

Nitroglycerine Maintenance (25 mg in 250 mL)					
mL/hr	mcg/min	mL/hr	mcg/min	mL/hr	mcg/min
3	5	21	35	39	65
6	10	24	40	42	70
9	15	27	45	45	75
12	20	30	50	48	80
15	25	33	55	51	85
18	30	36	60	54	90

Or mix: 50 mg in 250 cc D$_5$W (3.33 × rate = mcg/min)

Nitroglycerine Maintenance (50 mg in 250 mL)					
mL/hr	mcg/min	mL/hr	mcg/min	mL/hr	mcg/min
3	10	15	50	27	90
6	20	18	60	30	100
9	30	21	70	33	110
12	40	24	80	36	120

PRECAUTIONS
- Solution is stable only 24 hours.
- Tolerance develops in some patients over 1 to 2 days.

NITROPRUSSIDE *(see Nipride, p. 328)*

NORCURON *(see Vecuronium, p. 338)*

NOREPINEPHRINE *(see Levophed, p. 320)*

NORMODYNE *(see Labetalol, p. 320)*

PENTOBARBITAL (NEMBUTAL)

High-dose barbiturate coma is sometimes used in the ICU when increased intracranial hypertension is unresponsive to conventional therapy in hemodynamically stable patients.

INDUCTION OF COMA
LOAD with 10 mg/kg over 30 minutes, followed by 5 mg/kg every hour for three doses.

MAINTENANCE
- MAINTAIN at 1 to 3 mg/kg/hr by continuous infusion, adjusting to maintain control of ICP, burst suppression, and serum barbiturate levels.
- Burst suppression goal is one to five bursts/min. Zero bursts/min require holding the drug, whereas greater than five bursts/min may require upward titration.

(continued)

- Barbiturate serum levels of 30 to 40 mg/dL generally achieve adequate coma.
- If an ICP is maintained at lower than 20 mm Hg for 24 to 48 hours, then the drug should be tapered.

CONSIDERATIONS
- Patient must be mechanically ventilated.
- EEG monitoring is frequently used for assessment of coma depth.
- Normal neurologic assessment will be lost and cortical activity will be depressed.
- Barbiturate coma should have an almost immediate effective on lowering ICP.
- Major adverse reactions include hypotension, dehydration, myocardial depression, and erratic dose response.
- Because barbiturates are stored in body fat, attempting to determine brain death while the patient is receiving the drug is not possible.

PHENYLEPHRINE *(see Neo-Synephrine, p. 327)*

PRECEDEX (DEXMEDETOMIDINE)

Precedex is used in the ICU for the sedation of initially intubated and mechanically ventilated patients and can be used before, during, and after extubation. More recently, the FDA has approved it for use in nonintubated patients that require sedation prior to and/or during surgical and other procedures.

Mix: 2 mL of Precedex diluted in 48 mL of 0.9% NS, to a total of 50 mL (final concentration 4 μg/mL). Preparation of solution is the same whether for the loading or the maintenance dose.

Load: Initiate with a loading infusion of 1.0 μg/kg over 10 minutes.

Precedex Loading Infusion (10-Minute Infusion Only)

Weight (kg)	Load Infusion Rate (mL/hr for 10 minutes)	Weight (kg)	Load Infusion Rate (mL/hr for 10 minutes)
40	60	80	120
50	75	90	135
60	90	100	150
70	105	110	165

Maintain: Adjust between 0.2 and 0.7 μg/kg/hr to achieve desired effect.

Precedex Maintenance

Dose μg/kg/hr	0.2	0.3	0.4	0.5	0.6	0.7
Weight (kg)	Infusion Rate mL/hr					
40	2	3	4	5	6	7
50	2.5	3.75	5	6.2	7.5	8.7
60	3	4.5	6	7.5	9	10
70	3.5	5.2	7	8.7	10.5	12.2
80	4	6	8	10	12	14
90	4.5	6.7	9	11.2	13.5	15.7
100	5	7.5	10	12.5	15	17.5

(continued)

PRECAUTIONS

- Indicated for sedation and analgesia lasting less than 24 hours.
- Dosage reductions for patients with hepatic impairment.
- Use caution when administering to patients with advanced heart block.
- Adverse effects include significant bradycardia and sinus arrest; the most frequently observed are hypotension, hypertension (during loading dose), nausea, fever, vomiting, hypoxia, tachycardia, and anemia. Minimal effect on respirations.

PRIMACOR *(see Milrinone, p. 322)*

PROPOFOL (DIPRIVAN)

Propofol is a premixed lipid emulsion that serves as a rapid-acting sedative (onset approximately 30 seconds) with a short half-life (30–60 minutes). (It is **not** a paralytic.) Its use in the ICU allows frequent and ongoing neuro assessments as well as continuous sedation in adult patients receiving mechanical ventilation.

Infuse: Begin with 5 µg/kg/min for 5 minutes until onset of peak drug effect. When indicated, increase dosage by increments of 5 to 10 µg/kg/min over 5- to 10-minute intervals. Usual maintenance dosage is 5 to 50 µg/kg/min.

Continuous Infusion Flow Rates (mL/hr) for Propofol Maintenance

Dose (µg/min)	Weight (kg)																	
	45	50	55	60	65	70	75	80	85	90	95	100	105	110	115	120	125	130
5	1	1.5	2	2	2	2	2	2	3	3	3	3	3	3	3.5	4	4	4
10	3	3	3	4	4	4	4.5	5	5	5	6	6	6	7	7	7	7.5	8
15	4	4.5	5	5	6	6	7	7	8	8	9	9	9.5	10	10	11	11	12
20	5	6	7	7	8	8	9	10	10	11	11	12	13	13	14	14	15	16
25	7	7.5	8	9	10	10.5	11	12	13	13.5	14	15	16	16.5	17	18	19	19.5
30	8	9	10	11	12	13	13.5	14	15	16	17	18	19	20	21	22	22.5	23
35	9.5	10.5	12	13	14	15	16	17	18	19	20	21	22	23	24	25	26	27
40	11	12	13	14	16	17	18	19	20	22	23	24	25	26	28	29	30	31
45	12	13.5	15	16	18	19	20	22	23	24	26	27	28	30	31	32	34	35
50	13.5	15	16.5	18	19.5	21	22.5	24	25.5	27	28.5	30	31.5	33	34.5	36	37.5	39
55	15	16.5	18	20	21.5	23	25	26	28	30	31	33	35	36	38	40	41	43
60	16	18	20	22	23	25	27	29	31	32	34	36	38	40	41	43	45	47
65	18	19.5	21.5	23	25	27	29	31	33	35	37	39	41	43	45	47	49	51
70	19	21	23	25	27	29	31.5	34	36	38	40	42	44	46	48	50	52.5	55
75	20	22.5	25	27	29	31.5	34	36	38	40.5	43	45	47	49.5	52	54	56	58.5

(continued)

PROPOFOL INFUSION SYNDROME

PIS (propofol infusion syndrome), though rare, is a clinically devastating complication characterized by severe cardiac failure with bradycardia, metabolic acidosis, rhabdomyolysis, lipemia, and/or cardiac arrest. It seems to occur in the critically ill with SIRS and multiple organ failure in combination with high, prolonged doses of the drug. (High doses of propofol in the absence of other factors have not been reported to cause PIS.) If the range of >5 mg/kg/hr for 48 hours is exceeded, monitor for PIS by checking cardiac enzymes and myoglobin (pigment released by muscle cells when they die).

PRECAUTIONS

- Changes in rate should be made slowly (>5 minutes) to avoid hypotension and drug overdose.
- Propofol causes a substantial decrease in blood pressure in 25% to 40% of the patient population.
- A specific line should be dedicated for administration. Solution is capable of rapid growth of multiple organisms.
- Administration of bottle must be complete 12 hours after vial has been spiked. Tubing and unused portion must be discarded at that time.
- Tubing must be changed every 12 hours.

RT-PA *(see Alteplase, p. 298)*

REOPRO *(see Abciximab, p. 297)*

RESPIRATORY INHALATION MEDICATIONS *(see Part 3, p. 202)*

RETEPLASE *(see also Alteplase, p. 298; Tenecteplase, p. 334)*

Reteplase (Retavase) is a thrombolytic drug that converts plasminogen to fibrinolysin, a proteolytic enzyme with fibrinolytic effects. The onset is 30 minutes for coronary thrombolysis, peaking in 30 to 90 minutes. Begin therapy as soon as possible after onset of symptoms.

Therapy guidelines:

- Reconstitute as follows: Vials are packaged with sterile water for injection (without preservatives). **DO NOT use bacteriostatic water for injection.** Withdraw 10 mL of diluent and inject into vial, directing stream into powder. Slight foaming may occur; large bubbles will dissipate if left standing undisturbed for several minutes. Swirl gently until contents are completely dissolved. Solution should be colorless.
- Solution should be used within 4 hours of reconstitution.
- Protect from light.
- Overfill of 0.7 mL will remain in vial.

Infusion guidelines:

- Administer 10 U bolus IV over 2 minutes times two, 30 minutes apart.
- Potency is expressed in terms of units specific for reteplase that are not comparable to those of other thrombolytics.

HEPARIN THERAPY

Systemic anticoagulation may be started after completion of the therapy.

(continued)

Interventions:
- Carefully monitor ECG during treatment, and watch for reperfusion arrhythmias.
- Observe for bleeding, either internally or at external puncture sites. If local measures do not control bleeding, stop anticoagulation therapy and withhold second bolus of reteplase.
- Avoid IM injections and arterial punctures.
- Reteplase will have an adverse interaction with aspirin.
- Reteplase may precipitate out of solution if it is given with heparin in the same IV line. Therefore, each must be given separately. If a single IV line is used, it must be flushed thoroughly with sodium chloride before and after reteplase injection.

Contraindications:
- Hypersensitivity to reteplase products
- Active internal bleeding
- Severe uncontrolled hypertension
- Recent intracranial/spinal surgery or trauma
- Bleeding disorders
- History of stroke/aneurysm
- Intracranial neoplasm/arteriovenous malformation

RETAVASE *(see Reteplase, p. 333)*

t-PA *(see Alteplase, p. 298)*

TENECTEPLASE *(see also Alteplase, p. 298; Reteplase, p. 333)*

Tenecteplase (TNKase) is a thrombolytic agent (plasminogen activator) that converts plasminogen to the enzyme plasmin, which degrades fibrin clots, and lyses thrombi and emboli. It is most active at the site of the clot and causes little systemic fibrinolysis. The onset is immediate, and the peak occurs in 5 to 10 minutes. Begin therapy as soon as possible after onset of MI symptoms.

Preparation before infusion:
- Three large-bore IV sites.
- Initial lab work: complete blood count, coagulation panel, cardiac enzymes, group screen and hold.
- If arterial blood gases are required, use radial artery for puncture, and avoid brachial or femoral arteries.

Therapy guidelines:
- Reconstitute as follows: Vials are packaged with *sterile water* for injection (without preservatives). **Do NOT use bacteriostatic water for injection.** Reconstitute with 10 mL of diluent, yielding a concentration of 5 mg/mL. Swirl gently until contents are completely dissolved and a clear, transparent solution remains. Slight foaming may occur but large bubbles will dissipate if left standing undisturbed for several minutes.
- If not used immediately, the solution should be refrigerated and used within 8 hours.

Infusion guidelines:
Administer as a single IV bolus over 5 seconds (see table). Tenecteplase is NOT compatible with dextrose (precipitates). Therefore, if the IV injection line contains a dextrose solution, the line **must be flushed** with 10 mL normal saline before and after drug administration.

(continued)

Tenecteplase BOLUS 5 mg/mL		
<60 kg	6 mL	30 mg
61–70 kg	7 mL	35 mg
71–80 kg	8 mL	40 mg
81–90 kg	9 mL	45 mg
>90 kg	10 mL	50 mg

HEPARIN THERAPY
Systemic anticoagulation is usually begun several hours after the completion of thrombolytic therapy.

Interventions:
- Assess patients for bleeding every 15 minutes during the first hour and every 15 to 30 minutes during the next 8 hours, and at least every 4 hours for duration of therapy.
- Frank bleeding may occur from invasive sites or body orifices. If local bleeding occurs, apply pressure to site. If severe internal bleeding occurs, discontinue infusion.
- Clotting factors and/or blood volume may be restored through infusions of whole blood, packed red blood cells, fresh frozen plasma, or cryoprecipitate.
- Do not administer dextran because it has antiplatelet activity.
- Avoid IM injections and arterial punctures.
- Acetaminophen may be ordered to control fever.

Contraindications:
- Active internal bleeding
- History of CVA, recent trauma or surgery to central nervous system, neoplasm, or arteriovenous malformation (within 2 months)
- Severe uncontrolled hypertension
- Known bleeding tendencies
- Hypersensitivity

Use cautiously in:
- Recent major surgery, trauma, GI or GU bleeding
- Cerebrovascular disease
- Hypertension (blood pressure >180/110 mm Hg)
- Presence or high likelihood of thrombus on left side of heart
- Subacute bacterial endocarditis or acute pericarditis
- Hemostatic defect, especially those associated with severe hepatic or renal disease
- Severe hepatic dysfunction
- Geriatric patients (increased risk of intracranial bleeding)
- Hemorrhagic ophthalmic conditions
- Septic phlebitis
- Concurrent warfarin therapy or recent therapy with GP IIb/IIIa inhibitors
- Pregnant women, lactating women, or children (safety not established)

THROMBOLYTICS *(see Alteplase, p. 298; Reteplase, p. 333 Tenecteplase, p. 334, Thrombolytic Therapy in Part 2, p. 161)*

TIROFIBAN (AGGRASTAT)

Tirofiban is a GP IIb/IIIa inhibitor used in the treatment of acute coronary syndrome, including in patients who are to be managed medically and who are undergoing PTCA. It is intended to be used in combination with heparin and aspirin.

DOSAGE
- Supplied premixed as 500 mL 0.9% NaCl containing 2.5 mg Aggrastat (50 mcg/mL)
- Load: 0.4 mcg/kg/min over 30 minutes*
- Infuse: 0.1 mcg/kg/min through procedure and for 12 to 24 hours after angioplasty or atherectomy*

Patients with renal insufficiency (creatinine clearance <30 mL/min) should have the standard infusion rate decreased by 50%.

Tirofiban Dosing

Weight (kg)	Most Patients		Renal Insufficiency	
	30-Min Load Rate (mL/hr)	Maintenance Rate (mL/hr)	30-Min Load Rate (mL/hr)	Maintenance Rate (mL/hr)
30–37	16	4	8	2
38–45	20	5	10	3
48–54	24	6	12	3
55–62	28	7	14	4
63–70	32	8	16	4
71–79	36	9	18	5
80–87	40	10	20	5
88–95	44	11	22	6
96–104	48	12	24	6

CONSIDERATIONS
- Tirofiban and heparin can be administered through the same line.
- Tirofiban may be administered at the Y site with dopamine, famotidine, lidocaine, and potassium chloride.
- May cause bradycardia, thrombocytopenia, and increased risk of bleeding.
- Platelet function recovers within 4 to 8 hours after the drug is discontinued.

TISSUE PLASMINOGEN ACTIVATOR *(see Alteplase, p. 298)*

TNKASE *(see Tenecteplase, p. 334)*

TOBRAMYCIN *(see Therapeutic Drug Levels in Part 9, p. 357)*

TOCAINIDE *(see also Lidocaine, p. 321)*

Tocainide is the oral analogue of lidocaine.
Dose: 1,200 to 1,800 mg/day in three divided doses.

VANCOMYCIN *(see Therapeutic Drug Levels in Part 9, p. 357)*

VASODILATORS

Dilates arteries and veins to cause a decrease in preload and afterload, increase renal perfusion, and enhance cardiac output without increasing myocardial oxygen demands. Vasodilators can be classified based on their site of action (arterial vs. venous vs. mixed) or by mechanism of action (e.g., direct smooth muscle relaxants, ACE inhibitors, calcium channel blockers, alpha adrenergic blockers, vasopressors, etc.).

VASOPRESSIN

Vasopressin is a potent arterial vasoconstrictor indicated for use in (1) severe hypotension/shock that is nonresponsive to catecholamine (norepinephrine) therapy; (2) upper GI hemorrhages; and (3) as part of the ACLS protocol for restoring blood pressure in VF and pulseless VT.

Dose for cardiac arrest: A single injection of 40 units IV push

Dose for continuous infusion:

$$\text{Drip Calculation}: \frac{\text{Dose (in units/minute)} \times 60 \text{ (minutes)}}{\text{Solution concentration (units/mL)}} = \text{infusion rate in mL/hr}$$

- *For GI hemorrhage:*
  Standard mixture: **100 units** vasopressin/**100 cc** NS or D_5W (1.0 u/mL)* Infuse at 0.2 to 0.4 units/min. Increase by 0.2 units/min until bleeding is controlled to a maximum of 1.0 to 2.0 units/min. Continue infusion for 12 hours after bleeding is controlled, then cut dose by one half for 12 hours before cessation.

Vasopressin Dosing for GI Hemorrhage	
Units/Min	**Infusion Rate (mL/hr)**
0.20	12.0
0.40	24.0
0.60	36.0
0.80	48.0
1.00	60.0
2.00	120.0

- *For hypotension/shock:*
  Standard mixture of **100 units** vasopressin/**250 cc** NS or D_5W (0.4 u/mL)* Infuse at 0.01 to 0.04 units/min. This range reported effective in 85% of patients.

Vasopressin Dosing for Hypotension/Shock	
Units/Min	**Infusion Rate (mL/hr)**
0.01	1.5
0.02	3.0
0.03	4.5
0.04	6.0

While mixtures are institution specific, acceptable concentration must range between 0.1 to 1.0 units/mL.

(continued)

REMEMBER, REMEMBER, REMEMBER:

Watch the decimal points and zeroes in these doses, as well as the difference between *units/ minutes* (the way drug is ordered) and mL/hour (the way your pump will be set.) The hypotensive/shock dose is significantly smaller than the dose used for GI hemorrhage.

VECURONIUM (NORCURON)

Vecuronium is an intermediate-acting neuromuscular blockage agent, usually used during surgery to provide skeletal muscle relaxation. Off-label use in ICU patients is as a continuous infusion to facilitate mechanical ventilation.

Mix: 100 mg in 100 mL D_5W or 0.9% NS

Continuous infusion: 0.5 to 2 μg/kg/min (0.8–1.2 μg/kg/min average range)

PRECAUTIONS

- Vecuronium does **not** provide pain relief.
- Peripheral nerve stimulator should be used to monitor neurologic response.
- Continuous infusion raises the concern for drug-induced myopathies in ICU patients.
- Prolonged weakness persists in some patients after discontinuation of drug.
- Solution should be discarded 24 hours after reconstitution.

VERSED (MIDAZOLAM) *(see also Moderate Sedation, p. 323)*

Midazolam is a benzodiazepine used in the ICU for conscious sedation of mechanically ventilated patients.

Mix: 5 mg/mL formulation diluted to a concentration of 0.5 mg/mL in 0.9% NS or D_5W

Load dose: To rapidly initiate sedation: 0.01 to 0.05 mg/kg (approximately 0.5–4 mg for a typical adult) may be infused over several minutes and repeated at 10- to 15-minute intervals until adequate sedation is achieved.

Maintenance sedation: Usual initial infusion rate is 0.02 to 0.1 mg/kg/hr (1–7 mg/hr). Higher rates may occasionally be required in some patients.

PRECAUTIONS

Sedative effects are prolonged in patients who are obese, have decreased albumin, or renal failure.

XIGRIS (DROTRECOGIN ALFA)

Xigris is used for the reduction of mortality in adult patients with severe sepsis (sepsis associated with acute organ dysfunction) who have a high risk of death.

DOSAGE

Administered IV at a continuous rate of **24 mcg/kg/hr** (based on actual body weight at start of infusion with no adjustment for changes during infusion) for a total duration of **96 hours.**

- Complete each IV administration within 12 hours after the solution is prepared. Multiple infusion periods will be required to cover the entire 96-hour duration of administration.
- If the infusion is interrupted Xigris should be restarted at the initial infusion rate and continue to complete the 96-hour duration.

(continued)

- There is no load dose, no bolus, and no titration.
- A dedicated IV line must be used, and only NS, LR dextrose, or dextrose and saline solutions are compatible.
- There is no known antidote. In case of overdose, stop the infusion and monitor for signs of hemorrhagic complications.
- There is no standard mixture.

When using an *infusion pump* to administer: Typically, Xigris is diluted into an infusion bag containing NS to a final concentration of 100 to 200 mcg/mL.

When using a *syringe pump* to administer: Typically, Xigris is diluted with NS to a final concentration of 100 to 1,000 mcg/mL.

Dosing guidelines: Extensive dosing guidelines for 12-hour infusion bags and/or guidelines for fixed concentrations can be found at Xigris's website (**www.xigris.com).**

Contraindications: Since the most common adverse reaction to Xigris is an increased risk of bleeding, it is contraindicated in patients with active internal bleeding, recent hemorrhagic stroke (within 3 months), severe head trauma or intracranial or intraspinal surgery (within 3 months), trauma with an increased risk of life-threatening bleeding, presence of an epidural catheter, or intracranial neoplasm, mass lesion, or evidence of cerebral herniation.

ABG VALUES *(see also ABG Interpretation in Part 3, p. 168; Base Excess/Deficit in Part 3, p. 174; Mixed Venous ABGs in Part 3, p. 191)*

Normal Arterial Blood Gas Values

	Arterial Blood	Mixed Venous Blood
pH	7.35–7.45	7.33–7.43
PO₂	80–100 mm Hg	35–49 mm Hg
O₂ Sat	95% or greater	70%–75%
PCO₂	35–45 mm Hg	41–51 mm Hg
HCO₃	22–26 mEq/L	24–28 mEq/L
Base excess	−2 to +2	0 to +4

BILIRUBIN

Bilirubin is the pigmented end product of hemoglobin breakdown and a component of bile. Bilirubin is normally excreted with bile into the duodenum; then, it is broken down by bacteria in the lower intestines. When the hepatic or biliary ducts become blocked for any reason, bile is no longer excreted into the bowel. It is absorbed in the blood, causing jaundice, and is excreted by the kidneys.

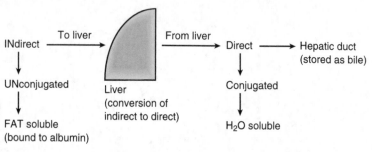

INdirect → To liver → Liver (conversion of indirect to direct) → From liver → Direct → Hepatic duct (stored as bile)

INdirect → UNconjugated → FAT soluble (bound to albumin)

Direct → Conjugated → H₂O soluble

■ Bilirubin conversion.

- Any increase in indirect bilirubin = liver disease (hepatitis or cirrhosis). Liver cannot convert bilirubin, and it remains unchanged.
- Any increase in direct bilirubin = biliary tract obstruction. Liver converts bilirubin, but obstruction is met, and direct bilirubin accumulates.
- Any increase in both direct and indirect bilirubin = hepatic failure.

BNP *(see also Chemistry Lab Values, p. 344; Heart Failure in Part 2, p. 110)*

B-type natriuretic peptide (BNP) is a neurohormone secreted from the cardiac ventricles in response to ventricular stretch and pressure overload. It counteracts the vasoconstriction that occurs as a compensatory mechanism in heart failure. Dyspnea associated with cardiac dysfunction is highly unlikely in patients with levels <100 pg/mL, whereas most patients with significant CHF have levels >400 pg/mL. **REMEMBER:** Natrecor (nesiritide) is a recombinant form of human BNP used to treat patients with acutely decompensated CHF. Many assays cannot differentiate between the infused BNP and the patient's natural BNP. Since the half-life of Natrecor is 20 minutes and is eliminated from the body within 2 hours, it is recommended that blood draws for BNP analysis not be done until a 2-hour suspension of the drug has been allowed.

C-DIFF *(see Clostridium Difficile, p. 346)*

C-REACTIVE PROTEIN

C-reactive protein (CRP) is an acute-phase protein produced by the liver during systemic inflammation or a bacterial infection, such as rheumatic fever. The test does not, however, indicate where the inflammation is or what is causing it. It may be used to monitor risk after a surgical procedure (rises within 2–6 hours after surgery, then decreases by the third day).
- Normal CRP (varies from lab to lab): Less than 10 mg/L

More recently, a special type of CRP test, the high-sensitivity CRP (hs-CRP) has been developed and is used as a risk predictor for recurrent cardiovascular and stroke events as well as indicating the increased risk of reclosure after angioplasty. (True independent association between hs-CRP and new cardiovascular events has not yet been established.)
- hs-CRP < 1.0 mg/L = low risk
- hs-CRP 1.0 to 3.0 mg/L = average risk
- hs-CRP > 3.0 mg/L = high risk

CALCIUM *(see also Calcium in Part 8, p. 306; Hypocalcemia in Part 9, p. 352; Hypercalcemia in Part 9, p. 350)*

TOTAL CALCIUM
Normal range 8.5 to 10.2 mg/dL

Approximately 40% of the body's serum calcium is loosely bound to proteins, rendering it unavailable for use by the body. 13% is chelated to anions, and the remaining 47% is UNbound or "ionized," and is metabolically active and readily available for use. Typical serum calcium measurements take into account all of these values (bound + ionized) to calculate the total calcium level.

REMEMBER:

Calcium has an *inverse* relationship with phosphorus and serum pH.

IONIZED CALCIUM
Normal range 4.7 to 5.1 mg/dL

Because albumin is responsible for 80% of the protein-bound calcium in plasma, any hypoalbuminemia will result in hypocalcemia reported on the total calcium value. However, as shown

(continued)

in the figure below, while total calcium in the plasma may decrease, the ionized (unbound) calcium that is metabolically active remains unchanged, and therefore, the hypocalcemia is not physiologically significant. To determine a true hypocalcemia in the face of a low albumin level, an ionized calcium level must be obtained from the laboratory.

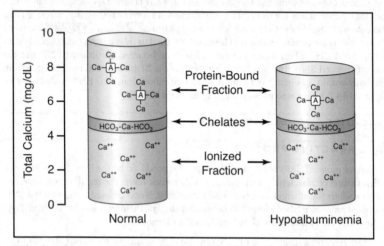

■ The three fractions of calcium in plasma and the contribution of each to the total calcium concentration. The column on the right shows how a decrease in plasma albumin can reduce the total plasma calcium without affecting the ionized calcium. (From Marino, P. L. [2007]. *The ICU book.* [3rd ed.]. Philadelphia: Lippincott Williams & Wilkins.)

CORRECTED CALCIUM

Corrected Ca (mg/dL) = (0.8 × [normal albumin − patient's albumin]) + serum calcium

While this correction factor has been used in the past for adjusting the calcium value in patients with low albumin levels, its reliability has come into question. **The use of direct laboratory testing of *ionized* calcium is recommended as the only method of identifying true hypocalcemia in the face of low albumin levels.** The correction factor can be employed as a quick "estimate" but therapy should not be based on the results.

CARDIAC MARKERS

The best marker to determine MI depends on the time from onset of symptoms. Earliest markers are myoglobin and the CK-MB isoforms. CK-MB and troponin are used in the intermediate period of 6 to 24 hours. Troponins are recommended in evaluating patients who present >24 hours after symptom onset. Lactic dehydrogenase (LDH) isoenzymes are rarely used.

(continued)

Cardiac Markers

Marker	Normal, Absent MI	In Presence of MI
CK	Males: 38–174 IU/L Females: 96–140 IU/L	Onset: 3–6 hours Peak: 24–36 hours Stays elevated 3–5 days
CK-MB*	Males: 0–4.2 ng/mL Females: 0–3.1 ng/mL	Onset: 3–6 hours Peak: 12–24 hours Stays elevated 2–3 days

CK-MB can be separated into two isoforms: CK-MB1 and CK-MB2. The normal ratio of the two is <1.0. Since CK-MB2 is initially released from the myocardium after an MI, a ratio that elevates >1.7 yields a positive result.

Myoglobin**	Males: 20–90 ng/mL Females: 10–75 ng/mL	Onset: 2–4 hours Peak: 8–12 hours Returns to normal 24–36 hours

**Myoglobin is a protein that is released into the circulation after damage to heart or skeletal muscle. Compared to CK, it is more sensitive in the evaluation of myocardial damage but is not as specific because of its release after skeletal muscle injury as well.*

Troponin I (TnI)***	0–2 ng/mL, but may be undetectable in normal healthy individual Rule in MI: >2.0 ng/mL with a serial rise Rule out MI: <0.6 with no rise	Onset: 3–4 hours Peak: 10–24 hours Stays elevated 1–2 weeks
Troponin T (TnT)***	0–3.1 ng/mL	Onset: 3–4 hours Peak: 10–24 hours Stays elevated 1–2 weeks

****Both troponins are found in the myocardium and will elevate in the event of myocardial infarction. However, because troponin I is found exclusively in the myocardium and has 100% sensitivity for MI, it is emerging as the most accurate test for confirming the presence of myocardial damage.*

CEREBROSPINAL FLUID (CSF) LAB VALUES

CSF Lab Values

Pressure	70–180	mm H_2O
Albumin	20–48	mg/dL
Ammonia	25–80	μg/dL
Bicarbonate	20–24	mEq/L
Calcium	2.1–3.0	mEq/L
Cell count	0–5	Cells
Chloride	116–122	mEq/L
Glucose	50–80	mg/dL
Magnesium	2.0–2.5	mEq/L
Osmolality	292–297	mOsm/L
Phosphorus	1.2–2.0	mEq/L
Potassium	2.7–3.9	mEq/L
Protein	20–45	mg/dL
Sodium	137–145	mEq/L
Urea	4.4–4.8	mmol/L
Uric acid	0.23–0.27	mg/dL

CHEMISTRY LAB VALUES

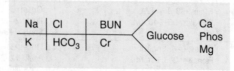

■ Medical schematic for chemistry values.

Chemistry Lab Values

Note: Values listed are guidelines only for the adult patient. Reference values are institution-specific

A/G ratio	1.2–2.3	
Acetone, serum	Negative	
Acid phosphatase	0–0.8	U/L
Albumin	3.8–5.0	g/dL
Alcohol, ethyl	Negative	
Alkaline phosphatase	36–120	U/L
ALT	0–35	U/L
Ammonia, plasma	11–35	μmol/L
Amylase, serum	23–85	U/L
Amylase, urine	4–37	U/2 hr
Anion gap	7–17	mEq/L
AST	17–59	U/L
Bilirubin direct	0–0.4	mg/dL
Bilirubin, indirect	0–1.1	mg/dL
Bilirubin total	0–1.5	mg/dL
BNP (see also BNP text)	5–1,300	pg/mL
	>2,300 pg/mL significant for CHF	
BUN	10–23	μg/dL
C-reactive protein (see also C-reactive protein text)	<10	mg/L
C-reactive protein (hs)	<3.0	mg/L
Calcium, ionized	4.7–5.1	mg/dL
Calcium, serum (see also hyper/hypocalcemia text)	8.5–10.2	mg/dL
Calcium, urine	30–200	mg/24 hr
Chloride, serum	99–111	mEq/L
Cholesterol, total	<300	mg/dL
Cholesterol, HDL	≥40	mg/dL
Cholesterol, LDL	<120	mg/dL
Cholesterol, HDLC ratio	<4.45	Calc
Cortisol, urine	20–90	μg/24 hr
Cortisol, serum AM	5–25	μg/dL
Cortisol, serum PM	2.5–12.5	μg/dL
Cortisol stimulation	10–50	μg/dL
Cortisol suppression	0–5	μg/dL

(continued)

Chemistry Lab Values (*Continued*)

Creatinine clearance		
Male	94–140	mL/min
Female	72–110	mL/min
Creatinine, serum	0.6–1.3	mg/dL
Creatinine, urine	1,000–2,000	mg/24 hr
Ferritin	20–300	ng/mL
Folate, serum	>2.0	ng/mL
Free thyroxine index	1.1–4.8	
Gastric fasting volume	20–100	mL
Gastric fasting pH	1.5–3.5	
Gastric unstim. free acid	0–40	mM
Gastric stim. free acid	10–130	mM
Gastric, 12-hr volume	150–1,000	mL
GGTP		
Male	11–63	U/L
Female	8–35	U/L
Glucose, fasting	70–115	mg/dL
Glucose, 2-hr PP	70–115	mg/dL
HgbA1C (see also HgbA1C text)	4.2–4.6	%
IgA	57–414	mg/dL
IgG	568–1,483	mg/dL
IgM	20–274	mg/dL
Iron, serum	42–135	μg/dL
Iron binding capacity, total	280–400	μg/dL
Iron saturation	12–50	%
Lactate (see also lactate text)	<2.0	mMol/L
Lipase	4–24	u/L
Magnesium (see also hypomagnesium text)	1.8–2.4	mg/dL
Osmolality, serum	280–295	mOsm/kg
Osmolality, urine	500–800	mOsm/L
Phosphorus (see also hyperphosphatemia text)	2.5–4.9	mg/dL
Potassium, serum (see also hyper/hypokalemia text)	3.5–5.0	mEq/L
Potassium, urine	25–120	mM
Protein, total serum	6.0–8.0	g/dL
Protein, total urine	40–150	mg/24 hr
Salicylate	0–29	mg/dL
Sodium, serum (see also hyper/hyponatremia text)	137–150	mEq/L
Sodium, urine random	40–220	mM
Sodium, urine timed	40–220	mM/L
T_3 uptake	25–40	%
T_4	4.5–12	μg/dL
TSH	0–7	μU/mL
Triglycerides	40–150	mg/dL
Uric acid, serum		
Male	3.0–7.4	mg/dL
Female	2.1–6.2	mg/dL
Vitamin B_{12}	180–960	ρg/mL

CLOSTRIDIUM DIFFICILE

C. diff is a gram-positive, anaerobic, spore-forming rod bacteria. It causes severe diarrhea after normal gut flora has been eradicated by the use of antibiotics and represents one of the most common nosocomial infections in the world. Generally appearing 4 to 9 days after beginning antibiotic intake, *C. diff* is most frequently linked to ampicillin, amoxicillin, clindamycin, and cephalosporins, although any antibiotic can be implicated.

Detection of *C. diff* in the stool is made by cytotoxicity assay. Since there is no correlation between the amount of bacteria found and the severity of the infection, results are reported only as "positive" or "negative." The drawback of this particular assay is that it requires 24 to 48 hours to read. Immunoenzymatic assays, which take just a few hours to run, are commercially available in the form of diagnostic kits. They are, however, relatively less sensitive and demonstrate lower specificity when compared with the cytotoxicity assay and should be used for rapid screening only.

Treatment includes placing the patient in isolation and strict handwashing (patient-to-patient spread is a major risk factor). Soap and water is preferred over alcohol-based hand rubs, as the soap is shown to be more effective against spore-forming bacteria. A 10- to 14-day regime of metronidazole or vancomycin is initiated in uncomplicated patients. Diarrhea should improve within 1 to 4 days, with complete resolution in 2 weeks. It is common for approximately 10% to 20% of the patients to experience relapse. The usual therapy for reappearance of the symptoms is another 1- to 4-day course of either metronidazole or vancomycin.

COAGULATION LAB VALUES

Coagulation Lab Values

ACT (see Hemochron text)		
Bleeding time	4–7	min
D-Dimer (see also D-Dimer text)	Negative	ng/mL
Fibrinogen (see also fibrinogen text)	200–400	mg/dL
Fibrin split products (see also FSP text)	<10	μg/dL
INR*	2.0–3.0*	
Platelets	150–400	$\times 10^3/mm^3$
Prothrombin time** (see also PT text)	11–14	sec
Partial thromboplastin time** (see also PTT text)	<40	sec
Thrombin clot time	8–10	sec

The INR (International Normalized Ratio) is intended for patients on stable, long-term oral anticoagulant therapy. Most thromboembolic conditions require the value at 2.0 to 3.0, with values at 2.5 to 3.5 for higher intensity of anticoagulation.

**REMEMBER:

PT measures Coumadin (warfarin). "PT boats were used in the war."
PTT measures heparin. The "TT" in PTT looks a bit like an "H" (for heparin).

D-DIMER

D-dimer is an end product derived from the degradation of fibrin clots. Increased levels in blood are a reliable clue that clotting has begun (i.e., when a clot is lysed by thrombolytic therapy) or that there are thrombolytic problems, such as deep vein thrombosis, pulmonary embolism, or sickle cell anemia. D-dimer is used as a highly sensitive and specific marker for DIC.

Normal findings: Negative (no D-dimer fragments present); <250 ng/mL

The D-dimer has a negative predictive value of 90% for pulmonary embolism. Thus, when results are <500 ng/mL, pulmonary embolism can be virtually excluded from the list of possible diagnosis. Conversely, when the value is >500 ng/mL and the patient is symptomatic, there is a 99% positive predictability of pulmonary embolism.

DRUG PEAKS AND TROUGHS (see Therapeutic Drug Levels, p. 357)

ERYTHROCYTE COUNT/INDICES

The erythrocyte (red blood cell) count is determined by estimating the number of red blood cells per cubic millimeter of blood. Hemoglobin (the amount of protein-iron compound in red blood cells) and hematocrit (the proportion of red blood cells in whole blood expressed as a percentage) are also measured. The hemoglobin and hematocrit concentration can be further used to calculate red blood cell indices, which define the size and hemoglobin content of an average red blood cell within a specific quantity of blood. Red blood cell indices are useful in determining the likely etiology of anemias.

The most common red blood cell indices are: mean corpuscular volume (MCV); mean corpuscular hemoglobin (MCH); and mean corpuscular hemoglobin concentration (MCHC).

ESBL (see Extended Spectrum Beta Lactamase, p. 347)

EXTENDED SPECTRUM BETA LACTAMASE

ESBLs are enzymes that are produced by some bacteria (most commonly gram negative rods, especially E. coli and Klebsiella) that cause the bacteria to be resistant to all beta lactam antibiotics (i.e., penicillins and cephalosporins). Treatment of ESBL infections is difficult, due to the limited selection of antibiotic choices. Contact precautions need to be implemented when a patient is colonized.

FIBRIN SPLIT PRODUCTS

FSP, also known as fibrin degradation products (FDP), are residual fragments of protein that are released after blood clot "breakdown." It is one of several tests done to evaluate blood clotting disorders, particularly DIC. An increase of FSP levels indicates primary fibrinolysis, the normal process of clot breakdown. Abnormally high levels, however, represent secondary fibrinolysis and are a result of disorders such as burns, DIC, hypoxia, infection/sepsis, leukemia, liver disease, or transfusion reactions.

FIBRINOGEN

Fibrinogen is a protein and coagulation factor that is produced in the liver and circulates in the plasma. In the presence of thrombin, fibrinogen converts to fibrin, and is responsible for clot formation. Fibrinogen concentrations may rise sharply in any condition that causes inflammation or tissue damage, such as seen in acute infections, hepatitis, cancer,

(continued)

stroke, trauma, coronary artery disease, or by drugs such as estrogens and oral contraceptives. Decreased levels may be the result of drugs such as anabolic steroids, androgens, phenobarbital, urokinase, or valproic acid. Acutely low fibrinogen levels are often related to DIC, and occur following rapid, large volume blood transfusions.

HEMATOLOGY LAB VALUES

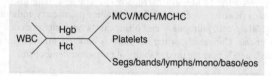

■ Medical schematic for CBC.

Hematology Lab Values

Erythrocyte count (RBC) (see also Erythrocyte Count/Indices)		
Males	4.7–6.1	$\times 10^6/mm^3$
Females	4.2–5.4	$\times 10^6/mm^3$
Leukocyte count (WBC)	4.8–10.8	$\times 10^3/mm^3$
Hemoglobin		
Males	14–18	g/dL
Females	12–16	g/dL
Hematocrit		
Males	42–52	%
Females	37–47	%
Reticulocyte count (see also Reticulocyte Count)	0.5–1.5	%
Platelet count	150–450	$\times 10^3/mm^3$
Circulating eosinophil	150–300	mm^3
Sedimentation rate		
Males	0–9	mm/hr
Females		
Erythrocyte indices (see also Erythrocyte Count/Indices)	0–20	mm/hr
MCV		
Males	80–94	μm^3
Females	81–99	μm^3
MCH	27–32	pg
MCHC	32–36	%
Leukocyte differential count (WBC)		
Neutrophils (first against bacteria)	40–80	%
*Bands (baby neutrophils)	0–6	%
*Segs (senior neutrophils)	50–62	%
Eosinophils (against parasites)	1–7	%
Basophils (chronic inflammation)	0–1	%
Lymphocytes (master immune cells)	24–44	%
Monocytes (second against bacteria)	3–10	%

REMEMBER:

*Neutrophils are illustrated from left to right. A "shift to the left" (bands → segs) indicates an increase in bands. The body is pumping out extra immature "baby" neutrophils in an attempt to respond to overwhelming infection.

HEMOCHRON, JR.

Hemochron, Jr. is a battery-operated, handheld instrument used to perform rapid activated clot time (ACT) tests at the bedside and in the OR for the monitoring and control of heparin therapy during cardiac surgery and cardiac angioplasty. *Each institution should establish its own normal range and target range of therapeutic anticoagulation based on its patient population.* In general, however, an ACT of <180 seconds is considered an acceptable result for the discontinuation of femoral access sheaths.

PROCEDURE

1. Bring all cuvettes to room temperature. This may require up to an hour.
2. Perform instrument quality control using the test cartridges.
3. Insert the cuvette into the analyzer. The instrument will display a number of messages (i.e., pump warming . . .) while performing a series of internal tests. Do *NOT* collect any blood sample until the analyzer display reads "ADD SAMPLE . . . PRESS START." Once displayed, you have 5 minutes to collect the fresh whole blood sample and add it to the cuvette.
4. Using a syringe, draw a blood waste, then obtain 0.2 cc for sampling. When utilizing indwelling blood lines, flush access port thoroughly following institutional procedures.
5. Immediately dispense one drop of blood in the sample well, filling from the bottom of the well up. A sufficient quantity of blood must be added directly to the center sample well to fill it flush to the top. Should a large drop of blood extend above the center sample well, push it over into the outer sample well. *Note:* If the blood sample is collected and added to the cuvette before the analyzer is ready, a fault message will be displayed, and the result will be invalid. If sample collection exceeds the 5-minute time limit, the analyzer will display a "START TIMEOUT" message, and you will need to discard the cuvette and replace it with a new one.
6. Depress the start key.

HgbA1C

Hemoglobin A1C is a minor component of hemoglobin to which glucose is bound; thus, the levels of HgbA1C depend on the blood glucose concentration. The higher the glucose concentration in blood, the higher the level of HgbA1C. Since the average lifespan of a red blood cell is 4 months, levels of HgbA1C are not influenced by *daily* fluctuations in the blood glucose concentration but *rather* reflect the average glucose levels over the prior 6 to 8 weeks. In healthy, nondiabetic patients, the HgbA1C level is less than 7% of the total hemoglobin. A range of 4.2% to 4.6%, which corresponds to blood sugars of about 83 to 90 mg/dL, is considered normal, as noted on the following table.

(continued)

NOTES

| Glycosylated Hemoglobin by the HgbA1C Method ||
Percent (%)	Blood Glucose (mg/dL)
4	60
5	90
6	120
7	150
8	180
9	210
10	240
11	270
12	300
13	330

HIT/HITT

Heparin-induced thrombocytopenia (HIT), with or without thrombosis (HITT), is an immune-mediated complication of heparin administration that contraindicates further heparin exposure. HIT/HITT occurs with a reported frequency of 1% to 5%; however, the reported frequency is increasing due to better recognition of the condition and more frequent testing for antibodies. HIT involves a decrease in circulating platelets (thrombocytopenia) with platelet counts falling by more than 30% within 5 to 12 days after initial exposure to heparin. This can have devastating clinical consequences, such as limb ischemia requiring amputation (10%–20%), myocardial infarction, stroke, pulmonary embolism, and even death (20%–30%). Treatment requires immediate discontinuation of all heparin products, including heparin infusions, heparin flushes, and heparin-coated catheters used for hemodynamic monitoring. The use of an effective anticoagulant (lepirudin, bivalirudin, argatroban, danaparoid) needs to be determined, focusing on either inhibiting thrombin formation, or direct thrombin inhibition.

HYPERCALCEMIA *(see also Calcium in part 8, p. 306; Calcium in part 9, p. 341)*

Normal calcium: 8.5 to 10 mg/dL. Inversely related to PO_4 level.

It is difficult to identify specific signs and symptoms as being due exclusively to increased calcium, because so many are common to other disease states: lethargy, anorexia, nausea, vomiting, constipation, dehydration. Hypercalcemia often occurs in multiple myeloma (related to lesions releasing calcium into the plasma), vitamin D overdose, Paget's disease, and other skeletal diseases.

TREATMENT

- Provide adequate hydration (to decrease the risk of renal damage) with normal saline (to produce saline diuresis); fluids up to 200 mL/hr followed by Lasix 40 mg IV every 4 hours (no thiazides).
- Administer phosphates (to promote calcium deposition in bone and decrease absorption from gastrointestinal [GI] tract).
- Administer corticosteroids, plicamycin (Mithramycin) (to lower serum calcium).

HYPERKALEMIA

Normal potassium: 3.5 to 5.0 mEq/L

Mild increase	5–6 mEq/L
Moderate increase	6–7 mEq/L
Severe increase (can result in cardiac arrest)	>7 mEq/L

Hyperkalemia usually occurs in patients with renal failure (no normal Na^+/K^+ exchange), hemorrhagic shock, Addison's disease (absence of aldosterone leads to heavy excretion of Na^+ and H_2O, leaving buildup of K^+), or massive cell damage (burns, myocardial infarction, crushing injury).

SIGNS AND SYMPTOMS
- Prolonged PR, wide QRS, tall tented T
- Ascending muscle weakness (legs to trunk)
- Lethargy

TREATMENT
Best treatment is to avoid the problem in the first place.

REMEMBER:

Patients with renal disease require a low-potassium diet. ACE inhibitors cause K^+ retention.
- Administer glucose and insulin to drive the K^+ back into the cells.
- Give $NaHCO_3$ to correct the underlying metabolic acidosis.
- Give Kayexalate enema: 15 to 50 g in 100 to 200 mL of 20% sorbitol. Repeat every 3 hours until diarrhea is produced.
- Peritoneal dialysis or hemodialysis may be indicated.

HYPERNATREMIA

Normal sodium: 135 to 145 mEq/L

Hypernatremia occurs when H_2O losses exceed Na^+ losses or when H_2O intake is inadequate. It usually reflects in dehydration and results in hyperosmolality. Over time, an actual gain in Na^+ is seen, as in hyperaldosteronism.

SIGNS AND SYMPTOMS
- Thirst, dry sticky mucous membranes
- Flushed skin, fever
- Oliguria
- Plasma osmolality >1.5 mOsm/L
- Urine specific gravity <1.015 if H_2O loss is nonrenal

TREATMENT
Administer salt-free solutions (usually D_5W) until level returns to normal, then ½ NS to avoid overcorrection. Be aware that the brain generates organic osmoles and "sucks up" fluid when aggressive fluid measures are taken, producing cerebral edema. Also, think of rhabdomyolysis in a patient who has been "down" for a long time (see Rhabdomyolysis).

HYPERPHOSPHATEMIA

Normal phosphorus: 2.5 to 5.0 mg/dL

Hyperphosphatemia is related to acute or chronic renal failure (kidney cannot excrete), hypoparathyroidism.

SIGNS AND SYMPTOMS
- Cramps to tetany; similar to hypocalcemia

TREATMENT
- Administer aluminum hydroxide gels to bind phosphate and reduce serum levels.
- Consider administration of acetazolamide (Diamox) to produce mild diuresis.
- Dialysis may be indicated.

HYPOCALCEMIA *(see also Calcium in Part 8, p. 306; Calcium in Part 9, p. 341; Hypoparathyroid in Part 6, p. 271)*

Normal calcium: 8.5 to 10 mg/dL

Hypocalcemia is related to chronic renal failure, multiple blood transfusions, excessive GI losses secondary to diarrhea or the effect of diuretics, or malabsorption syndromes. Because about 56% of serum calcium is bound to serum protein (and is therefore chemically inactive), any change in serum protein (as in renal disease) changes the total serum calcium (about 0.8 mg/dL of Ca^+ for each 1 g/dL change in albumin). The calcium value may be "corrected" by using the following formula:

$$(0.8 \times [\text{normal albumin} - \text{patient's albumin}]) + \text{serum Ca}$$

For example:

Patient = Ca^+ 9.0   Albumin 1.0
Normal albumin = 4.0 (ranges 3.5–5 g/dL)
$(0.8 \times 3.0) + 9.0 = 11.4$ mg/dL corrected Ca^+

The significance is that the patient's original lab test result indicates a normal calcium level, whereas the patient is actually hypercalcemic (see Hypercalcemia).

SIGNS AND SYMPTOMS
- Chvostek's and Trousseau's signs positive (see Part 1, Neurologic System)
- Seizures
- Laryngeal stridor (related to neuromuscular irritability)
- Bleeding abnormalities
- Prolonged QT interval

TREATMENT
IV administration of a Ca^+ salt, usually 10% calcium gluconate or calcium chloride.

HYPOKALEMIA

Normal potassium: 3.5 to 5.0 mEq/L

Hypokalemia is seen in patients with loss of body fluids (e.g., diuresis, excess vomiting, colitis, gastric damage, gastric suction, vomiting), adrenal disorders (aldosteronism, Cushing's disease, stress), congestive heart failure, or licorice candy addiction (glyceric acid has aldosterone-like effect).

(continued)

SIGNS AND SYMPTOMS
- Disturbed mental function
- Speech changes
- Cardiac dysrhythmias, flattened T wave, present U wave
- Rapid weak pulse
- Decreased blood pressure

TREATMENT
Provide K^+ replacement (be careful in patients with renal insufficiency).

HYPOMAGNESEMIA

Normal magnesium: 1.5 to 2.5 mEq/L

Hypomagnesemia frequently coexists with hypocalcemia and hypokalemia and is especially endemic in the ICU population. If the low calcium and potassium do not respond to treatment, it is more than likely related to the low magnesium, because magnesium interferes with K^+ replacement. Most hypomagnesemia disorders result from impaired absorption, excessive renal excretion, or fluid loss.

SIGNS AND SYMPTOMS
- Flushing, sweating
- Weak or absent deep tendon reflexes

TREATMENT
- Change in diet alone will usually correct a mild deficiency or may require oral administration of magnesium salts.
- For a life-threatening deficiency, magnesium is added to IV solutions with an IV infusion rate not to exceed 150 mg/min. It is contraindicated in patients with renal insufficiency. Calcium gluconate reverses magnesium overdose.

HYPONATREMIA

Normal sodium: 135 to 145 mEq/L

Severe decrease: <120 mEq/L

With hyponatremia, the amount of Na^+ in extracellular compartments is deficient in comparison with H_2O. It is related to
- Water intoxication
- Dilution (related to expansion of total body H_2O) as with CHF, renal failure, cirrhosis, SIADH. In this case, restrict intake.
- True hyponatremia (low body Na^+) is related to such conditions as burns, diarrhea, vomiting, adrenal insufficiency, drainage from fistulas.

SIGNS AND SYMPTOMS
- Weakness, irritability
- Weight loss or edema and weight gain
- Decreased blood pressure
- Decreased skin turgor
- Tremors, convulsions
- Serum osmolality decreased with retention; increased with diuresis
- Urine specific gravity <1.010 with diuresis; >1.010 with water retention

(continued)

TREATMENT

Administer normal saline at rapid rate (150 mL/hr), give Lasix 20 mg IV every 4 hours, run serial labs. However, if the patient is hyponatremic secondary to SIADH, IV saline can worsen the condition. If patient is having seizures, 3% saline ("hot salt") may be considered:

- 1 L 3% NaCl contains 513 mEq sodium.
- 500 cc 3% NaCl (available as premixed bag) contains 256 mEq sodium.
- One 3% salt tablet = 1 g NaCl.
- Replete at 1 to 2 mEq/L/hr until symptoms stop, 3 to 4 hours have elapsed and/or serum sodium has reached 120 mEq/L. Then slow down correction to 0.5 mEq/L/hr with 0.9 NS or simply restrict fluids.
- Aim for overall 24-hour correction to be <10 to 12 mEq/L/d to prevent myelinolysis.

There are potentially disastrous consequences of both living with hyponatremia and treating it. Caution is the watchword.

IDIOPATHIC THROMBOCYTOPENIC PURPURA (ITP)
(see Part 7, p. 290)

LAB DRAW PROTOCOLS

- Blood samples are obtained safely when a waste volume is drawn first. This discard amount is dependent on the "dead space" of the catheter and the lab study required, but a **5 to 10 mL waste** is generally adequate.
- When drawing blood samples from a multilumen catheter, all infusions should be stopped for optimal sampling and the **proximal lumen** used for the draw. If it is not feasible to temporarily halt infusions, contamination of the specimen can be avoided by ensuring adequate waste volume.
- For a **blood culture *line* draw, do NOT waste.** The waste is included in the 20 mL draw for the culture.
- All tubes require *gentle* mixing and should be sent back to the lab within 20 minutes for routine testing and immediately for stat results.
- Do not allow samples drawn in a syringe to sit before placing into vacutainer tubes. Have equipment ready, and transfer immediately.

What Sequence for Draw?

Whether the sample is from a peripheral vein, an IV catheter, or an arterial catheter, the same sequence of sample is required. With the use of a **vacutainer** (blood drawn directly into vacutainer tube), the following order is recommended by the National Committee for Clinical Laboratory Standards:

Tube	Additive
1. Blood culture tubes or vials	Not generally recommended for use with arterial catheters or central line catheters
2. Red top	Nonadditive or serum tubes
3. Light blue top	Citrate tubes
4. Green top	Heparin tubes
5. Lavender top	EDTA tubes
6. Tiger top/mottled top	Gel separator tubes and clot activator tubes
7. Other	Other

(continued)

Which Tube for Which Test?*		
Test	**Additive**	**Tube**
Waste, or tests requiring serum NOT from a gel tube (i.e., drug levels)	Clot activator (no gel)	Red
Coagulation testing (e.g., PT, PTT, D-dimer, fibrin split products)	Na Citrate	Blue
Ammonia	Heparin	Green (ON ICE)
Ionized calcium	Heparin	Heparinized syringe (ON ICE)
Hematology testing (e.g., CBC, hemogram, platelets, ESR, HgA1C, blood bank procedures)	EDTA	Lavender
X-match, type and screen (whole blood hematology determination)	EDTA	Pink or lavender
Chemistry (serum studies) (e.g., basic metabolic panel, amylase, TSH)	Silica clot activator	Institution-specific: Usually tiger top, mottled top, or gold
Lactate	K-oxylate	Gray (ON ICE)

*General guidelines only. Reader is advised to verify institution-specific protocols.

LACTATE

A normal lactate level in a nonstressed patient is <1.0; however, a patient with a critical illness can often be considered normal at <2.0. High lactate levels are typically present in patients with severe sepsis or septic shock and may be secondary to anaerobic metabolism due to hypoperfusion. Hyperlactemia is defined as 2.0 to 5.0 *without metabolic acidosis*. A level >5.0 *with metabolic acidosis* is considered actual lactic acidosis. A level of >15, especially in the elderly, puts the patient at a high risk of death. However, the interpretation of blood lactate levels in septic patients is not always straightforward. Elevated lactate levels may result from cellular metabolic failure in sepsis (rather than from hypoperfusion) or from decreased clearance by the liver. General recommendations for the use of lactate are to follow trends rather than a single measurement and to first rule out causes of tissue hypoxia before assuming that other factors are responsible. The technique of obtaining serum lactate by venipuncture typically carries a 24- to 48-hour turnaround time and will not be suitable to care for septic patients. Serum lactate with rapid turnaround time (minutes) can be accomplished by an arterial gas analyzer.

MRSA

Methicillin-resistant staph aureus (MRSA) is a bacterial strain that has developed resistance to methicillin and similar antibiotics such as nafcillin and cefazolin. As many as 40% of inpatients colonized with MRSA will later develop a MRSA infection. Unrecognized MRSA colonization can easily spread the infection to others, particularly to individuals that are immunocompromised. Spread is generally caused by inadequate handwashing by healthcare workers or via unclean equipment such as stethoscopes.

- **Colonized** means that the MRSA is "on" the patient's skin but *not* "in" the patient's system and is *not* causing the patient any harm (asymptomatically colonized). A colonized patient requires contact isolation, but specific antibiotic therapy is typically not required. People that are "colonized" with MRSA were usually previously infected. Their infection is now cured, but the germ is still "on" them (since antibiotics do not work on the surface of the skin) and could cause another infection later on.

(*continued*)

- **Infected** means that the MRSA is *both* "on" and "in" the patient and is causing harm. Infection may take the form of a locally infected wound or the bacteria may spread systemically causing hemodynamic instability due to sepsis. Contact isolation is required.

  Eradication protocols are institution-specific, and reader is advised to refer to specific in-house policies. In general, however, the protocol will likely include:
- Contact isolation, strict handwashing
- Daily wash/shower with chlorhexidine topical (Hibiclens)
- Mupirocin ointment to the anterior nares
- Antibiotics/antimicrobials (oral or IV) until clinically cleared of infection
- Proof of decolonization established by three sets of negative cultures of the anterior nares, as well as negative cultures of all previously positive sites (unless healed or amputated). Each set of cultures to be obtained at least 1 week apart, 48 hours after all therapy has been stopped.

PARTIAL THROMBOPLASTIN TIME

PTT is a blood test that measures the time it takes the blood to clot. The clotting cascade, usually triggered by tissue injury, has three pathways: extrinsic, intrinsic, and common. The PTT test evaluates the factors found in the *intrinsic* and *common* pathways (PT evaluates the extrinsic). An elevated PTT may be caused by medications such as heparin, or by medical conditions such as liver failure or DIC.

REMEMBER:

PTT reflects the action of heparin. The two "T's" in PTT resemble an "H" (for heparin).

PEAKS/TROUGHS *(see Therapeutic Drug Levels, p. 357)*

PROTHROMBIN TIME

PT is a test to evaluate the *extrinsic* system of coagulation (PTT evaluates intrinsic and common). An elevated PT may be caused by medications such as warfarin and/or medical conditions such as bile duct obstruction, cirrhosis, DIC, hepatitis, or a vitamin K deficiency.

REMEMBER:

PT reflects the action of warfarin. The "PT boat" was used in a "war."

RETICULOCYTE COUNT

A "retic count" measures the percentage of reticulocytes (slightly immature red blood cells) in the blood, which normally comprises approximately 1% of the circulating red blood cells. The test is done to determine if red blood cells are being created in the bone marrow at an appropriate rate, based on the body's need for RBCs. The count may help diagnose the cause of and classify anemia. A higher than normal percentage of reticulocytes may indicate bleeding (acute or chronic) or hemolytic anemia. A lower than normal percentage of reticulocytes may indicate bone marrow stress as seen in toxicity, tumor or sepsis, cirrhosis, folate/iron deficiency, radiation therapy, kidney failure with decreased erythropoietin production, or B_{12} deficiency.

THERAPEUTIC DRUG LEVELS (PEAKS/TROUGHS)

Drug	Level	Next Draw or Staging
Acetaminophen	<150 mcg/mL <0.5 mcg/mL	4 hours after ingestion 12 hours after ingestion
Amikacin	Peak: 20–35 mcg/mL Trough: <5 mcg/mL	30 minutes after infusion Just prior to next dose
Amitriptyline	120–250 ng/mL	Just prior to next dose
Aspirin	>500 ng/mL	Toxic
Carbamazepine	Trough: 4–12 mcg/mL	Just prior to next dose
Cyclosporine	Trough: 50–300 ng/mL	Just prior to next dose
Digoxin	0.8–2.0 ng/mL	Just prior to next dose
Dilantin	Trough: 10–20 mcg/mL 20–30 mcg/mL >40 mcg/mL	Just prior to next dose Toxic Severely toxic
Ethanol	>2.4 ng/mL 100–200 mg/100 mL 150–300 mg/100 mL 250–400 mg/100 mL 350–500 mg/100 mL >500 mg/100 mL	Toxic Legally drunk Confusion Stupor Coma Death
Gentamicin	Peak: 5–10 mcg/mL Trough: <2.0 mcg/mL	30 minutes after infusion Just prior to next dose
Ibuprofen	>100 mcg/mL	Toxic
Lidocaine	1.5–5.0 mcg/mL	12–24 hours after start of infusion
Lithium	Trough: 0.6–1.2 mEq/L	Just prior to first morning dose
NAPA	10–30 mcg/mL	Just prior to next procainamide dose
Phenobarbital	Trough: 15–40 mcg/mL	Just prior to next dose
Procainamide	4–10 mcg/mL	Just prior to next dose
Quinidine	2–5 mcg/mL	Just prior to next dose
Tegretol	8–12 mcg/mL	Just prior to next dose
Theophylline (po)	5–15 mcg/mL	8–12 hours after once daily dose
Tobramycin	Peak: 5–10 mcg/mL Trough: <2 mcg/mL	30 minutes after infusion Just prior to next dose
Valproic acid	50–100 mcg/mL	Just prior to next dose
Vancomycin	Peak: No longer utilized Trough: 5–15 mcg/mL	Just prior to third or fourth dose

NOTES

URINE LAB VALUES

Urine Lab Values

Specific gravity	1.003–1.030
pH	4.5–7.5
Protein	Negative
Leukocytes	Negative
Glucose	Negative
Ketones	Negative
Nitrate	Negative
Bilirubin	Negative
Blood	Negative
Urobilinogen	0–4 mg/24 hr
Epithelial cells	
Male	Small number
Female	Large number
WBC	
Male	1–5 hpf
Female	1–10 hpf
RBC	Negative
Casts	Negative
Occult blood, fecal	Negative

SEROLOGY

Mono screen	Negative
RA screen	Negative
RA titer	<1:20
ASO screen	Negative
ASO titer	<125 Todd units
VDRL/RPR	Nonreactive
Bacteria	Negative

24-HOUR URINE

Amylase	280–1,100	IU/24 hr
Calcium	100–240	mg/24 hr
Chloride	140–250	mEq/24 hr
Creatinine	1.0–2.0	g/24 hr
Creatinine clearance		
Male	100–130	mL/min
	18–25	mg/kg/24-hr total
Female	85–125	mL/min
	12–20	mg/kg/24-hr total
Magnesium	24–255	mg/24 hr
Osmolality	500–850	mOsm/kg
Phosphorus	0.9–1.3	g/24 hr
Potassium	26–123	mEq/24 hr
Protein	0–150	mg/24 hr
Sodium	43–217	mEq/24 hr
Urea nitrogen	12–21	g/24 hr
Uric acid	250–750	mg/24 hr

VRE

Vancomycin-resistant *Enterococcus* is a type of *Enterococcus* bacteria that has become resistant to antibiotics such as penicillin, gentamicin, and vancomycin. The resistant enterococci behave in the same way as the nonresistant enterococci and can cause the same range of infections. Thus, the problem is how to treat the resistant strain, as there is a limited arsenal of treatment options, and predicting the antibiotics to which the strain will be sensitive is difficult. The drug regime typically involves *combinations* of antibiotics.

- Contact isolation (gown and gloves required) since VRE is transmitted by direct contact. Strict handwashing is imperative.
- VRE can survive on inanimate objects for a considerable length of time.
- Healthy people rarely get ill if they become colonized; the danger is to the already compromised patient (i.e., renal dialysis patients, ICU patients, etc.)
- The optimal time to discontinue isolation is unknown, as VRE colonization can persist for long periods.

NOTES

PART 10

Imaging

ANGIOGRAPHY, CEREBRAL (*see Part 1, p. 7*)

ANGIOGRAPHY, CORONARY (*see Part 2, p. 71*)

ADENOSINE STRESS TEST (*see Stress Testing, p. 366*)

CHEST X-RAY

As an x-ray beam passes through a structure, different levels of absorption of the beam by different tissues occurs. The quality of the film, therefore, is dependent upon the amount of contrast between the tissues and different radiodensities. (The thickness of tissue through which the beam has to penetrate is a factor as well, i.e., the heart, a large structure, will appear more opaque than the much smaller right or left pulmonary artery.)

> **REMEMBER:**

The structure that absorbs the most x-rays will appear the lightest.
Thus:

1. Bony structures, lightest (absorb most x-rays)
2. Fat, somewhat darker
3. Body fluids (includes soft tissue, muscle, blood, heart), medium contrast
4. Gas or air, darkest (absorb minimal x-rays)

Accordingly, when a lung is referred to as being "whited out," this means that air density of the lung has been replaced (or displaced) by a tissue or water-density disease process, and has resulted in increased opacity.

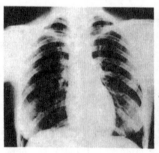 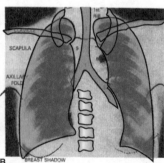

■ A, Normal posteroanterior chest radiograph. B, Outline of structures visible on normal posteroanterior chest radiograph. (Adapted from Fraser, R. G., Pare, J. A. P., et al. [1988]. *Diagnosis of disease of the chest* [pp. 288–290]. Philadelphia: WB Saunders. Reprinted with permission.)

(*continued*)

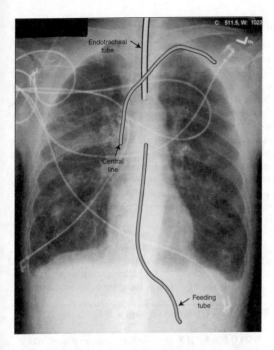

■ Radiograph depicting proper tube placements. Courtesy: Wausau Heart Institute, Wausau, WI.

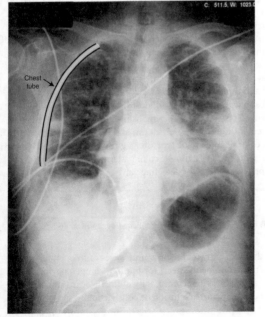

■ Radiograph denoting chest tube placement. Courtesy: Wausau Heart Institute, Wausau, WI.

CT SCAN (COMPUTED TOMOGRAPHY)

Computed refers to the fact that the information obtained from the procedure is reconstructed by a computer, and *tomography* refers to the method of producing images on a plane. CT imaging is particularly useful because it can show several types of tissue with great clarity—lung, bone, soft tissue, and blood vessels. (Very fine soft tissue areas, such as the knee and shoulder, are better served by magnetic resonance imaging. See MRI.) As with conventional x-rays, dense objects (bone) will appear bright, while less dense material (tissue) will appear darker.

Inside the CT scanner is a rotating gantry that has an x-ray tube mounted on one side and an arc-shaped detector on the opposite side. An x-ray beam is emitted in a fan shape as the rotating frame spins the x-ray tube and detector around the patient. Each time the x-ray tube and detector make a 360-degree rotation and the x-ray passes through the body, an image is acquired. Think of the scan as a meat loaf cut into thin slices. When the "slices" are reassembled by the computer, a very detailed multi-dimensional view of the structure is obtained.

A relatively new technique, **spiral CT,** has improved CT scanning even more. It allows for faster scanning and higher resolution by advancing the examination table through the gantry at a constant rate while having the x-ray tube rotate continuously around the patient. Most common are 4 or 16 slice systems. With a 16 slice system, the radiologist can obtain 32 image slices per second, allowing for a complete scan of the chest or abdomen in 10 seconds or less.

DOBUTAMINE STRESS TEST *(see Stress Testing, p. 365)*

DOPPLER ECHOCARDIOGRAPHY *(see also Echocardiography, p. 362)*

The newest innovation in echocardiography is Doppler echocardiography. It is based on the principle that the frequency of sound reflected from a moving object is changed in a predictable way by the motion of that object. When the object moves toward the detector, the frequency increases; when it moves away from the detector, the frequency decreases. (Think of an approaching train: The whistle is loud, then recedes as the train passes). In a like manner, Doppler echocardiography consists of recording sound waves reflected from moving red blood cells, displayed as an audible signal or as a spectral image, graphed with frequency on the vertical axis and time on the horizontal axis.

Color Doppler is the most sophisticated form of echocardiography, making it possible to turn flow signals into different colors and then superimposing the image on the real-time 2-D image. Red denotes movement toward the transducer, and blue denotes movement away from it. The intensity of color denotes velocity: Faster signals are lighter, and slower signals are darker. Turbulence is indicated by a mosaic color pattern. Because an entire sector can be imaged, this is the preferred mode for detecting valvular regurgitation.

EBUS *(see Endobronchial Ultrasound, p. 363)*

ECHOCARDIOGRAPHY *(see also Doppler Echocardiography, p. 362; Transesophageal Echocardiography, p. 366)*

Echocardiography is a study that uses ultrasound, or sound waves of frequencies higher than the human ear can detect, to examine the heart for motion, competency of cardiac valves, size of cardiac chambers, thickness and contractility of the myocardium, presence of structural abnormalities, and/or pericardial effusion or constriction.

(continued)

M-MODE (MOTION)

A hand-held transducer is applied to the front of the chest. High-frequency sound waves (2.5–5 mHz) are generated in short bursts (e.g., 1 microsecond), after which the transducer operates as a receiver (e.g., 1 millisecond). The returned echoes are then converted to impulses and transmitted to a machine for display and recording on videotape. The patient does not feel or hear the sound waves, and no tissue damage is produced.

TWO-DIMENSIONAL (2-D) MODE

Two-dimensional (2-D) echocardiography is a further refinement of the M-mode. The transducer crystal rotates through an arc, or many crystals emit pulses, to provide a tomographic "slice" of cardiac structures, more closely resembling actual cardiac anatomy. The problem with 2-D echocardiography, however, is that incorrect positioning or beam angulation can significantly alter the appearance of the heart and can obscure diagnostic information. Thus, M-mode echocardiography continues to be used in addition to 2-D echocardiography, because the resolution is significantly better.

ENDOBRONCHIAL ULTRASOUND
(see also Transbronchial Needle Aspiration, p. 366)

EBUS is a relatively new, minimally invasive, lung cancer diagnosis technique that allows physicians to perform transbronchial needle aspiration (TBNA) via the use of ultrasound. A special endoscope, fitted with an ultrasound processor and a fine gauge aspiration needle, is utilized to obtain tissue or fluid samples from the lungs and surrounding lymph nodes. Using EBUS guidance for TBNA, real-time imaging of the surface of the airways, blood vessels, lungs, and lymph nodes is possible. The physician can view difficult to reach areas and access more and smaller lymph nodes for sampling. EBUS is performed under moderate sedation or general anesthesia, in usually less than half an hour.

ERCP (ENDOSCOPIC RETROGRADE CHOLANGIOPANCREATOGRAPHY)

ERCP is a test used to diagnose and treat conditions in the liver, gallbladder, pancreas, and bile ducts such as gallstones, inflammatory strictures, leaks, and obstructing masses. It combines the use of x-rays and endoscopy. Initially, the test starts with the patient lying on their left side, and the endoscope is passed orally to the point where visualization of the biliary tree is possible. Once the scope is positioned correctly, the patient is placed supine and a small plastic tube is passed through the scope to facilitate injection of dye into the biliary and pancreatic ducts. X-rays are taken at the point dye is injected to reveal narrowing or blockages. Tissue biopsies may be taken via the endoscope and abnormalities addressed, such as stone retrieval.

The most common complication of ERCP is pancreatitis, and more rarely, infection, bleeding, and perforation of the duodenum. Discomfort may be experienced post procedure due to the fact that air and dye are injected during the test.

HIDA SCAN

Formally known as a hepatobiliary iminodiacetic acid scan, this test is a nuclear scan that utilizes an injection of a radioactive tracer to track the production and flow of bile from the liver to the small intestine. Traditionally used to diagnose gallbladder disease, it has a sensitivity of 95% and a specificity of 90%.

MRI

Magnetic resonance imaging (MRI) uses powerful magnets to set the nuclei of atoms in cells vibrating. The sensitive scanner measures the minute oscillations of the atoms and converts them via computer into either still or moving 3-D images. MRI scanning is superior to CT scanning in many instances, in that it can create a graphic image of bone, fluid, and soft tissue structures and give a defined image of anatomical details (CT scanning can only give information about structure of tissues, not about functional status). While MRI is superior in the evaluation of soft tissue (i.e., knee, shoulder), it unfortunately cannot detect calcium deposits, which could signal dangerously narrowed vessels.

Patients with pacemakers, stents, aneurysm clips, or other metal implants are prohibited from having an MRI due to the intense magnetic field of the scanner. All caregivers must remove all metal objects from their person before taking the patient into the scanning area. The procedure is noisy (earplugs or a headset is usually provided) and can be difficult if the patient is claustrophobic, as older MRI tubes are confining.

MUGA SCAN

Multigated acquisition scan (MUGA), also known as a nuclear ventriculogram, is a tool for measuring the function of the heart and is performed on patients suspected to have dilated cardiomyopathy, CHF, or who are status post MI. The test is performed by withdrawing blood from the patient, injecting the sample with a radioactive substance (Technetium 99), and then returning the sample to the patient's bloodstream. The patient is then placed under a special gamma camera, which is able to detect the low-level radiation given off by the technetium-labeled red blood cells. With computer assistance, the end result is a "movie" of the heart beating. The test is referred to as "multi-gated" because the gamma camera takes several images at very specific times.

Several important cardiac functions can be evaluated by a MUGA scan. If a patient has had an MI (or any other disease that affects the heart muscle), the MUGA scan can localize the portion of the heart muscle that has sustained damage and can assess the degree of damage. But, more importantly, it gives an accurate and reproducible means for evaluating left ventricular ejection fraction (normal EF is 50%–55%).

PERSANTINE STRESS TEST (see Stress Testing, p. 366)

PET SCAN

Positron emission tomography (PET) is an imaging technique that uses positively charged particles (radioactive positrons) to detect subtle changes in the body's metabolism and chemical activity. As opposed to the CT or MRI, which produce images of body structure, the PET scan provides a color-coded image of the body's function. Based on the principle that when disease strikes, the biochemistry of tissues and cells change, it is the most accurate, non-invasive way to tell whether a tumor is benign or malignant or to stage a cancer by showing metastases anywhere in the body. In the heart, PET can quantify the extent of disease and determine after a heart attack if the heart muscle would benefit from surgery. In the brain, PET can locate tumors and distinguish them from scar tissue, diagnose Alzheimer's for early intervention, or locate the focus of seizures for epileptic patients.

The PET scanner is a ring-shaped apparatus with an attached table. The patient lies on the scanning table, and the table slides slowly through the opening in the scanner ring. PET works by injecting the patient with small amount of a tracer drug (typically, a chemical

(continued)

that is normally found in the body such as carbon, nitrogen, or oxygen and that has been altered to allow it to emit positrons). The tracer travels through the body, emitting signals, and eventually collecting in the organs targeted for examination. The PET scanner records these signals, then transforms them into pictures of chemistry and function. Different colors or degrees of brightness on a PET image represent different levels of tissue or organ function.

RADIOFREQUENCY ABLATION

Radiofrequency ablation (RFA) is a procedure that utilizes electrodes to generate heat and destroy tissue.

For use in tumors: Done under CT, MRI, or ultrasound guidance, RFA may be employed to destroy or "ablate" a tumor, usually of the lung, liver, kidney, breast, or bone. It is used as an alternative treatment for patients with small, early stage tumors who wish to avoid conventional surgery, or for those that are too ill to undergo surgery. It is not intended to replace surgery, radiation, or chemotherapy, but is most effective when used in conjunction with them. The procedure consists of inserting a thin needle electrode through the skin and directly into tumor tissue. Radiofrequency energy, in the form of high-frequency alternating current, is passed through it. The energy causes the tissues around the needle electrode to heat up, and effectively kills nearby cancer cells. At the same time, heat from the radiofrequency energy closes small blood vessels and lessens the risk of bleeding. During the subsequent months, the dead cells turn into a harmless scar. The procedure is typically done on an outpatient basis under conscious sedation, although general anesthesia is preferred by many clinicians to minimize procedural pain.

For use in cardiology: RFA is also useful in cardiology to destroy an abnormal electrical pathway in heart tissue that is contributing to a cardiac arrhythmia. The procedure is primarily used in A-fib, SVT, and some types of ventricular arrhythmia. An energy emitting probe at the tip of a specialized catheter is threaded into the heart via a vein. The errant electrical pathway is then identified and eliminated via the use of radiofrequency current.

SESTAMIBI STRESS TEST *(see Stress Testing, p. 366)*

STRESS TESTING

Stress tests are done to evaluate blood flow to the heart during periods of exertion versus rest. In general, they answer two questions: is there underlying coronary artery disease that is apparent only when the heart is stressed? And, if disease is present, how severe is it likely to be? There are several different types of stress tests, which can be divided into four categories:

Exercise Echo (ECG) Stress Test: The most straightforward of all stress tests. Patient walks on a treadmill while 12-lead EKG and blood pressure are monitored. Incline and speed are increased at 3 minute intervals until the patient reaches target heart rate (85% of maximum predicted heart rate based on age) or until chest pain or fatigue occurs.

Pharmacologic Stress Test (Dobutamine): Resting echocardiography images are taken in four different views. The patient is then injected with dobutamine (an escalating dose every 3 minutes) until the heart rate reaches its predicted maximum based on age. Echo images are taken at each increasing dose of medication and again at peak heart rate. Atropine is sometimes given if the heart rate does not reach its predicted maximum

(continued)

from the dobutamine. The heart rate is then allowed to return to normal, and a final set of echo images are completed.

Nuclear Stress Test (Sestamibi, Thallium):   The patient is placed on a treadmill (or bicycle) and instructed to exercise as vigorously as possible. When the maximum exertion is obtained, a small amount of radioactive substance (radiotracer) is injected. The tracer will travel through the coronary arteries and into the heart muscle as the exercise is completed. The patient will then be placed on an x-ray table and the gamma camera will scan the heart. This first set of films will show circulation during exercise. The patient will then be required to lie quietly for 2 to 3 hours, and at that point, the scanner will take another series of fills to show circulation during rest.

Interpretation: When a normal amount of tracer arrives into all areas of the heart, the test is considered normal. Peak exercise films are compared with resting films. If both show normal uptake, blood flow through the coronary arteries is considered normal. However, if any area on the film lacks radiotracer and shows a spot of a different color (termed a defect), poor blood flow to that area is diagnosed. When a defect occurs at peak exercise and not at rest, the most likely cause is a significant blockage of a coronary artery. When a defect is observed both at rest and with exertion, there is indication that previous damage from heart attack has occurred and that the heart muscle has a scar.

Nuclear Stress Test Combined with Pharmacologic (Adenosine, Persantine):   This test is indicated if there are contraindications to exercise or the patient is unable to do so. First, a small dose of radioactive tracer is given. The patient is placed on the x-ray table for the first gamma camera scan. After the "resting" heart images are complete, adenosine or Persantine are given by slow IV to cause vasodilation and to elicit the feeling of having vigorously exercised. A second radioactive tracer is then injected, and a second gamma camera scan of the heart is done to obtain "stress" images.

TBNA *(see Transbronchial Needle Aspiration, p. 366)*

THALLIUM STRESS TEST *(see Stress Testing, p. 366)*

TRANSBRONCHIAL NEEDLE ASPIRATION
(see also Endobronchial Ultrasound, p. 363)

TBNA is a non-surgical procedure used to collect tissue from an area of the lung or airway for diagnosis and staging of disease. It is done by inserting an aspiration needle through the bronchoscope and applying a vacuum to draw tissue into the needle tip. It is different from a transbronchial biopsy in that it allows the physician to obtain samples from organs or tumors *outside* the airway, such as enlarged lymph nodes or deep submucosal lesions.

TRANSESOPHAGEAL ECHOCARDIOGRAPHY
(see also Echocardiography, p. 362)

In most cases, echocardiograms are obtained using a transthoracic approach; that is, the transducer is positioned on the wall of the anterior part of the chest. However, because ultrasound loses its clarity as it passes through tissue, lung, and bone, a more recent technique is the transesophageal (TEE) approach. It involves threading a small transducer, mounted on an endoscope (replacing fiberoptics used by the gastroenterologist), through the mouth and into the esophagus. This places the transducer in close proximity to the left atrium. As a result, the images are clearer and more accurate than those obtained with

(continued)

transthoracic echocardiography. The patient is given adequate sedation to be relaxed, but not asleep, because assistance in swallowing and changes in position are necessary during the procedure. Obviously, this method is more invasive than transthoracic, and complications are related primarily to esophageal intubation; trauma to the oropharynx, esophagus, or stomach; hypoxemia; aspiration; and rare vagal reaction.

ULTRASOUND *(see also Transcranial Doppler Studies in Part 1, p. 60; Esophageal Doppler Monitoring in Part 2, 107; Doppler Echocardiography, p. 362; Echocardiography, p. 362)*

Ultrasound imaging, also known as sonography, is a method of obtaining images from inside the human body through the use of high-frequency sound waves (no ionizing radiation is involved). Since the sound wave echoes are recorded and displayed as a real-time visual image, physicians are able to see and evaluate the actual movement of internal organs, blood flow, and valves The test is of diagnostic use with the liver, gallbladder, spleen, pancreas, kidneys, and bladder. Obstetrically, ultrasound may be used to visualize the fetus. The technique does have its limitations, however, and if visualization of bone is required, ultrasound may not be the imaging technique of choice. Sound waves have difficulty penetrating bone, and in this case, an MRI would be more appropriate. In addition, ultrasound waves do not pass through air. Therefore, evaluation of the stomach, small intestine, and large intestine may be of limited value.

The principles involved in ultrasound imaging are the same as those used by ships at sea or by bats. As sound passes through the body, echoes are produced that can be used to identify an object's distance, how large it is, its shape, and its consistency. The ultrasound transducer functions as both a generator of sound and a detector. When the transducer is pressed against the skin, sound "echoes" from the body's fluids and tissues, producing waves that the transducer records. With Doppler ultrasound, a microphone captures and records tiny changes in the sound wave pitch and direction.

VENTRICULOGRAM *(see MUGA Scan, p. 364)*

NOTES

PART 11

Miscellaneous

ALDRETE SCORING SYSTEM

A scale commonly used to determine when postsurgical patients can be safely discharged from the Post Anesthesia Recovery Unit.

Aldrete Scoring System

Assessment	Postprocedure Aldrete Scoring System	
Activity	Able to move four extremities voluntarily or on command	2
	Able to move two extremities voluntarily or on command	1
	Not able to move extremities voluntarily or on command	0
Respiration	Able to deep breathe and cough freely	2
	Dyspnea, shallow or limited breathing	1
	Apneic	0
Circulation	Blood pressure ±20 mm Hg of presedation level: stable pulse/pediatrics: return to VS baseline	2
	Blood pressure ±20–50 mm Hg of presedation level: abnormal dysrhythmia	1
Consciousness	Blood pressure ±50 mm Hg of presedation level: symptomatic dysrhythmia	0
	Fully awake	2
	Arousable on calling	1
	Not responding	0
O_2 Saturation	Able to maintain SaO_2 >90% on room air	2
	Needs O_2 to maintain SaO_2 >90%	1
	SaO_2 <90% even with O_2 supplement	0

More recently, the system has been modified, and two additional criteria were added, to create the modified Aldrete score:

Modified Aldrete Score Criteria

Postoperative pain assessment	None or mild discomfort	2
	Moderate to severe pain controlled with IV analgesics	1
	Persistent severe pain	0
Postoperative emetic symptoms	None or mild nausea with no active vomiting	2
	Transient vomiting or retching	1
	Persistent moderate to severe nausea and vomiting	0

ANTI-EMBOLISM STOCKINGS

Proper fit is required to obtain maximum benefit from compression hose. Improper fit will produce a reversed pressure gradient and is associated with a statistically higher incidence of DVT compared with stockings that produce a proper gradient.

MEASUREMENT FOR KNEE LENGTH TED COMPRESSION STOCKINGS

1. Measure calf circumference at the greatest portion to determine size;
2. Measure the distance from the bend of the knee to the bottom of the heel to determine length.

Knee Length TED Compression Hose		
Calf Circumference	**Length**	
	Regular	**Long**
Small >10" but <12"	Less than 16"	16" and over
Medium 12"–15"	Less than 17"	17" and over
Large 15.1"–17.5"	Less than 18"	18" and over
X-Large 17.6"–20"	Less than 18"	18" and over

MEASUREMENT FOR THIGH LENGTH TED COMPRESSION STOCKINGS

1. Measure upper thigh circumference at the buttock fold;
2. Measure calf circumference at greatest portion to determine size;
3. Measure distance from the base of the heel to determine length.

Thigh Length TED Compression Hose				
Thigh Circumference	**Calf Circumference**	**Length**		
		Short	**Regular**	**Long**
Less than 25" (If >25" but <32" consider XL thigh length with belt, or knee length)	Small <12"	<29"	29"–33"	29"–33"
	Medium 12"–15"	<29"	29"–33"	29"–33"
	Large 15.1"–17.5"	<29"	29"–33"	29"–33"

APACHE SCORING SYSTEM

The Acute Physiology and Chronic Health Evaluation (APACHE) score is a tool used to calculate a patient's risk of hospital mortality after the first day of ICU, based on severity of disease. It compares each individual's medical profile against nearly 18,000 cases in its memory before reaching a prognosis that is, on average, 95% accurate. The system consists of 4 components:

1. Age;
2. Major disease category (reason for ICU admission);
3. Acute (current) physiology;
4. Prior site of healthcare (emergency room, general floor, etc.).

Within 24 hours of admission, the physician must enter a number for each of several easily obtained facts. The sum of these numbers results in a score ranging from 0 to 71. (After the initial score has been determined, no new score can be calculated during the hospital stay. If a patient is discharged from the ICU and readmitted, a new APACHE score needs to be calculated.) Higher scores imply a more severe disease and a higher risk of death. A score of >50 is associated with increased mortality in nonpregnant cardiac and trauma patients.

ASA (AMERICAN SOCIETY OF ANESTHESIA) CLASSIFICATION SCALE *(see Moderate Sedation in Part 8, p. 324)*

BRADEN SCALE

The Braden scale is used to assess for risk of development of pressure ulcers; the lower the numeric score, the higher the patient's probability for development of pressure ulcers.

Braden Risk Interpretation	
Total Score	**Potential Risk**
9 or less	Very high risk
10–12	High risk
13–14	Moderate risk
15–18	Low risk
19–23	No risk

Braden Skin Assessment Scale			
SENSORY PERCEPTION Ability to respond meaningfully to pressure-related discomfort	1. **Completely Limited:** Unresponsive (does not moan, flinch, or grasp) to painful stimuli due to diminished level of consciousness or sedation. OR limited ability to feel pain over most of body surface.	2. **Very Limited:** Responds only to painful stimuli. Cannot communicate discomfort except by moaning or restlessness. OR has a sensory impairment that limits the ability to feel pain or discomfort over the half of body.	3. **Slightly Limited:** Responds to verbal commands but cannot always communicate discomfort or needs to be turned. OR has some sensory impairment that limits ability to feel pain or discomfort in one or two extremities.
MOISTURE Degree to which skin is exposed to moisture	1. **Constantly Moist:** Skin is kept moist almost constantly by perspiration, urine, etc. Dampness is detected every time patient is moved or turned.	2. **Very Moist:** Skin is often but not always moist. Linen must be changed at least once a shift.	3. **Occasionally Moist:** Skin is occasionally moist, requiring an extra linen change approximately once a day.
ACTIVITY Degree of physical activity	1. **Bedfast:** Confined to bed.	2. **Chairfast:** Ability to walk severely limited or nonexistent. Cannot bear own weight and/or must be assisted into chair or wheelchair.	3. **Walks Occasionally:** Walks occasionally during the day, but for very short distances, with or without assistance. Spends majority of each shift in bed or chair.
MOBILITY Ability to change and control body position	1. **Completely Immobile:** Does not make even slight changes in body or extremity position without assistance.	2. **Very Limited:** Makes occasional slight changes in body or extremity position but unable to make frequent or significant changes independently.	3. **Slightly Limited:** Makes frequent though slight changes in body or extremity position independently.

(continued)

Braden Skin Assessment Scale (*Continued*)

NUTRITION *Usual* food intake pattern	1. **Very Poor:** Never eats complete meal. Rarely eats more than one third of any food offered. Eats two servings or less of protein (meat or dairy products) per day. Takes fluids poorly. Does not take a liquid dietary supplement. OR is NPO and/or maintained on clear liquids or IVs for more than 5 days.	2. **Probably Inadequate:** Rarely eats a complete meal and generally eats only about half of any food offered. Protein intake includes only three servings of meat or dairy products per day. Occasionally will take a dietary supplement. OR receives less than optimum amount of liquid diet or tube feeding.	3. **Adequate:** Eats over half of most meals. Eats a total of four servings of protein (meat, dairy products) each day. Occasionally will refuse a meal but will usually take a supplement if offered, OR is on a tube feeding or TPN regimen that probably meets most of nutritional needs.
FRICTION AND SHEAR	1. **Problem:** Requires moderate to maximum assistance in moving. Complete lifting without sliding against sheets is impossible. Frequently slides down in bed or chair, requiring frequent repositioning with maximum assistance. Spasticity, contractures, or agitation lead to almost constant friction.	2. **Potential Problem:** Moves feebly or requires minimum assistance. During a move, skin probably slides to some extent against sheets, chair, restraints, or other devices. Maintains relatively good position in chair or bed most of the time but occasionally slides down.	3. **No Apparent Problem:** Moves in bed and in chair independently and has sufficient muscle strength to lift up completely during move. Maintains good position in bed or chair at all times.

▌ BURNS

The rule of nines is a clinical calculation used to determine the percentage of body surface area burned on an adult. It provides a useful guide for fluid resuscitation and further treatment decisions.

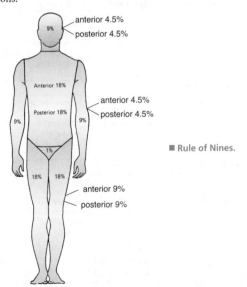

■ Rule of Nines.

(continued)

FLUID RESUSCITATION

Fluid resuscitation is the major goal during the initial treatment of a burn patient. There are two common methods to determine this number:

Parkland (also known as the Baxter or Consensus) formula:

Lactated Ringer's solution: $4\ mL$ × kg body weight × % BSA burned

Half to be given over the first 8 hours postburn; remainder over the next 16 hours

Modified Brooke formula:

Lactated Ringer's solution: $2\ mL$ × kg body weight × % BSA burned

Half to be given over the first 8 hours postburn; remainder over the next 16 hours

There is a large difference in the amount of fluid between these two formulas. Which one to use will depend upon the needs of the patient. Remember, formulas *are a guide only,* and the goals are response to fluid administration and tolerance of the patient during therapy. For example, patients with inhalation injury or electrical burns, and those who were burned while intoxicated may require additional fluid, yet fluid overload can easily cause pulmonary or cerebral edema. However, if an inadequate amount of fluid is used in resuscitation, it may result in further insult to the pulmonary, renal, and mesenteric vascular bed. Ultimately, the fluid resuscitation effort will be determined by the patient's response to it and needs to be reassessed hourly. Urine output of 0.5 to 1 cc/kg/hr for adults is commonly used as a resuscitation goal.

The addition of colloids during resuscitation is the subject of much controversy. Some clinicians assert that adding colloids to the fluid regime decreases the amount of fluid needed and also prevents massive edema formation. Others believe that after 24 hours, the integrity of the capillaries begins to be restored and the use of colloids during that time has no advantage at all. Further investigational studies are required.

Characteristics of Burns According to Depth

Depth of Burn and Causes	Skin Involvement	Symptoms	Wound Appearance	Recuperative Course
SUPERFICIAL (FIRST DEGREE)				
Sunburn Low-intensity flash	Epidermis	Tingling Hyperesthesia (super sensitivity) Pain that is soothed by cooling	Reddened; blanches with pressure Minimal or no edema	Complete recovery within a week Peeling
PARTIAL THICKNESS (SECOND DEGREE)				
Scalds Flash flame	Epidermis and part of dermis	Pain Hyperesthesia Sensitive to cold air	Blistered, mottled red base; broken epidermis; weeping surface Edema	Recovery in 2 to 3 wk Some scarring and depigmentation Infection may convert it to third degree
FULL THICKNESS (THIRD DEGREE)				
Flame Prolonged exposure to hot liquids Electric current	Epidermis, entire dermis, and sometimes subcutaneous tissue	Pain free Shock Hematuria (blood in the urine) and, possibly, hemolysis (blood cell destruction) Possible entrance and exit wounds (electrical burn)	Dry; pale white, leathery, or charred Broken skin with fat exposed Edema	Eschar sloughs Grafting necessary Scarring and loss of contour and function Loss of digits or extremity possible

CALCULATING DRUG DOSES *(see Drug Dose Calculations, p. 381)*

CENTRAL VENOUS CATHETERS

A central venous catheter is any infusion device whose distal end is placed in the central venous system (superior vena cava or right atrium). Major types of vascular access catheters are:

- Nontunneled
- Tunneled
- PICC (peripherally inserted central catheter)
- Implanted

NONTUNNELED CATHETERS

These catheters are common in hospitalized patients and are useful because of their larger caliber. They are designed to be inserted into a relatively large central vein such as the internal jugular, subclavian, or femoral. Some types of nontunneled catheters are:

- Single, double, triple, or quad lumen central venous catheters
- Swan-Ganz catheters (see Swan-Ganz: Catheter Information in Part 2, p. 152)

Frequently, these catheters are used to monitor central venous pressure and/or pulmonary artery pressures and have an in-line flush device.

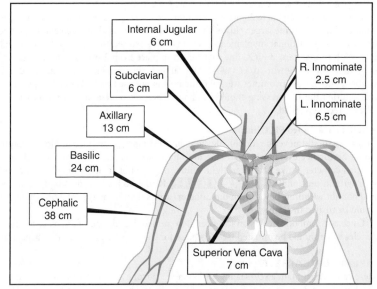

Internal Jugular
6 cm

Subclavian
6 cm

Axillary
13 cm

Basilic
24 cm

Cephalic
38 cm

R. Innominate
2.5 cm

L. Innominate
6.5 cm

Superior Vena Cava
7 cm

■ Central venous catheter lengths. (From Marino, P. L. [2007]. *The ICU book* [3rd ed.]. Philadelphia: Lippincott Williams & Wilkins.)

(continued)

To remove a nontunneled central venous catheter:
1. Place the patient in a *supine position to prevent emboli.*
2. Wash hands, and put on clean gloves and a mask.
3. Turn off all infusions, and prepare a sterile field, using a sterile drape.
4. Remove and discard the old dressing, and change to sterile gloves.
5. Clean the site with alcohol sponge or povidone-iodine solution.
6. Clip the sutures, and remove the catheter in a slow, even motion. *Have the patient perform a Valsalva maneuver to prevent emboli.*
7. Apply povidone-iodine ointment to the site to seal it, then cover with a gauze pad and transparent dressing. Keep site covered for 48 hours.
8. Inspect the catheter to see if any portions have broken off during removal. If so, notify the physician immediately, and monitor the patient closely.

TUNNELED CATHETERS
These catheters travel under the skin before going into a vein, and contain a Dacron cuff that allows the surrounding tissue to grow in and secure the catheter in place. A tunneled catheter is usually the best choice when long-term access is required, and is more stable than a PICC. These catheters require flushing with normal saline before and after administration of a medication as well as a heparin flush. Examples of tunneled catheters are:
- Hickman
- Broviac
- Groshong

PICC (PERIPHERALLY INSERTED CENTRAL CATHETERS)
PICC lines can be from 20 to 25 inches in length and are inserted in the arm and threaded to a location deep in the large veins of the chest. Frequently used to receive fluids, blood products, and nutritional supplements, they may also be used to withdraw blood for lab tests. With proper care, a PICC line may be left in place from 2 weeks to 6 months. The line requires flushing with 10 cc's of normal saline before and after medication administration, and at least two times weekly if the port is not used daily. While it is generally accepted that the site dressing should be changed weekly, referral to institution-specific policy is recommended.

To declot an occluded PICC line:
A catheter should never be forcibly flushed, and resistance or absence of blood aspirate should be further evaluated. First, rule out any *nonthrombotic* cause of the occlusion: clamped catheter, kinked catheter, tight suture, migrated or malpositioned catheter tip, or drug/lipid precipitate. **REMEMBER:** Partial occlusions (the ability to infuse fluid but not withdraw blood from the catheter) are as significant as a total occlusion and should be treated the same.

Once a thrombotic occlusion has been determined, instillation of alteplase for catheter clearance should be initiated (see Alteplase for Catheter Clearance in Part 8, p. 300)

IMPLANTED CATHETERS
These catheters contain a self-sealing, disk-shaped silicone septum that is connected to a metal or plastic port. This catheter is useful in patients who require long-term scheduled infusions.
- Medi-Port
- Infuse-A-Port
- Port-A-Cath

(continued)

These ports require flushing with normal saline before and after administration of a medication as well as a heparin flush. When the port is not in use, it must be flushed every 4 weeks with normal saline and heparin to prevent clot formation.

To access an implanted port:
1. Prepare the site by cleaning with povidone-iodine swabs, according to institution policy.
2. Put on sterile gloves and a mask, and flush the needle and tubing to ensure patency. Remove air from tubing.
3. Stabilize the port between the thumb and forefinger and insert a noncoring needle (Huber) through the skin at a 90-degree angle until bottom of port is reached (needle will hit metal). Do not rotate the needle, and do not insert the needle at any other angle because this will damage the septum of the port.
4. After insertion, the needle's upper portion should lie just above the skin surface. If it lies more than 0.5 cm above, support it with a folded 2 × 2 pad.
5. Check placement by aspiration. If there is no blood return, have the patient cough, turn, and raise the arm to take a breath. If this does not produce backflow, remove the needle, and repeat the process at a different site.
6. Aseptically anchor the needle and tubing, and apply transparent dressing.

To deaccess site:
1. Wearing sterile gloves, flush the port with saline and then heparin, per institution policy.
2. Stabilize the port with the thumb and forefinger, and remove needle.
3. Little or no bleeding should occur.

CIWA SCORE

The Clinical Institute Withdrawal for Alcohol Score (more recently referred to as the CIWA-Ar Score because it has been expanded to include "Alcohol Revised") is a clinical assessment tool consisting of 10 common withdrawal symptoms. Each symptom is scored from 0 (not present) to 7 (most extreme), with the exception of the category "Orientation and Clouding of Sensorium," which is rated 0 to 4.

While there are 67 possible points, any patient with a score of 8 or greater should be started on withdrawal medication, and for a score of 15 or greater (impending DTs) additional PRN medication should be included. Since alcohol withdrawal symptoms can change rapidly, the CIWA Score is used continually throughout the initial withdrawal period. The timing of reassessments is institution specific, although during primary withdrawal, scoring every 2 to 4 hours is a common practice.

(continued)

NOTES

CIWA-Ar Scoring

Nausea/Vomiting—Rate on scale 0–7
0   None
1   Mild nausea with no vomiting
2
3
4   Intermittent nausea
5
6
7   Constant nausea and frequent dry heaves and
    vomiting

Anxiety—Rate on scale 0–7
0   No anxiety, patient at ease
1   Mildly anxious
2
3
4   Moderately anxious or guarded, so anxiety is inferred
5
6
7   Equivalent to acute panic states seen in severe
    delirium or acute schizophrenic reactions.

Paroxysmal Sweats—Rate on scale 0–7.
0   No sweats
1   Barely perceptible sweating, palms moist
2
3
4   Beads of sweat obvious on forehead
5
6
7   Drenching sweats

Tactile Disturbances—Ask, "Have you experienced
any itching, pins & needles sensation, burning or
numbness, or a feeling of bugs crawling on or under
your skin?" Rate on scale 0–7
0   None
1   Very mild itching, pins & needles, burning, or
    numbness
2   Mild itching, pins & needles, burning, or
    numbness
3   Moderate itching, pins & needles, burning, or
    numbness
4   Moderate hallucinations
5   Severe hallucinations
6   Extremely severe hallucinations
7   Continuous hallucinations

Visual Disturbances—Ask, "Does the light appear
to be too bright? Is its color different than normal?
Does it hurt your eyes? Are you seeing anything that
disturbs you or that you know isn't there?" Rate on
scale 0–7
0   Not present
1   Very mild sensitivity
2   Mild sensitivity
3   Moderate sensitivity
4   Moderate hallucinations
5   Severe hallucinations
6   Extremely severe hallucinations
7   Continuous hallucinations

Tremors—have patient extend arms and spread
fingers. Rate on scale 0–7.
0   No tremor
1   Not visible, but can be felt fingertip to fingertip
2
3
4   Moderate, with patient's arms extended
5
6
7   Severe, even w/ arms not extended

Agitation—Rate on scale 0–7
0   Normal activity
1   Somewhat normal activity
2
3
4   Moderately fidgety and restless
5
6
7   Paces back and forth, or constantly thrashes about

Orientation and Clouding of Sensorium—Ask,
"What day is this? Where are you? Who am I?" Rate
scale 0–4
0   Oriented
1   Cannot do serial additions or is uncertain about date
2   Disoriented to date by no more than 2 calendar days
3   Disoriented to date by more than 2 calendar days
4   Disoriented to place and/or person

Auditory Disturbances—Ask, "Are you more
aware of sounds around you? Are they harsh?
Do they startle you? Do you hear anything that
disturbs you or that you know isn't there?" Rate
on scale 0–7
0   Not present
1   Very mild harshness or ability to startle
2   Mild harshness or ability to startle
3   Moderate harshness or ability to startle
4   Moderate hallucinations
5   Severe hallucinations
6   Extremely severe hallucinations
7   Continuous hallucinations

Headache—Ask, "Does your head feel different
than usual? Does it feel like there is a band
around your head?" Do not rate dizziness or
lightheadedness. Rate on scale 0–7.
0   Not present
1   Very mild
2   Mild
3   Moderate
4   Moderately severe
5   Severe
6   Very severe
7   Extremely severe

COMPARTMENT SYNDROME

A condition classified as acute if from injury or surgery, or chronic if due to repetitive activities such as running or cycling, where pressure from swelling within the fascial compartment compresses blood vessels, nerves, and/or tendons, and results in a decreased blood supply to that area. The syndrome typically involves the lower leg, although it can also occur in the hand, foot, thigh, or upper arm. Symptoms include the 5 Ps:

1. Pain which is severe, deep, and constant and out of proportion to the injury;
2. Paresthesia described as "pins and needles" in the affected area;
3. Paralysis of the limb (usually a late finding);
4. Pulse will be present, as pressures in the compartment are below arterial pressure;
5. Paleness of skin (tense, swollen, shiny).

A definitive diagnosis is obtained by attaching a needle to a pressure meter and inserting directly into the affected area. If the pressure is >45 mm Hg, or when the pressure is within 30 mm Hg of the diastolic pressure, compartment syndrome is confirmed.

Acute compartment syndrome is a medical emergency and requires a fasciotomy, which involves making long surgical cuts in the fascia to relieve the pressure. The wounds are initially left open, and closed with a second surgery usually 48 to 72 hours later. Chronic compartment syndrome typically employs conservative treatment first: rest, anti-inflammatory drugs and limb elevation. Ultimately, however, a fasciotomy may still be required.

NOTES

COMPATIBILITY CHART

KEY

- ▨ Compatible
- 4 Compatible only for hours indicated
- ▨ Incompatible
- ? Questionable compatibility
- ☐ Data unavailable

All other numbers signify the number of hours that the drugs are compatible

	acyclovir	albumin	amikacin	aminophylline	amiodarone	ampicillin	calcium gluconate	cefazolin	cefoxitin	ceftazidime	cimetidine	ciprofloxacin	clindamycin	dexamethasone sodium phosphate	dextrose 5% in water (D₅W)	D₅W in lactated Ringer's	D₅W in normal saline solution	diazepam	diphenhydramine	dobutamine	dopamine	epinephrine	erythromycin lactobionate	esmolol	gentamicin	heparin sodium	hydrocortisone sodium succinate
acyclovir			4			4		4	4	4	4		4	4					4					4	4	4	4
albumin																											
amikacin	4			8	4		24	8	48		24	48	48	?	24	24	24		24		24		24		24		24
aminophylline			8							48			24	24	24	24	24					24	24			24	24
amiodarone			4								4				24				24	24		4		24	4		
ampicillin	4											24		24										24		4	?
calcium gluconate			24						3		2				24	24	24			3							
cefazolin	4						3							48	24	24	24								24	6	
cefoxitin	4		48								24			48	24	24	24								24	8	
ceftazidime	4									2			4	48	24		24								24	6	
cimetidine	4		24	48				?			24		24	24	24	48	48	48	4	4			24	24	24	24	6
ciprofloxacin			48				2				24							2	4	24	24				48		
clindamycin	4		48	4	24			48	48	48	24				24	24	24								24	24	24
dexamethasone sodium phosphate	4		?	24							24				24											6	4
dextrose 5% in water (D₅W)	4		24	24	24		24	24	24	24	48		24							24	24	24		24		24	48
D₅W in lactated Ringer's			24	24			24	24	24		48		24							24	48	24		24			
D₅W in normal saline solution			24	24			24	24	24	24	48		24							24	48	24		24			48
diazepam																											
diphenhydramine	4		24								4	24								24	24		24			4	24
dobutamine					24						24				24	24	24		24		24					24	
dopamine				24							24				24	48	48			24				24	6	24	18
epinephrine			24				3				24				24	24	24			24					4	4	
erythromycin lactobionate	4		24	4	4						24				24	24	24							24			
esmolol			24	24	24	24		24		24	24				24	24	24			24					24	24	24
gentamicin	4			4					24		24	48	24		24							6		24			
heparin sodium	4					4		6	8	6	6		24	6	24			4		24	4		24				?
hydrocortisone sodium succinate	4		24	24		?					24		4	48	24	48	24		24		18	4		24		?	
insulin (regular)				24			2	2	24		24															2	2	4
isoproterenol				24							24				24	24	24			24						4	4
lactated Ringer's	4		24	24			24	24	24				48	24						24	48	24	18	24	24		24
lidocaine			24	24		24					24		24		24					24	24				24		
methylprednisolone sodium succinate	4		?								24		24		?		?			18						?	?
mezlocillin											24																
midazolam			24		24		24	24			24	24	24					4	4	4	4	24	24	24	24		
morphine sulfate	4		4		24	4		4	4	4			4	4					¼	4	4	4	4	8	1	1	4
nafcillin	4		24					2						4		24				24					24		
norepinephrine			24	24											24		24		4			24					24
normal saline solution			24	24		8	24	24	24	24	48		24							24	48	24	22	24	24		24
ondansetron			4					4	4	4	4		4		4	4	48		48	4					4	4	4
oxacillin			8																					24		4	4
oxytocin															6							24					4
penicillin G potassium	4		8		4						24		24		24	24	24		24						24	1	?
phenylephrine				24																	24						
phenytoin																									24		
phytonadione			24				3				24												3			4	4
piperacillin	4									2			4	48		24			24						24	6	24
potassium chloride	4		4	4	24	4	4				24	24	24	4	24	24	24		4	?	24	4		24		6	24
procainamide											24															4	4
ranitidine	4		24	24		?		?		?	24		24	24	48			?	1		48	48	24	24	24	24	
sodium bicarbonate	4		24	24		?			24	6		24	4	24						24					24	24	24
ticarcillin	4									2				4											6		
tobramycin	4			4		1			24	48		24						48							24		
vancomycin	4		24	4		?		?			24		24											24			
verapamil			24			48	24	24			24	24	24	24	24	24	24		24	24	24	24	24	24	24	24	24

■ Compatibility Chart. © 2007 by Lippincott Williams & Wilkins.

(continued)

Compatibility chart (values indicate hours of compatibility; "?" indicates conflicting data).

	insulin (regular)	isoproterenol	lactated Ringer's	lidocaine	methylprednisolone sodium succinate	mezlocillin	midazolam	morphine sulfate	nafcillin	norepinephrine	normal saline solution	ondansetron	oxacillin	oxytocin	penicillin G potassium	phenylephrine	phenytoin	phytonadione	piperacillin	potassium chloride	procainamide	ranitidine	sodium bicarbonate	ticarcillin	tobramycin	vancomycin	verapamil
acyclovir			4		4			4	4				4		4		4		4	4		4	4	4	4	4	4
albumin																											
amikacin			24				24	4		24	24		4		8		8		24			4	24	24		24	24
aminophylline		24	24	?			24				24								24			4	24		4	4	24
amiodarone	24	24		24			24	24			24				4		24		24	24					4	4	24
ampicillin	2						4	8										3		?	?					?	24
calcium gluconate			24	24			24				24								4			1					48
cefazolin	2		24				24	4			24	4							?						?		24
cefoxitin	24		24				4				24	4							2			4		24			24
ceftazidime							4				24	4							?			6					24
cimetidine	24	24		24	24		24				48	4			24				24						24	24	
ciprofloxacin		48	24	18		24					24						24		24	24		?	24	48			24
clindamycin		24		24		24	4				24	4			24				48	24		?	24	48			24
dexamethasone sodium phosphate							4				4								4	24	4						24
dextrose 5% in water (D5W)		24		24	?	24				24	24		48	6	6	24			24	24	24	48	24	24	24	24	24
D5W in lactated Ringer's		24		24							24			24		24				24							24
D5W in normal saline solution		24		24	?				24			48	?		24				24	24			24	48			24
diazepam																				?							24
diphenhydramine				4	¼						4				24				4		1						
dobutamine	24	24	24				4	4			24			24					?	24	48						24
dopamine		48	24	18			4	4			48		24							24	48						24
epinephrine		24					4	4		4	24							3	4	24							24
erythromycin lactobionate	18						4	4			22									24	24						24
esmolol		24					24	8	24	24	24				24	24			24	24				24	24	24	24
gentamicin	2		24				24	1			24	4			1					24							24
heparin sodium	2	24		24	?		24	1			4	4	4	4	?		4	6	24	4	24	24	6				24
hydrocortisone sodium succinate	4	4	24		?		4			24	4	4		4	24	4			24	3	2	2	48				24
insulin (regular)			24				24	1						2					4			24			24	24	24
isoproterenol	24			24	?	72			24		24			24		24			24	24				24	24		24
lactated Ringer's	24			24			4	48			24					?			24		?	48	2				24
lidocaine																											24
methylprednisolone sodium succinate	24			24	48				24	24	24								24	24				24	24		
mezlocillin	1		4	4		24		4	4		4	4		4	1	4		4	4		1	3	4	1	4	24	
midazolam	24	48						4			24				24				24			24					24
morphine sulfate		24		?	48		24		24			48	24		24				24	24		24	48	24			24
nafcillin							24	4			48								4		4						
norepinephrine		24		24			4	1												4							24
normal saline solution		24		24	?	48	24												4	24				24	24	24	24
ondansetron							4	48			4		2														24
oxacillin																			4								24
oxytocin	2						1												4			24					24
penicillin G potassium		24		24			4				24								24					24	24		24
phenylephrine											24								24								48
phenytoin											24	24							4					24	24		48
phytonadione																			4			4					24
piperacillin		24		24	4			24			24									24	4						24
potassium chloride	4		24	?			24	4	24		24	4		4		4			24		4	48	24				24
procainamide			24								24									4							48
ranitidine	24	24		24	48			1			4	48	4		4				24		4	48	24		24	24	24
sodium bicarbonate	3			24	2			3	24		24			24	24	24	24		24								24
ticarcillin	2		24								24	4			4				2			4					24
tobramycin	2		24				24	1			48								24								24
vancomycin	2		24				4	4			4	4							2		4						24
verapamil	48	24	24	48	24			24		24	24				24	24	48					24	24	24	24		

COMPRESSION HOSE (*see Anti-Embolism Stockings, p. 369*)

CONVERSION AND EQUIVALENT REFERENCES

Height
- 1 inch = 2.54 cm
- Convert inches to centimeters → inches × 2.54
- Convert centimeters to inches → centimeters ÷ 2.54

Weight
- 1 kg = 2.2 lb
- 1 lb = 0.453 kg or 454 g
- 1/150 grain = 0.4 mg
- 5 grains = 325 mg
- 15 grains = 1 g
- Convert kilograms to pounds → kilograms × 2.2
- Convert pounds to kilograms → pounds ÷ 2.2*

REMEMBER

*The rule for quick approximation of this conversion:
Divide pounds by 2 and subtract 10%

Temperature (37°C = 98.6°F)
- Convert Fahrenheit to centigrade → temperature − 32 × 0.5555
- Convert centigrade to Fahrenheit → temperature × 1.8 + 32

Length
- 2.54 cm = 1 inch
- 1 cm = 0.4 inch
- 1 m = 39.4 inches
- 1 km = 0.6 mile

Volume
- 1 fluid dram = 4 cc
- 1 teaspoon = 5 cc
- 1 tablespoon = 15 cc
- 1 fluid ounce = 30 cc
- 1 quart = 946 cc
- 1 L = 1,000 cc

NOTES

DERMATOMES *(see also Epidural Analgesia in Part 1, p. 28)*

Dermatomes are patches of skin innervated by a given spinal cord level, with each dermatome having a specific point recommended for testing. After injury, dermatomes can expand or contract, depending on the plasticity of the spinal cord.

DRUG DOSE CALCULATIONS

- **Know rate of infusion, want to know mcg/kg/min**

  Example: Nipride drip (100 mg/250 cc) running at 20 mL/hr. Patient weight 65 kg.
  Use this equation:

$$\frac{\text{Unknown mcg/kg/min} \times \text{weight (kg)} \times 60 \text{ (min/hr)} \times \text{mL of solution}}{\text{mcg of drug in bag}} = \text{rate of infusion}$$

  Plug in numbers:

$$\frac{(x) \times 65 \times 60 \times 250}{100,000} = 20 \text{ mL/hr}$$

$$9.75x = 20 \text{ mL/hr}$$

$$x = 2.05 \text{ mcg/kg/min}$$

- **Know mcg/kg/min, want to know rate of infusion (mL/hr)**

  Example: Dobutamine drip (500 mg/250 mL). Patient weight 70 kg.
  Want to start drip at 3 mcg/kg/min. How many mL/hr is that?
  Use this equation:

$$\frac{\text{mcg/kg/min} \times \text{weight (kg)} \times 60 \text{ (min/hr)} \times \text{mL of solution}}{\text{mcg of drug in bag}} = x \text{ mL/hr}$$

  Plug in numbers:

$$\frac{3 \times 70 \times 60 \times 250}{500,000} = 6.3 \text{ mL/hr}$$

(continued)

NOTES

- **Calculating drug doses using a "constant"** (Great for titration!)

    Once a "constant" has been determined for a specific solution, you only need to multiply the drip rate by the "constant" to obtain the mcg/kg/min value. Every time the drip rate changes, simply multiply the new drip rate by the "constant" to obtain the new mcg/kg/min value.

REMEMBER:

The "constant" will remain *valid only as long as the patient's weight and drip concentration do not change*. If either of these varies, a new "constant" will need to be calculated.

> **Example:** Dopamine drip (800 mg/500 cc). Patient weight 70 kg. Drip infusing at 13 cc/hr, and is titrated up to 16 cc/hr, and increased again to 20 cc/hr.

First calculate the "constant" using this equation:

$$(\text{mg of drug in solution} \div \text{mL of solution}) \div \text{weight (kg)} \div 60 \text{ (min/hr)} \times 1{,}000 \text{ (mcg/mg)} = \text{"constant"}$$

Plug in numbers:

$$(800 \div 500) \div 70 \div 60 \times 1{,}000 = 0.380 \text{ "constant"}$$

Multiply the drip rate by the calculated "constant":

$$13 \text{ cc/hr} \times 0.380 = 4.95 \text{ mcg/kg/min}$$
$$16 \text{ cc/hr} \times 0.380 = 6.08 \text{ mcg/kg/min}$$
$$20 \text{ cc/hr} \times 0.380 = 7.6 \text{ mcg/kg/min}$$

EQUIVALENT REFERENCES *(see Conversion and Equivalent References, p. 380)*

FRACTURES

There are four general classifications of fractures:
- Simple (closed): Bone fragments DO NOT penetrate the skin.
- Compound (open): Bone fragments DO penetrate the skin.
- Incomplete (partial): Bone continuity IS NOT completely interrupted.
- Complete: Bone continuity IS completely interrupted.

    Fractures are further divided by defining fracture position and fracture line, as denoted in the following figure.

(continued)

NOTES

Comminuted: Bone breaks into separate small pieces.

Impacted: One bone fragment is forced into another.

Nondisplaced: The two sections of bone maintain essentially normal alignment.

Overriding: Fragments overlap, shortening the total bone length.

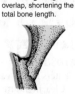

Angulated: Fragments lie at an angle to each other.

Displaced: Fracture fragments separate and are deformed.

Segmental: Fractures occur in two adjacent areas with an isolated central segment.

Avulsed: Fragments are pulled from normal position by muscle contractions or ligament resistance.

Linear: The fracture line runs parallel to the bone's axis.

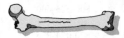

Spiral: The fracture line crosses the bone at an oblique angle, creating a spiral pattern.

Longitudinal: The fracture line extends in a longitudinal (but not parallel) direction along the bone's axis.

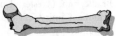

Transverse: The fracture line forms a right angle with the bone's axis.

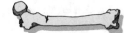

Oblique: The fracture line crosses the bone at roughly a 45-degree angle to the bone's axis.

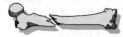

■ Fractures. (From Springhouse. [2008]. *Visual nursing.* Philadelphia: Lippincott Williams & Wilkins.)

(*continued*)

NOTES

HOTLINE PHONE NUMBERS *(see also Website Help, p. 392)*

Help is just a phone call away.

AIDS/HIV

Centers for Disease Control and Prevention/AIDS Clearinghouse	800-458-5231
Sexually Transmitted Disease Hotline	800-227-8922

BEHAVIORAL HEALTH

Depression and Bipolar Support Line	800-826-3632
Substance Abuse and Mental Health Services (federal)	800-662-HELP
National Alliance on Mental Illness	800-950-NAMI
Smoking Cessation	800-QUIT NOW
Suicide Prevention Hotline	800-SUICIDE

BLIND

American Council of the Blind	800-424-8666
American Foundation for the Blind	800-232-5463
Braillegrams (Western Union)	800-325-6000
National Library Service for the Blind and Physically Handicapped	800-424-8567
Random House Audio Books	800-733-3000
Recorded Books	.800-638-1304
Recordings for the Blind & Dyslexic (Learning through Listening)	800-221-4792

CARDIOVASCULAR

American Heart Association	800-242-8721
American Stroke Association	800-553-6321

DIABETES

American Diabetes Foundation	800-232-3472
Juvenile Diabetes Research Foundation	800-223-1138

DISABILITY

The Arc of the United States	800-433-5255

EPILEPSY

Epilepsy Foundation of America	800-332-1000

GASTROINTESTINAL

Crohn's and Colitis Foundation of America	800-343-3637
National Digestive Diseases Information Clearinghouse	301-654-3810
Simon Foundation for Continence	900-23-SIMON
United Ostomy Association	800-826-0826

HEARING

American Speech, Language and Hearing Association	800-638-TALK
Captioned Media Program (Captioned Films for the Deaf)	800-237-6213
International Hearing Society	800-521-5247

(continued)

HOTLINE PHONE NUMBERS *(Continued)*

HEPATIC
American Liver Foundation 800-223-0179

IMMUNOLOGY
Lupus Foundation 800-558-0121
West Nile Hotline 888-246-2675

MISCELLANEOUS
Arthritis Foundation 800-283-7800
Jehovah's Witnesses Hospital Information Service 718-560-4300
Job Accommodation Network 800-526-7234
Malignant Hyperthermia Hotline 800-644-9737
National Health Information Center 800-336-4797
The Living Bank (organ donation) 800-528-2971

NEUROLOGICAL
American Parkinson Disease Association 800-223-2732
Amyotrophic Lateral Sclerosis (ALS) Association 800-782-4747
Christopher Reeve Foundation (paralysis) 800-225-0292
International Dyslexia Association 800-222-3123
Multiple Sclerosis Foundation 800-441-7055
National Brain Injury Information Center 800-444-6443
National Brain Tumor Society 800-034-2873
National Organization for Rare Disorders 800-999-6673
National Spinal Cord Association 800-962-9629

ONCOLOGY
American Cancer Society 800-ACS-2345
Cancer Information and Counseling 800-525-3777
Cancer Information Service 800-4-CANCER

PULMONARY
American Lung Association 800-586-4872
National Jewish Health Lung Line
  (asthma and respiratory disorders) 800-222-5864
National Cystic Fibrosis Foundation 800-344-4823

RENAL
American Kidney Fund 800-638-8299

TOXICOLOGY
American Association of Poison Control Centers 800-222-1222

IV FLUID THERAPY (*see also Body Fluid Compartments in Part 7, p. 280*)

CRYSTALLOIDS

Crystalloids are solutions composed of electrolytes and water. Because of their composition, they will equalize across the vascular membrane and pass into the interstitial spaces, resulting in only 10% to 25% of the crystalloid solution remaining within the vascular space. There are three types: hypotonic, hypertonic, and isotonic.

1. *Hypotonic.* Provides salt and H_2O. Moves fluid into cell to hydrate cell; results in intracellular expansion; decreases intravascular osmolality.

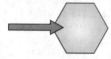

- ½ NS   77 mEq/L Na^+, 77 mEq/L Cl^-, 154 mOsm/L
- 2.5% Dextrose   130 mOsm/L
- D_5W Provides hydration

2. *Hypertonic.* Replaces sodium. Pulls fluid from cell and shifts into intravascular space, resulting in interstitial dehydration. Increases intravascular osmolality.

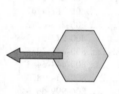

- 3% NS   512 mEq/L Na^+, 513 mEq/L Cl^-, 1026 mOsm/L
- D_5½ NS   Provides Na^+, Cl^-, 406 mOsm/L
- D_5¼ NS   Provides Na^+, Cl^-
- D_5 NS   565 mOsm/L
- D_5 LR   575 mOsm/L
- D_{10} LR   Maintains volume; supplies blood lactate ions
- $D_{50}W$ Increases blood sugar when given rapidly
- $D_{10}W$, $D_{20}W$ Provides calories in small amount of fluid

REMEMBER:

Hypertonic solutions are commonly given to all postoperative patients to prevent severe cellular edema.

3. *Isotonic.* Provides hydration. Maintains same osmotic pressure as blood; therefore, cellular components are unchanged.

- 0.9% NS   154 mEq/L Na^+, 154 mEq/L Cl^-, 308 mOsm/L
- LR   130 mEq/L Na^+, 109 mEq/L Cl^-, 4 mEq/L K, 27 mEq/L lactate, 274 mOsm/L
- D_5W Isotonic in bag only

REMEMBER:

Never use Lactated Ringer's if the patient is alkalotic (a normal liver converts the lactate to bicarbonate) or if the patient has liver disease (a diseased liver produces lactic acid and ammonia as by-products).

COLLOIDS

Colloids are known as plasma expanders or volume expanders and can be artificial (dextran, Hespan) or made from blood products (albumin, Plasmanate). Because colloid solutes are as large as the solutes in blood plasma, they cause an increase in osmotic pressure. This increased osmotic pressure causes fluid to be drawn from the interstitial compartment into

(*continued*)

the intravascular space and results in an increase in total vascular blood volume. Their effect is limited, however, lasting only 24 to 48 hours. Although colloids are plasma expanders, they do not have the oxygen-carrying capacity of red blood cells and cannot be used as such.

MALIGNANT HYPERTHERMIA

Caused by an autosomal dominant trait (that requires only one parent to carry the disease), malignant hyperthermia is an inherited disease seen when the infected person undergoes general anesthesia. The best course of action for MH is *prevention,* as it can be fatal if not treated promptly.

SIGNS
- Rapid rise in body temperature to 105°F or higher after anesthesia is given
- Trunk or total body rigidity after anesthesia is given
- Tachycardia
- Tachypnea (increased $ETCO_2$)
- Acidosis
- Dark brown urine (rhabdomyolysis) with elevated myoglobin levels
- Eventual kidney failure due to destruction of muscle tissue
- Chemistry panel showing increased levels of CPK, potassium, uric acid, and phosphate

ACUTE TREATMENT
- Procedure must be aborted.
- Hyperventilate with 100% oxygen at flows of 10 L/min or more.
- Dantrolene 2.5 mg/kg rapid IV, repeated until there is control of the signs of MH. Sometimes more than 10 mg/kg (up to 30 mg/kg) is necessary.
- Bicarbonate for metabolic acidosis, 1 to 2 mEq/kg if blood gas values are not yet available.
- Cool the patient with core temp >39°C, and lavage open body cavities, stomach, bladder, or rectum. Apply ice to the surface, and infuse cold saline IV. Stop cooling if temperature is <38°C and falling to prevent drift to <36°C.
- Dysrhythmias usually respond to treatment of acidosis and hyperkalemia. Use standard drug therapy EXCEPT calcium channel blockers (in the presence of dantrolene, cardiac arrest may occur).
- Treat hyperkalemia with bicarbonate, glucose, insulin, and calcium.

MALLAMPATI AIRWAY CLASSIFICATION
(see Moderate Sedation in Part 8, p. 324)

NEGATIVE PRESSURE WOUND THERAPY
(see Vacuum-Assisted Wound Closure, p. 392)

ORGAN DONATION *(see also Brain Death Criteria in Part 1, p. 10)*

Under contract with the U.S. Department of Health and Human Services, the United Network for Organ Sharing (UNOS) maintains a centralized computer network that links all transplant hospital and organ procurement organizations in a secure, real-time environment. When a deceased organ donor is identified, a transplant coordinator will access the system and enter all pertinent medical information about the donor. This information is

(continued)

then used to match the medical characteristics of the donor against potential candidates. A list is generated, called a "match run," and all patients who may be suitable recipients are listed and ranked. Factors that affect ranking may include:

1. Tissue match
2. Blood type
3. Length of time on the waiting list
4. Immune status
5. Distance between the potential recipient and the donor
6. Degree of medical urgency (for heart, liver, lung, and intestines)

Because laws that oversee donation vary from state to state, the reader is advised to access the United Network for Organ Sharing website for more specific information and for the names of organ procurement organizations in their region.

PAP SMEAR CLASSIFICATIONS

- **Class 1**   Normal cells
- **Class 2**   Atypical cells, probably normal
- **Class 3**   Doubtful, may be malignant
- **Class 4**   Probably malignant
- **Class 5**   Definite malignancy

PICC LINE *(see Central Venous Catheters, p. 374)*

PRESSURE ULCERS *(see also Wound Care/Dressings, p. 393)*

Stage I: (Closed) Intact skin with nonblanchable redness of a localized area, usually over a bony prominence. Darkly pigmented skin may not have visible blanching; its color may differ from the surrounding area. The area may be painful, firm, soft, and warmer or cooler as compared to adjacent tissue. May be difficult to detect in individuals with dark skin tones.

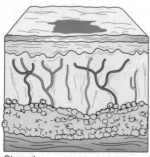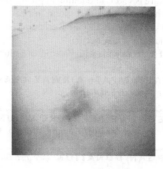

Stage 1

■ Stage I Pressure Ulcer. (From Carter, P. J. [2008]. *Lippincott's textbook for nursing assistants* [2nd ed.]. Philadelphia: Lippincott Williams & Wilkins.)

(continued)

Stage II: (Open) Partial thickness loss of dermis presenting as a shallow, open ulcer with a red/pink wound bed, without slough. May also present as an intact or open/ruptured serum- filled blister. Should NOT be used to describe skin tears, tape burns, maceration, or excoriation.

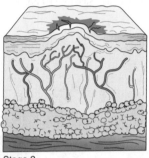 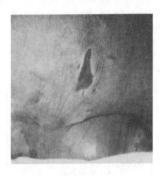

Stage 2

■ Stage II Pressure Ulcer. (From Carter, P. J. [2008]. *Lippincott's textbook for nursing assistants* [2nd ed.]. Philadelphia: Lippincott Williams & Wilkins.)

Stage III: Full thickness tissue loss. Subcutaneous fat may be visible, but bone, tendon, or muscle are not exposed. Slough may be present but does not obscure the depth of tissue loss. May include undermining and tunneling. The depth of a stage III pressure ulcer varies by anatomical location. The bridge of the nose, ear, occiput, and malleolus do not have subcutaneous tissue and stage III ulcers there can be shallow. In contrast, areas of significant adiposity can develop extremely deep stage III pressure ulcers. Bone/tendon is not visible or directly palpable.

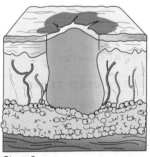 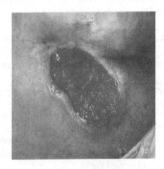

Stage 3

■ Stage III Pressure Ulcer. (From Carter, P. J. [2008]. *Lippincott's textbook for nursing assistants* [2nd ed.]. Philadelphia: Lippincott Williams & Wilkins.)

(*continued*)

Stage IV: Full thickness tissue loss with exposed bone, tendon, or muscle. Slough or eschar may be present on some parts of the wound bed. Often includes undermining and tunneling. Depth of stage IV pressure ulcers (like stage III) vary by anatomical location. The bridge of the nose, ear, occiput, and malleolus do not have subcutaneous tissue and stage IV ulcers can be shallow. Stage IV ulcers can extend into muscle and/or supporting structures (e.g., fascia, tendon, or joint capsule) making osteomyelitis possible. Exposed bone/tendon is visible or directly palpable.

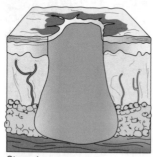 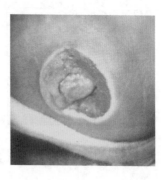

Stage 4

■ Stage IV Pressure Ulcer. (From Carter, P. J. [2008]. *Lippincott's textbook for nursing assistants* [2nd ed.]. Philadelphia: Lippincott Williams & Wilkins.)

Unstageable: Full thickness tissue loss in which the base of the ulcer is covered by slough (yellow, tan, gray, green, or brown) and/or eschar (tan, brown, or black) in the wound bed. Until enough slough and/or eschar is removed to expose the base of the wound, the true depth (and therefore, stage) cannot be determined. Stable (dry, adherent, intact without erythema or fluctuance) eschar on the heels serves as "the body's natural (biological) cover" and should not be removed.

RAMSEY SCALE *(see Part 1, p. 49)*

RIKER SEDATION-AGITATION SCALE *(see Part 1, p. 50)*

SIGNS, SYNDROMES, FREQUENTLY USED TERMS

Babinski's reflex is dorsiflexion of the big toe upon scratching bottom of foot. It indicates upper motor neuron dysfunction.

Battle's sign is ecchymosis behind the ear associated with basilar skill fracture.

Brudzinski's sign is flexion of the neck, causing flexion of the legs. It is seen in meningitis (see also Kernig's sign).

Chvostek's sign is evidenced by tapping over the facial nerve, causing facial twitching in hypocalcemic states (see also Trousseau's sign).

Cullen's sign is a bluish color around the umbilicus. It is seen in hemorrhagic pancreatitis.

De Musset's sign is a head bob with each heartbeat, signaling aortic regurgitation.

Duroziez's sign is a biphasic femoral murmur heard with mild pressure, indicating aortic insufficiency.

(continued)

Fremitus is a vibration palpated when the patient speaks. Sound is best conducted through solid material; therefore, fremitus is increased in atelectasis and lung tumors. Sound is poorly conducted through fluid and air; therefore, fremitus is decreased in pneumothorax, pleural effusions, and emphysema.

Grey Turner's sign is ecchymosis in the flank associated with retroperitoneal bleeding.

Hill's sign is accentuated leg systolic pressure <40 mm Hg from brachial artery systolic pressure. It is indicative of severe aortic insufficiency.

Janeway lesions are slightly raised, irregular, nontender, erythematous lesions on palms and soles. They are a possible indication of infective endocarditis.

Kehr's sign is seen in 50% of splenic injuries. Pain is referred to left shoulder.

Kerley's B lines are seen on chest x-ray films and are indicative of pulmonary edema.

Kernig's sign is seen with thigh flexed at a right angle; complete extension of the leg is not possible. It is seen in meningitis.

McBurney's point is located one third of the distance from the anterior superior iliac spine to the umbilicus. McBurney's sign is tenderness of the site and is associated with appendicitis.

Muller's sign is a bobbing of the uvula with each pulse that indicative of aortic insufficiency.

Murphy's sign is severe pain and inspiratory arrest with palpation of the right upper quadrant.

Psoas sign occurs when extension and elevation of the right leg produces pain in cases of inflammation of the psoas muscle. The sign is positive with appendicitis.

Quincke's sign is alternating blushing and blanching of the fingernail bed after light compression. It is seen in aortic regurgitation.

Romberg's sign is seen when the patient stands with feet close together and eyes closed; unsteadiness is associated with cerebellar damage.

Roth's spots are round or oval white spots seen in the retina, indicating possible subacute bacterial endocarditis.

Somogyi effect is rebound hyperglycemia (insulin causing high glucose level).

Traube's sign is described as a "pistol shot" sound auscultated over the femoral arteries in aortic insufficiency.

Trousseau's sign is carpopedal spasm after restriction of circulation in the arm by a blood pressure cuff and is indicative of hypocalcemia (see also Chvostek's sign).

TED HOSE *(see Anti-Embolism Stockings, p. 369)*

TUMORS, GRADING/STAGING

The *grade* of a tumor indicates its degree of malignancy:

Grade I	Least malignant, slow growing. Surgery alone is an effective treatment.
Grade II	Slightly abnormal microscopic appearance. Slow growing with invasion of adjacent tissue.
Grade III	Malignant. Actively reproducing with a tendency to recur.
Grade IV	Highly malignant. Reproducing rapidly with areas of necrosis in the center of the cells.

The *stage* of a tumor indicates the extent of the cancer:

T (Primary tumor)	T0-T4	The higher the number, the larger the tumor
N (Regional lymph node involvement)	N0-N3	The higher the number, the greater the involvement
M (Distal metastasis)	M0	No metastasis
	M1	Positive metastasis

VACUUM-ASSISTED WOUND CLOSURE

Also known as negative pressure wound therapy, this is a wound closure system whereby negative pressure is applied to the wound bed to stimulate granulation of tissue by dilating the arterioles, decompressing interstitial spaces, and removing stagnant materials. The wound bed is filled with a sterile foam sponge material, and a vacuum is applied via a closed system. Continuous or intermittent cycling pressures (usually intervals of 5 minutes on and 2 minutes off) are selected at a level **between 50 and 200 mm Hg (125 mm Hg standard),** depending on the amount of exudate and granulation tissue within the wound and the type of foam used. If wound has stalled, pressure can be adjusted rather than discontinuing therapy. Best if placed on wound without necrotic tissue or minimal necrosis.

TIPS AND CAUTIONS

- Dressing changes are typically done every 48 hours; however, some infected wound beds require changes at least every 12 hours, and conversely, dressings over grafts may be changed less frequently, as rarely as every 3 to 5 days.
- Use protective barriers (i.e., Hydrofiber or Vaseline gauze) to protect weakened, irradiated, or sutured blood vessels or organs that are close to areas being treated with vacuum therapy.
- Change and date the collection cannister every 7 days; mark drainage every shift, and record I&O.
- Assess patient for preexisting bleeding disorders or use of anticoagulants, as these will predispose to hemorrhage.
- Air leaks most often occur around tubing and create a soft, whistling noise. Gently press around the tubing to better seal the drape. Excess drape can also be used to patch over leaks.
- If the sponge collapses and an area of the wound isn't covered, turn off the unit, make an opening in the drape, and insert extra foam from the dressing kit to fill the wound. Reseal the area with additional drape, and turn on the unit.
- Occasionally ointments may be used "off label" to aid in adding moisture to a wound.
- If the wound appears overly wet or macerated at dressing changes, request an increase in pressure.
- Optimally, therapy should be used at least 22 hours a day to aid in wound healing.
- Newer "VACs" have set-ups to assist in finding leaks.

WEBSITE HELP *(see also Hotline Phone Numbers, p. 384)*

To view this list of over 70 web resources, visit http://thepoint.lww.com/Diepenbrock4e.

NOTES

WOUND CARE/DRESSINGS (see also Pressure Ulcers, p. 388)

Alginates	Derived from brown seaweed and composed of soft, nonwoven fibers shaped as ropes or pads. The alginate, when in contact with wound exudate, converts to a gel. Used for wounds that have moderate to heavy exudate. Facilitates autolytic debridement and is also hemostatic. Usually requires a secondary dressing. *Examples:* **Sorbsan, Kaltostat, MediHoney** (available since 2008, a debriding agent in alginate form, hydrocolloid or wound gel. Can be used from beginning to end of wound healing), **Tegagen**
Antimicrobials	Contain ionic silver to provide broad spectrum bactericidal activity in the management of infected wounds and antimicrobial activity against a variety of pathogens, including MRSA and VRE. *Examples:* **Aquacel AG, Acticoat, Contreet, Silvercel, PolyMem Silver, Silvasorb**
Collagen	Stimulates new tissue development and wound debridement. Absorb exudate and maintain a moist healing environment and may be used in combination with topical agents. *Examples:* **Fibracol Plus Collagen, Promogran, Skin Temp**
Composites	To be classified as a composite, the dressing must include a bacterial barrier, an absorptive layer, and a semi- or nonadherent covering for the wound. *Examples:* **Alldress, Combiderm ACD, Covaderm Plus, Tegaderm Plus, CovRSite Plus, Visasorb**
Foams	Used to create a moist environment and to provide thermal insulation to the wound. May require a secondary dressing, tape, wrap, or net to anchor in place. Appropriate for a variety of wounds, including leg ulcers and pressure sores. *Examples:* **Allevyn, Hydrasorb, Hydrofera Blue (bacteriostatic), Lyofoam, Mepilex, PolyMem, Sof-Foam**
Hydrocolloids	Provide a moist healing environment that allows clean wounds to granulate and necrotic wounds to debride autolytically. May be left in place for 3 to 5 days. *Examples:* **Comfeel, Duoderm CGF, MediHoney** (available since 2008, a debriding agent in alginate form, hydrocolloid or wound gel. Can be used from beginning to end of wound healing), **Replicare, Tegasorb**
Hydrofibers	A sterile, nonwoven pad or ribbon composed of sodium carboxymethyl cellulose fibers. The fibers interact with exudate to form a gel, maintaining a moist wound environment for healing, debridement, and easy dressing removal. Hydrofiber dressings require a secondary dressing. *Examples:* **Aquacel, Cutinova Hydro, Versiva with Hydrofiber**
Hydrogels	Water- or glycerin-based amorphous gels. Because of their high water content, they do not absorb large amounts of exudate. They rehydrate the wound bed, facilitate autolytic debridement, fill in dead space, and promote granulation. *Examples:* **Elasto-Gel, Flexi-Gel, Granugel, MediHoney** (available since 2008, a debriding agent in alginate form, hydrocolloid or wound gel. Can be used from beginning to end of wound healing), **Nu-Gel, Transi-Gel**

Index

Abbreviations Key

ABGs — arterial blood gases
ABI — ankle-brachial index
ACE — angiotensin converting enzyme
ARDS — acute respiratory distress syndrome
ARF — acute renal failure
AV — arteriovenous
CABG — coronary artery bypass graft
CHF — congestive heart failure
CK — creatine kinase
COPD — chronic obstructive pulmonary disease
CSF — cerebrospinal fluid
CT — computed tomography
CVA — cerebral vascular accident
CVP — central venous pressure
D5W — 5% dextrose in water
DBP — diastolic blood pressure
DDAVP — desmopressin
DIC — disseminated intravascular coagulation
DVT — deep venous thrombosis
EDV — end-diastolic volume
EMD — electromechanical dissociation
ESV — end-systolic volume
ET — endotracheal tube
FFP — fresh frozen plasma
Fr — french
FRC — functional residual capacity
GCS — Glasgow coma scale
HHNK — hyperglycemic hyperosmolar nonketotic
ICS — intercostal space
ID — internal diameter
IJ — internal jugular
IM — intramuscular
INR — international normalized ratio
IPPB — intermittent positive-pressure breathing
IVPB — intravenous piggyback
JVD — jugular venous distention

kCAL — kilocalorie
LOC — level of consciousness
mA — milliamp
MAP — mean arterial pressure
MI — myocardial infarction
MRI — magnetic resonance imaging
mV — millivolt
$M\dot{V}O_2$ — myocardial oxygen
NG — nasogastric tube
NS — normal saline
NSAIDs — nonsteroidal anti-inflammatory drugs
PAC — premature atrial contraction
PAD — pulmonary artery diastolic
PAWP — pulmonary artery wedge pressure
PCWP — pulmonary capillary wedge pressure
PE — pulmonary embolism
PEA — pulseless electrical activity
PEEP — positive end-expiratory pressure
PET — positron-emission tomography
PSVT — paroxysmal supraventricular tachycardia
PT — pulmonary toilet
PTCA — percutaneous transluminal coronary angioplasty
PVC — premature ventricular contraction
RBCs — red blood cells
RSI — rapid sequence intubation
RV — right ventricular
SAH — subarachnoid hemorrhage
SBP — systolic blood pressure
SC — subcutaneous
SVR — systemic vascular resistance
SVT — supraventricular tachycardia
TEE — transesophageal echocardiogram
TPN — total parenteral nutrition
UTI — urinary tract infection
V tach — ventricular tachycardia
VT — tidal volume
WPW — Wolff-Parkinson-White syndrome